# Structure and Function of
# the Genetic Apparatus

# NATO ASI Series

## Advanced Science Institutes Series

*A series presenting the results of activities sponsored by the NATO Science Committee, which aims at the dissemination of advanced scientific and technological knowledge, with a view to strengthening links between scientific communities.*

The series is published by an international board of publishers in conjunction with the NATO Scientific Affairs Division

| | | |
|---|---|---|
| **A** | **Life Sciences** | Plenum Publishing Corporation |
| **B** | **Physics** | New York and London |
| | | |
| **C** | **Mathematical** | D. Reidel Publishing Company |
| | **and Physical Sciences** | Dordrecht, Boston, and Lancaster |
| | | |
| **D** | **Behavioral and Social Sciences** | Martinus Nijhoff Publishers |
| **E** | **Engineering and** | The Hague, Boston, and Lancaster |
| | **Materials Sciences** | |
| | | |
| **F** | **Computer and Systems Sciences** | Springer-Verlag |
| **G** | **Ecological Sciences** | Berlin, Heidelberg, New York, and Tokyo |

*Recent Volumes in this Series*

*Volume 93*—Biology of Invertebrate and Lower Vertebrate Collagens
 edited by A. Bairati and R. Garrone

*Volume 94*—Cell Transformation
 edited by J. Celis and A. Graessmann

*Volume 95*—Drugs Affecting Leukotrienes and Other Eicosanoid Pathways
 edited by B. Samuelsson, F. Berti, G. C. Folco, and G. P. Velo

*Volume 96*—Epidemiology and Quantitation of Environmental Risk in Humans
 from Radiation and Other Agents
 edited by A. Castellani

*Volume 97*—Interactions between Electromagnetic Fields and Cells
 edited by A. Chiabrera, C. Nicolini, and H. P. Schwan

*Volume 98*—Structure and Function of the Genetic Apparatus
 edited by Claudio Nicolini and Paul O. P. Ts'o

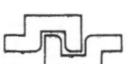

*Series A: Life Sciences*

# Structure and Function of the Genetic Apparatus

Edited by

## Claudio Nicolini

Temple University
Philadelphia, Pennsylvania

and

## Paul O. P. Ts'o

Johns Hopkins University
Baltimore, Maryland

Plenum Press
New York and London
Published in cooperation with NATO Scientific Affairs Division

Proceedings of a NATO Advanced Study Institute,
held September 18–30, 1983,
in Erice, Italy

Library of Congress Cataloging in Publication Data

NATO Advances Study Institute (1983: Sept. 18–30: Erice, Sicily)
  Structure and function of the genetic apparatus.

  (NATO ASI series. Series A, Life sciences; vol. 98)
  "Proceedings of a NATO Advanced Study Institute, held September 18–30,
1983, in Erice, Italy"—T.p. verso.
  "Published in cooperation with NATO Scientific Affairs Division."
  Includes bibliographies and index.
  1. Cytogenetics—Congresses. I. Nicolini, Claudio A. II. Ts'o, Paul O. P. (Paul On
Pong), 1929-     . III. North Atlantic Treaty Organization. Scientific Affairs Divi-
sion. IV. Title. V. Series: NATO ASI series. Series A, Life sciences; v. 98) [DNLM: 1.
Cytogenetics—congresses. QH 605 N2785s 1983]
QH426.N38   1983                       574.87′3223                       85-24806
ISBN-13: 978-1-4684-5026-2        e-ISBN-13: 978-1-4684-5024-8
DOI: 10.1007/978-1-4684-5024-8

© 1985 Plenum Press, New York
A Division of Plenum Publishing Corporation
233 Spring Street, New York, N.Y. 10013

Softcover reprint of the hardcover 1st edition 1985

PREFACE

    The Fourth Course of the International School of Pure and Applied Biostructure, a NATO Advanced Study Institute, was held September 18-31, 1983 at the Ettore Majorana Center for Scientific Culture in Erice, Sicily. The subject of the Fourth Course, which was co-sponsored by national and international agencies, was "Structure and Function of the Genetic "Apparatus." Participants from 15 countries around the world attended the course.

    The study of the genetic apparatus is one of humanity's most challenging problems, and it has been approached in the tradition of the School from many different points of view, among them biochemistry, genetic engineering, cell biology, oncology, biophysics and other fields. It has been most difficult to confine such diverse points of view, as well as their proponents, within the four walls of one room, in front of one audience - especially since the heterogeneity of background and the inherent difficulties encountered in communication could overshadow the true spirit of scientific exchange. We are once again pleased to say the outcome of the 1983 Course has matched the success of the previous course held in Erice on the same subject five years ago.

    This book is the result of the 1983 Advanced Study Institute, and aims to present a cohesive, interdisciplinary view of the current knowledge on the structure and fuction of the genetic apparatus. The book has been edited in a tutorial format, with the cooperation of several leading scientists. We wish to take this opportunity to express our gratitude to all who have contributed to the success of the course and the contents of this book. Our gratitude is also expressed to Drs. Pinola and Gabriele for their invaluable cooperation during the Institute. The preparation of the manuscripts for the publication of the book was done professionally by Ms. Audrey DeBaugh and Ms. Dorothy Lindstrom. For their excellent work and cooperation we wish to express our gratitude.

Claudio Nicolini  
Paul O.P. Ts'o

CONTENTS

HYDRODYNAMICS, THERMODYNAMICS AND SCATTERING PROPERTIES: NUCLEIC ACIDS,

NUCLEOSOMES AND CHROMATIN

Henryk Eisenberg

Polymer Research Department
The Weizmann Institute of Science
Rehovot 76100 Israel

INTRODUCTION

Though the progress of both experimental and theoretical chemistry has been steady since the eighteenth century, it was only in our lifetime that the nature of the macromolecular state was clearly established. Until about fifty years ago it was generally believed that large, covalently bonded, well defined macromolecules do not exist, and only ill-defined colloidal structures and complexes are formed[1]. Thus DNA, known since 1869, was considered to be a colloidal aggregate of tetranucleotides of unknown structure and function[2]. Once the basic principle was recognized that various atoms (such as carbon, nitrogen, oxygen, phosphorous and others) can join to form long chains, the macromolecular state could be defined and studied. The very important functional properties of biological macromolecules were quickly recognized and the classical contribution of Watson and Crick[3] provided the link between structure and function. Today we again stand at the threshold of a major revolution. We are witnessing the possibility to interfere with genetic, developmental and regulatory features of the biological machinery, in which macromolecules play a major role[4].

Linear double stranded helical DNA threads of higher order eukaryotic organisms may be centimeters long but only nanometers across. For proper packaging in nuclei of microscopically sized cells, DNA complexes with proteins, mostly histones. Hierarchies of structures arise, culminating in the chromosome. Though packaged, DNA must be instantly available for transcription and replication. The exact details are under active investigation[5]. DNA, histones and non-histone proteins play both structural and functional roles.

A complex of about 160 base pairs of DNA wound in two superhelical turns around eight (twice four) inner, or core, histones constitutes the nucleosome, the basic repeating unit in chromatin structure discovered not so long ago[6]. Long strings of nucleosomes, separated by stretches of linker DNA and complexed with one additional H1(H5) linker histone, form irregularly unfolded "10 nm" fibers at low ionic strength, yet fold apparently regularly into "30 nm" solenoids upon addition of monovalent salt or small amounts of divalent ions[7]. Work from our laboratory to be presented here focuses on understanding some basic aspects of the transition from free DNA in solution to the DNA-histone nucleosome complex and

1

thence to the characterization of the formation and significance of the chromatin higher order structure.

The methodology applied to study structural features of biological macromolecules in solution has developed over many years. For two-component non-ionic systems (one macromolecule, one solvent) simple particle or thermodynamic approaches are equivalent for the successful interpretation of information devised from an ultracentrifugation or scattering experiment. Biological macromolecular systems on the other hand often comprise more than one macromolecular component but always a number of low molecular weight buffer components. Strong interactions between macro-macro, micro-micro and macro-micro components make the use of multicomponent thermodynamic and fluctuation theory imperative[8]. The ionic character of both macro and micro components prescribes use of polyelectrolyte and ionic solution theory for proper evaluation of experimental data[9,10].

DNA CONFORMATION IN SOLUTION

The conformation of DNA in solution is best described by the Porod-Kratky model of the wormlike, or persistent chain[11,12]. Intuitively we expect that over short distances along the Watson-Crick B double helix rodlike behavior is indicated, whereas over larger distances bending occurs due to the large size of chains, the natural flexibility of the multiply bonded structure, and thermal disorganizing motion. The type of behavior encountered depends on the nature of the probe used. Small angle scatterring of X-rays (having a typical wavelength $\lambda$ = 0.154 nm) is analogous to scattering with visible light (typical $\lambda$ = 514.5 nm) but is more sensitive to the rodlike nature of the DNA structure over short distances. From its use we may derive the radius of gyration of the cross-section ($R_{gc}$) and the mass per unit length ($M_L$) along the chain. From the angular dependence of the scattered light, on the other hand, information may be derived on global properties, such as the molar mass (M) and the radius of gyration ($R_g$), allowing evaluation of the bending of DNA molecules over larger, macromolecular distances[13]. At this lower resolution, details of molecular structure cannot be inferred.

The Porod-Kratky model envisages a stiff chain which, at short lenghts of the chains, approximates rodlike behavior. With increasing chain lengths coiled conformations come into play, and at very long chain lengths the model asymptotically approaches the Gaussian chain. The persistent chain is characterized by a continuous curvature of the chain skeleton, the direction of curvature at distant points on the trajectory being random.

For evaluation of the basic features of the persistent chain, one may start[14] with a hypothetical freely rotating chain constructed of $\underline{n}$ bonds of length $\ell$ each, joined at fixed bond angles $\pi-\theta$; the average projection of the kth bond on the direction of the first bond is $\ell\alpha^{k-1}$, where $\alpha = \cos\theta$. The persistence length, $\underline{a}$, is defined by the sum of all these projections, for an infinitely long chain ($n \to \infty$), $a = \ell/(1-\alpha)$. The freely rotating chain, with fixed bond length and angle, is transformed into a continuously curving chain (the wormlike chain) by letting both $\ell$ and $\theta$ go to zero, while keeping the total contour length $L = \alpha n\ell$ of the chain constant. One derives for the mean square end-to-end distance ($<r^2>$)

$$<r^2>/L^2 = 2(a/L) \ [1 - (a/L) \ (1-e^{-L/a})] \tag{1}$$

For very short stiff chains ($L/a \ll 1$) the exponential in eq. (1) may be expanded to yield the limiting value $<r^2> = L^2$, which is the relationship applicable for a rigid rod; for very long chains ($L/a \gg 1$), eq. (1) simplifies to $<r^2> = 2aL$ which is the relationship applicable to Gaussian

2

coils when the persistence length $\underline{a}$ is just one half the length of the Kuhn statistical element A. We can thus refer to L/a persistence lengths or L/2a Kuhn statistical elements per chain. For an intuitive feeling for chain bending, we note that for L = a eq. (1) yields $\langle r^2 \rangle / L^2 = 2/e$ and $\langle r^2 \rangle^{1/2}/L = 0.86$, whereas unity would correspond to a straight rod.

A derivation of eq. (1) based on the elastic properties of a curving chain provides a physical basis for the rather abstract statistical concept of the persistence length, in terms of the energy changes invovled in fluctuations (in a Brownian field) in the curvature of long-chain molecules[15]. It is assumed that the chain is originally straight and undergoes weak bending in the sense that the curvature $\rho$ is small at every point. The free energy of the elastically bent molecule is then given as a linear function in the square of the curvature vector. Statistical considerations lead to

$$\langle \cos\theta(\ell) \rangle = \exp(-\ell kT/b) \tag{2}$$

where $\theta(\ell)$ denotes the angle between two tangents to the curve separated by a distance $\ell$ along the chain, and b is the force constant in the relationship $\Delta F = 0.5\, b^2 \rho$. Eq. (2) shows that for large values of $\ell$ the mean values of $\langle \cos\theta(\ell) \rangle$ approach zero, that is, distant sections along the macromolecule are statistically independent. (In this treatment torsion is neglected and the average cosine of the angles between planes of successive tangents to the chain equals zero.) In the final step of the calculation a result identical to eq. (1) is obtained for $\langle r^2 \rangle$ with the persistence length $\underline{a}$ in the previous derivation equal to a = b/kT. Thus we expect $\underline{a}$ to decrease with increasing temperatures; at low temperatures, on the other hand, a more rodlike behavior is expected.

The mean square end-to-end distance $\langle r^2 \rangle$ of polymer chain is not a measurable quantity. A measurable quantity (from the angular dependence of the scattering of radiation, light, X-rays or neutrons) is the root-mean-square radius of gyration, $\langle R^2 \rangle^{1/2} \equiv R_g$. From it the persistence length $\underline{a}$ can be evaluated by[16]

$$\frac{R_g^2}{L^2} = \frac{1}{6X} - \frac{1}{4X^2} + \frac{1}{4X^3} - \frac{1-e^{-2X}}{8X^4} \tag{3}$$

where X = L/2a, the number of Kuhn statistical segments per chain. For short stiff chains (X << 1) the exponential in eq. (3) may be expanded to yield the limiting value $12R_g^2 = L^2$, which is the relationship applicable to a rigid rod; for very long chains (X >> 1) eq. (3) simplifies to $6R_g^2 = 2aL$, which applies to Gaussian coils. In Figure 1 we have plotted the coiling ratio $\sqrt{12}\, R_g/L$ calculated for reasonable values of $\underline{a}$, applicable to DNA, as a function of log M (or log number of base pairs, bp) to indicate the transition from typical, almost rodlike, DNA fragments to Gaussian coils[17]. For nucleosome length DNA (about 165 bp), the coiling ratio is around 0.9.

All considerations presented above for the analysis of the persistent chain neglects excluded volume. At low concentrations of low molecular weight salt, volume exclusion is large, and mostly due to electrostatic repulsion within highly charged DNA chains. Excluded volume of electrostatic origin is much reduced and vanishes at high enough concentrations of salt, the remaining volume exclusion being due to physical crossing of chains and van der Waals repulsion. Many years ago Flory[1] showed that, in poor solvents, attraction may outweight repulsion, leading to a vanishing of the excluded volume. Under these conditions eq. (3) applies. We have, some time ago, been able to show that such circumstances can be conveniently realized in poly A solutions at neutral pH[18]. In the case of NaDNA in

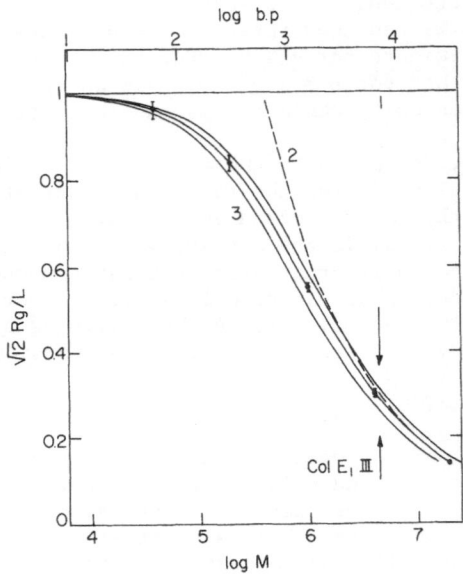

Fig. 1: Coiling ratio $\sqrt{12}R_g/L$ of NaDNA chains against log M (or log number of base pairs, bp). Curve 1, rigid rod; curve 2, Gaussian coil with statistical element 2a equal to 100 nm; set of curves 3, Kratky-Porod wormlike chains without excluded volume, for (in descending order) persistence lengths a equal to 60, 50, and 40 nm. Experimental points have been simulated for a = 50 nm, assuming a combined error in $R_g$ and L. of ±2%; a repeat length 0.34 nm/bp and M/L = 1950 g $mol^{-1}nm^{-1}$ have been assumed for the B-form of NaDNA[17].

NaCl the excluded volume does not vanish at the highest NaCl concentrations, as monitored by nonvanishing values of the second virial coefficients, $A_2$, which constitutes a measure of intermolecular chain interactions. Flory[1] has shown that intermolecular chain interactions, as expressed in $A_2$, are a good measure of the intramolecular chain interactions leading to expansion of the polymer chains at finite excluded volume. He and others[19] have indicated ways for correcting experimental values to vanishing excluded volume, by equating intermolecular to intramolecular excluded volume. We have used these procedures[20] to correct values for the persistence length a of DNA, obtained over a wide range of NaCl concentrations, to the absence of excluded volume. Fearful of overcorrection, we have also used approximate scattering equations of chains with excluded volume for the same intent[17]. At high enough NaCl concentrations (above 0.2 M), the outcome is not sensitive to the procedure employed even though, as pointed out by Manning[21], equating the intermolecular to intramolecular excluded volume is restricted to infinitely long chains. Post[22] has recently compared the various procedures used to correct for excluded volumes in finite chains to a Monte Carlo evaluation of this correction.

To overcome the difficulties involved in correcting for excluded volumes in DNA solutions, we have recently studied scattering and hydrodynamic properties of monodisperse linear Col $E_1$ plasmid LiDNA in LiCl solutions[23]. LiDNA is believed to undergo chain condensation followed by precipitation at very high concentrations of LiCl[24]. We were pleasantly surprised to note that up to about 9M LiCl concentration conformational parameters decreased smoothly reaching a limiting value at high salt[23]. Virial coefficients vanished, allowing use of equations without excluded volume. Since it had been recently shown that contrary to previous views, LiDNA remains in the B conformation even at these high LiCl concentrations[25], we could calculate from our data limiting persistence lengths for LiDNA at high salt. We found a value of 28.5 nm, which is in good agreement with values previously obtained for NaDNA at high NaCl concentrations[17,20] and can be identified with the high salt limit of DNA flexibility, with long range electrostatic interactions effectively screened. At 0.2 LiCl we find 38.7 nm, rather close to 36.6 nm obtained for NaDNA in NaCl by the correction procedure[20] equating intermolecular to intramolecular volume exclusion (the alternate procedure[17] yielded 40.8 nm for NaDNA in 0.2 M NaCl). These numbers at 0.2 M NaCl are close enough to indicate significantly higher flexibility for DNA than previously accepted (with the persistence length $a$ around 50 nm at 0.2 M NaCl) and the reader is referred to the original publications for a detailed discussion[17,20,23]. Higher DNA flexibility is a desirable attribute if we focus, as we shall below, on the folding of DNA in nucleosome and chromatin structures.

The study of DNA flexibility has literally gone through many ups and downs since this question could be properly posed. I have summarized the early work in 1974[26]. Doubts that the Kratky-Porod treatment yields a reliable value of $a$ for very short chains[27] could be put aside once proper corrections for optical anisotropy were applied to classical light scattering experiments[28]. Yet a true turning point in this type of study came about with the present day possibility to investigate uniform DNA samples of appropriate size by modern laser light scattering techniques, at low angles of scattering[29]. Laser light scattering, in addition to the classical elastic scattering technique, now also provides dynamic information by quasielastic scattering of light. Therefore, in conjunction with hydrodynamic measurements (by viscosity and ultracentrifuge) we now dispose of a broad spectrum of experimental methods to characterize well defined DNA conformations. Though our discussion here has been limited to the classical B form DNA, much work is yet to be done on the conformation of Z and other conformational DNA forms[5] under various experimental conditions.

EQUILIBRIUM SEDIMENTATION AND FORWARD SCATTERING OF RADIATION

It is a deeply ingrained feeling in many that molecular weights, or rather, molar masses (in g/mole) using modern parliance, are determined by equilibrium sedimentation in the ultracentrifuge. Perhaps no such strong feelings exist for quantities derived from a scattering process, such as the intensity of the scattered light, for instance, yet it seems intuitive that a centrifugal field weighs particles, and therefore directly yields the molar mass. Nothing could be further from the truth and I have spent many years to dispel this erroneous notion[8]. Both equilibrium sedimentation and the intensity of light, of neutrons and X-rays, extrapolated into the forward direction, are colligative methods, counting particles, rather than weighing them. We thus derive through experiments the number of particles, or moles, per unit volume (ml) from which a molar mass may be derived, based on the knowledge of the particle concentration in g/ml, or some other suitable unit. As we shall soon see in a brief summary of working equations, both the distribution in a centrifugal field and the intensity of radiation scattered in the forward direction depend on the second derivative of the free energy with respect to particle concentration (equivalent to the first derivative of the osmotic pressure $\Pi$ with respect to concentration), at constant chemical potentials $\mu$ of low molecular weight components. In the simplest case for discussion, yet sufficient to describe even considerably more complex situations, we consider a three-component system where component 1 is the principal solvent, component 2 is a homogeneous macromolecule and component 3 is a low molecular weight neutral component, or salt. In the latter case, and if component 2 is composed of charged species, we stipulate a common ion between components 2 and 3.

A brief summary of equations follows. The exact expression for the equilibrium distribution of component 2 in the centrifugal field is given by

$$\frac{d\ell n c_2}{dr^2} = \frac{\omega^2}{2} \; (\frac{\partial \rho}{\partial c_2})_\mu \; (\frac{d\Pi}{dc_2})^{-1} \tag{4}$$

where r is the distance from the center of rotation, $\omega$ is the angular velocity, $(\partial \rho / \partial c_2)_\mu$ is the density increment, at constant chemical potential $\mu$, of all components ($\mu_1$ and $\mu_3$ in this case) diffusible through a semipermeable membrane, and can be determined in a separate experiment. Eq. (4) is symmetrical with respect to all electroneutral components of the system and applies at each level $\underline{r}$ in the ultracentrifuge. Constant temperature is assumed throughout and will not be specified in the subscripts.

Under the conditions discussed above, the osmotic pressure derivative in eq. (4) can be expanded in a virial series in powers of $c_2$ to yield

$$\Pi/c_2 \, RT = M_2^{-1} + A_2 c_2 + A_3 c_2^2 + \ldots \tag{5}$$

where $M_2$ is the molar mass (g/mole) and the $A_i$ are the virial coefficients. (This expansion is not allowed in the absence of a supporting simple screening electrolyte component 3, if component 2 is charged and the electrostatic potential is long ranged. In the presence of any amount of screening electrolyte it is required for the concentration of component 2 to be such that the ionic strength contributed by it be smaller than that due to component 3.)

At vanishing concentration $c_2$, eq. (4) reduces to

$$\frac{d\ell n c_2}{dr^2} = \frac{\omega^2}{2RT} \; (\frac{\partial \rho}{\partial c_2})_\mu \; M_2 \tag{6}$$

The formulations, eqs. (4) and (6), clearly indicate that multiplication of $c_2$ and $M_2$ by scale factors leaves the equations unchanged; the dimensions of $c_2/M_2$ are moles/ml. We thus confirm the conclusion that this colligative method 'counts' molecules per unit volume and molar masses enter in units commensurate to the concentrations units chosen.

All forward scattering experiments lead to similar results[30]. I dramatize this conclusion by asking, if a sample of NaDNA is dissolved in a solution of CsCl, is the molecular weight of NaDNA, or of CsDNA, or of a mixed entity, determined at equilibrium in the ultracentrifuge? Or do we determine the molecular weight of the macroion without or with only a partial condensed layer of counterions? The question is irrelevant, following the argument above. If we express the concentration in the density increment (in the experimental medium) in grams of NaDNA per ml then the molecular weight is given in grams of NaDNA per mole. Any other concentration unit (moles of phosphate per ml for instance) will lead to a self-consistent result for M (moles of phosphate per mole of macromolecules in this case). No additional "primary" information beyond the number of particles and the thermodynamic interactions between them (as expressed in the virial coefficients) is derivable from equilibrium sedimentation and from all forward scattering experiments. We will soon discuss how, nevertheless, information on binding of component 3 and of component 1 can be obtained from this type of experiment.

6

In conventional equilibrium sedimentation, the density $\rho°$ of the solvent medium (in the absence of solute) is constant throughout the ultracentrifuge cell; this leads to constant $(\partial\rho/\partial c_2)_\mu$ at vanishing $c_2$. On the other hand, if $\rho°$ increases with r, $(\partial\rho/\partial c_2)_\mu$ decreases in the density gradient. A macromolecular 'band' will form around the position at which the density increment vanishes. The position and shape of the band discloses information about buoyancy properties and molecular weight of macromolecules banded. The relation to contrast variation in X-ray and neutron forward scattering is immediate[30].

The derivative in eq. (4) of the osmotic pressure with respect to $c_2$ appears because, in order to create a concentration gradient of component 2 in the centrifugal field, osmotic work must be expended, even though a semipermeable membrane is absent. A powerful way to analyze scattering phenomena uses statistical mechanics to relate time average fluctuating scattering inhomogeneities in small volumes of solution to the intensity of the scattered forward radiation. Osmotic work is required to produce the fluctuations and refractive index increments $(\partial n/\partial c_2)_\mu$ in light scattering, electron density increments $(\partial\rho_{el}/\partial c_2)_\mu$ in X-ray scattering, and scattering length density increments $(\partial\rho_n/\partial c_2)_\mu$ in neutron scattering replace the density increments encountered in ultracentrifugation.

At finite concentration the equivalent equations are

$$(\frac{\partial n}{\partial c_2})^2_{P,\mu_3} \frac{Kc_2}{\Delta R(0)} = \frac{1}{RT} \frac{d\Pi}{dc_2} \tag{7}$$

for light scattering (K is an optical constant and $\Delta R(0)$ refers to forward [extrapolated to zero angle] scattering in excess of solvent scattering).

For small angle X-ray scattering

$$(\frac{\partial\rho_{el}}{\partial c_2})^2_{P,\mu_3} \frac{I_{el}c_2}{\Delta I(0)} = \frac{1}{kT} \frac{d\Pi}{dc_2} \tag{8}$$

where $I_{el}$ is the scattering of an electron and $\Delta I(0)$ is the forward excess scattering of X-rays.

Finally, for neutrons

$$(\frac{\partial\rho_n}{\partial c_2})^2_{P,\mu_2} \frac{c_2}{\Delta I_o(0)} = \frac{1}{kT} \frac{d\Pi}{dc_2} \tag{9}$$

where $\Delta I_o(0)$ is the forward excess scattering of neutrons per unit incident neutron flux, with proper corrections for geometrical factors and detector configuration. Details have been given elsewhere[30]. At vanishing concentration $c_2$, the osmotic pressure derivative, is replaced everywhere by $RT/M_2$ and all considerations presented in the context of equilibrium sedimentation apply. The increments of $\rho$, and of $n$, are experimentally accessible quantities, whereas those of $\rho_{el}$ and of $\rho_n$ are derived indirectly, though it may have recently become possible to determine the concentration increment of $\rho_n$[30].

CONTRAST VARIATION FOR THE DETERMINATION OF BINDING OF COMPONENTS 2 AND 1 (HYDRATION)

From the variation of the density increments $(\partial\rho/\partial c_2)_\mu$ with solution density $\rho°$ in three component systems, information may be derived on the interaction of component 2 with both components 1 and 3. I will restrict myself here to a brief discussion of the increments of mass only, yet the considerations apply equally to the other increments mentioned and interesting complementarities result following combination of more than one method. The increments may be determined experimentally, where applicable, or extracted from sedimentation, or scattering, experiments[8,30].

For the three component system under consideration

$$(\partial\rho/\partial c_2)_\mu = (1 - \bar{v}_2\rho) + \xi_1 (1 - \bar{v}_1\rho) \tag{10a}$$

$$= (1 + \xi_1) - \rho° (\bar{v}_2 + \rho_1\bar{v}_1) \tag{10b}$$

where $\xi_1$ is a formal interaction parameter (g of component 1 "preferentially" excluded per g of component 3), the $\bar{v}_i$ are partial specific volumes, and symmetry considerations require validity of substitution of subscript 1 by subscript 3 in eqs. (10); $\xi_1$ and $\xi_3$ are related by

$$\xi_1 = - \xi_3/w_3 \tag{11}$$

where $w_3$ is a weight molality in g of component 3 per g of component 1.

It is often found that $(\partial\rho/\partial c_2)_\mu$ decreases linearly with $\rho°$, yet this does not imply constancy of $\xi_1$ or $\xi_3$. As a matter of fact $\xi_1$ and $\xi_3$ vary strongly with $\rho°$ (or $w_3$). If we assume that component 2 'excludes' $B_1$ g/g of component 1 as well as $B_3$ g/g of component 3 then one easily derives

$$(\partial\rho/\partial c_2)_\mu = (1 - \bar{v}_2\rho°) + B_1 (1 - \bar{v}_1\rho°) + B_3 (1 - \bar{v}_3\rho°) \tag{12a}$$

$$= (1 + B_1 + B_3) - \rho° (\bar{v}_2 + B_1\bar{v}_1 + B_3\bar{v}_3) \tag{12b}$$

(If component 2 is charged we should write $B_3' = B_3 - E_3$, where $E_3$ is g/g of component 3 excluded by a Donnan mechanism.)

The equivalence of eqs. (10) and (12) is established by deriving

$$\xi_1 = B_1 - B_3/w_3 \tag{13}$$

From eq. (12b) we conclude that component 2 can be redefined as an equivalent particle, for all intents and purposes, of mass $M_2(1 + B_1 + B_3)$ and volume $M_2(\bar{v}_2 + B_1\bar{v}_1 + B_3\bar{v}_3)$ per mole. Thus it is proven that contrast variation allows the determination of 'binding' of low molecular weight to the macromolecular component from the measurements of density increments, equilibrium sedimentation, combination of velocity sedimentation and diffusion or, equivalently, forward scattering of light, X-rays and neutrons.

From the linear dependence of $\xi_1$ on $w_3$, $B_1$ and $B_3$ may be calculated. This has been done for a number of systems. With Donnan exclusion duly considered, we derive a value of $B_1 = 3.7$ water molecules per nucleotide for NaDNA in NaCl and 5.9 water molecules per nucleotide for CsDNA in CsCl, an average of 5 water molecules, with an uncertainty of one[31,32]. This compares well with the value of 5 (three phosphate and one each in the major and minor grooves) with an uncertainty of one, recently estimated by Kopka et al.[33] from X-ray diffraction studies of a B-DNA dodecamer. This is about half of other estimates arrived at by various procedures.

Above I have demonstrated that, probing by varying the concentration of 'small' probes (NaCl, CsCl) we determine volumes of component 2 'excluded' to the probe, and qualified as hydration, in this operational definition. Using the 'small' neutral probes (sucrose, raffinose, glycerol) we could show[34] that hydration of nucleosome core particles derived from equilibrium sedimentation, agrees with the corresponding quantity derived from neutron scattering by varying glycerol concentration. Different excluded volumes may be probed by contrast variation with larger probes which do not, or only partially, penetrate the nucleosome. We initially demonstrated this procedure by studying equilibrium sedimentation of nucleosome core particles of various concentrations of dextran, a soluble branched polysaccharide[34]. We have now extended this work to sedimentation and small angle X-ray scattering studies of nucleosome core particles, probing with cyclodextrin, a well defined cycloocta-amylase[35]. Whereas, by the determination of frictional parameters and of parameters from small angle scattering only gross dimensional outlines can be established, contrast variation with suitable probes may, in favorable circumstances, distinguish between interior excluded volumes and surface convolutions[35].

## NUCLEOSOME CORE PARTICLE STABILITY AND CONFORMATIONAL CHANGE

The methods discussed above have been applied to the study of the reversible dissociation of core size DNA from chicken erythrocyte nucleosome core particles in solutions containing 0.1 M to 0.6 M NaCl[36]. It was found that dissociation increases with increasing NaCl concentration, increasing temperature and decreasing particle concentration. At high particle concentrations, below 0.3 M NaCl, no free DNA is observed, whereas above 0.3 M NaCl a lower limit of dissociation is reached. The data were analyzed on the basis of the migrating octamer mechanism of Stein[37] involving core particles (C), free DNA (D) and histone octamer (O). The octamers O may leave a core particle C and remain free in solution, or associate with another core particle C (Stein[37] did not allow for free O in solution). The two equilibria

$$D + O \rightleftharpoons C \tag{14}$$

and

$$C + O \rightleftharpoons CO \tag{15}$$

are characterized by two equilibrium association constants

$$K_1 = [C]/[D] [O] \tag{16}$$

and

$$K_2 = [CO]/[C] [O] \tag{17}$$

Furthermore,

$$K \equiv K_1/K_2 = [C]^2/[D] [CO] \tag{18}$$

characterizes the migration of histone octamers between two core particles

$$D + CO \rightleftharpoons 2C. \tag{19}$$

Strictly speaking, at the NaCl concentrations (0.5 and 0.6 M) at which the analysis was performed the core histones are not in the octamer complex (when free in solution) but appear rather as H3, H4 tetramers and H2A, H2B dimers, yet a detailed analysis taking all subspecies into consideration is far too complex for kinetic analysis. From the inability, though, of H2A,

H2B dimers to bind to nucleosome core particles (in distinction to the H3, H4 tetramers)[34] we assume the determining step in DNA histone association under these conditions to be with the H3, H4 entity, the H2, AB dimers then fitting into the preformed site. The H3, H4 tetramer and nominal histone octamer concentrations are identical.

The migrating octamer mechanism provides a good explanation for our observations, and those of others, up to 1 M NaCl concentration. In particular it explains why, at the higher NaCl concentrations, free DNA remains at the highest concentrations of nucleosome core particles. It appears from the analysis that the core particle is not primarily stabilized by electrostatic interactions. DNA length is not critical for core particle stabilization. The conformation of remaining intact nucleosome core particles changes only moderately within the range (0.1 to 0.7 M) of NaCl concentrations studied. We note that though frictional parameters increase moderately in this range of NaCl concentrations, the radius of gyration $R_g$, as determined by small angle X-ray scattering[35,38], is totally unchanged over the whole range of NaCl concentrations. Considering that the intensity of X-ray scattering under the conditions of the experiment is essentially determined by the nucleic acid, rather than the protein moiety, we conclude that DNA conformation is unchanged between 0.1 and 0.7 M NaCl. The change in frictional coefficients must therefore be rationalized in terms of changes in histone conformation involving increasing mobility of histone tails with increasing concentration of salt[39]. The conformational stability of the nucleosome core particles has been further confirmed by monitoring essentially identical hydrodynamic properties between 0.1 and 0.6 M NaCl, following in situ crosslinking by copper phenantroline of the Cys-110 histone H3 single sulfhydryl groups in intact nucleosome core particles[36]. The frictional properties of nucleosome core particles at 0.1 M NaCl are well described[34] in terms of a flat cylinder model (diameter 11 nm, height 5.7 nm) as derived by neutron scattering and X-ray diffraction[40-42].

INTERACTION OF CHROMATIN WITH NaCl AND $MgCl_2$, SOLUBILITY AND BINDING STUDIES, TRANSITION TO, AND CHARACTERIZATION OF THE HIGHER ORDER STRUCTURE

In distinction to uniform plasmid DNA[29] and nucleosome core particles[36] even well characterized chromatin samples are not of uniform size and the polydispersity of the chromatin must be taken into account in the evaluation of hydrodynamic and light scattering results. Chicken erythrocyte chromatin containing histones H1 and H5 was carefully separated into a number of well characterized fractions[43]. Distinction could be made between chromatin insoluble in NaCl above about 80 mM, and chromatin soluble at all NaCl concentrations. Both chromatin forms were indistinguishable electrophoretically and both underwent the transition from the low salt "10 nm" coil to the "30 nm" higher order structure solenoid[7], by either raising the $MgCl$ concentration to about 0.3 mM or NaCl concentration to about 75 mM. The transitions were examined in detail by elastic light scattering procedures. It could be shown that the "10 nm" form is a flexible coil. The "30 nm" solenoid assumption of rigid cylindrical structure was in good agreement with 5.7 nucleosomes per helical turn. However, disagreement of calculated frictional parameters with values derived from quasielastic light scattering and sedimentation introduced the possibility that the higher order structure, under these conditions, is more extended, flexible, or maybe a mixture of structures[43]. The study of small angle X-ray scattering presently in progress in our laboratory[44] extends the resolution achievable by light scattering to the probing of details of local structure. In particular, it allows reinterpretation of data in terms of a more extended, flexible, "higher order" structure. This is not unreasonable considering that the "higher order" structure is only one step in a plethora of further stages of chromatin condensation.

ACKNOWLEDGEMENTS

This research is the result of collaboration with many colleagues over many years, their names appearing in the appropriate references. Recent work was supported by a grant from the United States-Israel Binational Science Foundation (BSF), Jerusalem, Israel.

To understand the interaction of chromatin with NaCl and with $MgCl_2$, a number of experiments were undertaken to study solubility, precipitation, conformational transitions and binding of ions over a wide range of experimental conditions, including chromatin concentration[43]. We have also investigated the interaction of other divalent ions with chromatin towards a closer understanding of the role of metal ions in the nucleus[45]. The first row transition metal ion chlorides $MnCl_2$, $CoCl_2$, $NiCl_2$, and $CuCl_2$ lead to precipitation of chicken erythrocyte chromatin at a significantly lower concentration than the alkali earth metal chlorides $MgCl_2$, $CaCl_2$ and $BaCl_2$. A similar distinction can be made for the compaction of chromatin to "30 nm" solenoid higher order structure, which occurs at lower $MeCl_2$ concentration in the first group, but at the same $MeCl_2$ concentration within each group. In other experiments in which mixed solutions of NaCl and of $MgCl_2$ were examined, it could be shown that increasing NaCl concentration leads to increasing solubility in the presence of $MgCl_2$. Best compaction of chromatin was obtained at 40 mM NaCl and 0.8 mM $MgCl_2$ at a value $A_{260}$ approximately 0.8. Similar experiments were undertaken with mixtures of NaCl and $MnCl_2$.

REFERENCES

1. P. J. Flory, "Principles of Polymer Chemistry," Cornell University Press, Ithaca (1953).

2. A. Kornberg, "DNA Replication," W.H. W. H. Freeman and Company, San Francisco (1980).

3. J. D. Watson and F. H. C. Crick, Molecular structure of nucleic acids, Nature 171:737 (1953).

4. Recombinant DNA, Science 209:]3]7-]438 (1980).

5. Structures of DNA, Cold Spring Harbor Symposium on Quantitative Biology, Vol. 47, Cold Spring Harbor, New York (1982).

6. Chromatin, Cold Spring Harbor Symposium on Quantitative Biology, Vol. 42, Cold Spring Harbor, New York (1977).

7. J. T. Finch and A. Klug, Solenoidal model for superstructure in chromatin, Proc. Natl. Acad. Sci. USA 73:1897-1901 (1976).

8. H. Eisenberg, "Solutions of Biological Macromolecules and Polyelectrolytes," Clarendon Press, Oxford (1976).

9. G. S. Manning, The molecular theory of polyelectrolyte solutions with applications to the electrostatic properties of polynucleotides, Q. Rev. Biophys. 11:179-246 (1978).

10.  M. T. Record, Jr., C. F. Anderson, and T. M. Lohman, Thermodynamic analysis of ion effects on the binding and conformational equilibria of proteins and nucleic acids:  The roles of ion association on release, screening, and ion effects on water activity, Q. Rev. Biophys. 11:103-178 (1978).

G. Porod, X-ray and light scattering by chain molecules in solution, J. Polymer Sci. 10:157-167 (1953).

12.  O. Kratky and G. Porod, X-ray investigation of dissolved chain molecules, Rec. Trav. Chim. Pays-Bas. 68:1106-1122 (1949).

13.  H. Eisenberg, Light scattering and some aspects of small angle X-ray scattering, in: "Procedures in Nucleic Acid Research," Volume 2, G. L. Cantoni and D. R. Davies, eds., Harper and Row, New York, pp. 137-175 (1971).

14.  P. J. Flory, "Statistical Mechanics of Chain Molecules,"  Interscience Publishers, New York, pp. 401-403 (1969).

15.  L. D. Landau and E. M. Lifshitz, "Statistical Physics," Pergamon Press, London, pp. 478-482 (1959).

16.  H. Benoit and P. Doty, Light scattering from non Gaussian chains, J. Phys. Chem. 57:958-963 (1953).

17.  Z. Kam, N. Borochov, and H. Eisenberg, Dependence of laser light scattering of DNA on NaCl concentration, Biopolymers 20:2671-2690 (1981).

18.  H. Eisenberg and G. Felsenfeld, Studies of the temperature dependent conformation and phase separation of polyriboadenylic acid solutions at neutral pH, J. Mol. Biol. 30:17-37 (1967).

19.  H. Yamakawa, "Modern Theory of Polymer Solutions," Harper and Row, New York, pp. 372-379 (1971).

20.  N. Borochov, H. Eisenberg, and Z. Kam, Dependence of DNA conformation on the concentration of salt, Biopolymers 20:231-235 (1981).

21.  G. S. Manning, A procedure for extracting persistence lengths from light scattering data on intermediate molecular weight DNA, Biopolymers 20:1751-1755 (1981).

22.  C. B. Post, Excluded volume of an intermediate molecular weight DNA. A Monte Carlo analysis, Biopolymers 22:1087-1096 (1983).

23.  N. Borochov and H. Eisenberg, Conformation of LiDNA in solutions of LiCl, Biopolymers 23:1757-1769 (1984).

24.  B. Wolf, S. Berman, and S. Hanlon, Structural transitions of calf thymus DNA in concentrated LiCl solution, Biochemistry 16:3655-3662 (1977).

25.  S. B. Zimmerman and B. H. Pheiffer, Does DNA adopt the C form in concentrated salt solutions or in organic solvent/water mixtures?  An X-ray diffraction study of fibers immersed in various media. J. Mol. Biol. 142:315-330 (1980).

26. H. Eisenberg, Hydrodynamic and thermodynamic studies, in: "Basic Principles in Nucleic Acid Chemistry," Volume 2, Paul O. P. Ts'o, ed., Academic Press, New York, pp. 171-264 (1974).

27. H. Eisenberg, On the inherent flexibility of DNA chains, Biopolymers 8:545-551 (1969).

28. J. E. Godfrey and H. Eisenberg, The flexibility of low molecular weight double stranded DNA as a function of length, Biophysical Chem. 5:301-318 (1976).

29. G. Voordouw, Z. Kam, N. Borochov, and H. Eisenberg, Isolation and physical studies of the intact supercoiled, the open circular and the linear forms of Col $E_1$ plasmid DNA, Biophysical Chem. 8:171-189 (1978).

30. H. Eisenberg, Forward scattering of light, X-rays and neutrons, Q. Rev. Biophys. 14:141-172 (1981).

31. E. Reisler, Y. Haik, and H. Eisenberg, Bovine serum albumin in aqueous guanidine hydrochloride solutions. Preferential and absolute interactions and comparison with other systems, Biochemistry 16:197-203 (1977).

32. G. Cohen and H. Eisenberg, Deoxyribonucleate solutions: sedimentation in a density gradient, partial specific volumes, density and refractive index increments, and preferential interactions, Biopolymers 6:1077-1100 (1968).

33. M. L. Kopka, A. V. Fratini, H. R. Drew, and R. E. Dickerson, Ordered water structure around a B-DNA dodecamer, J. Mol. Biol. 163:129-146 (1983).

34. H. Eisenberg and G. Felsenfeld, Hydrodynamic studies of the interaction between nucleosome core particles and core histones, J. Mol. Biol. 150: 537-555 (1981).

35. K. O. Greulich, J. Ausio, and H. Eisenberg, J. Mol. Biol., submitted.

36. J. Ausio, D. Seger, and H. Eisenberg, Nucleosome core particle stability and conformational change: effect of temperature, particle and NaCl concentration, corsslinking of H3 histone sulfhydryl groups. J. Mol. Biol. 176:77-104 (1984).

37. A. Stein, DNA folding by histones: The kinetics of chromatin core particles reassembly and the interaction of nucleosomes with histones, J. Mol. Biol. 130:103-134 (1979).

38. M. Reich, Small angle X-ray scattering from biological macromolecules, Thesis, The Weizmann Institute of Science, Rehovot (1982).

39. P. D. Cary, T. Moss, and E. M. Bradbury, High resolution proton-magnetic-resonance studies of chromatin core particles, Eur. J. Biochem. 89:475-482 (1978).

40. J. R. Pardon, D. L. Worcester, J. C. Wooley, K. Tatchell, K. E. van Holde, and B. M. Richards, Low angle neutron scattering from chromatin subunit particles, Nucl. Acids Res. 2:2163-2176 (1975).

41.  P. Suau, G. G. Kneale, G. W. Braddock, J. P. Baldwin, and E. M. Bradbury, A low resolution model for the chromatin core particle by neutron scattering, Nucl. Acids Res. 4:3769-3786 (1977).

42.  J. T. Finch, L. C. Lutter, D. Rhodes, R. S. Brown, B. Rushton, M. Levitt, and A. Klug, Structure of nucleosome core particles of chromatin, Nature 269:29-36 (1977).

43.  J. Ausio, N. Borochov, D. Seger, and H. Eisenberg, Interaction of chromatin with NaCl and $MgCl_2$, solubility and binding studies, transition to, and characterization of the higher order structure, J. Mol. Biol. 177:373-398 (1984).

44.  K. O. Greulich, E. Wachtel, J. Ausio, D. Seger and H. Eisenberg, in preparation.

45.  N. Borochov, J. Ausio, and H. Eisenberg, Interaction and conformational changes of chromatin with divalent ions, Nucl. Acids Res. 12: 3089-3096 (1984).

# SIGNIFICANT LOCAL MOBILITY IN DOUBLE STRANDED DNA AND RNA

Stephen R. Holbrook* and Sung-Hou Kim

Department of Chemistry and
*Lawrence Berkeley Laboratory
University of California
Berkeley, California 94720

ABSTRACT

An analysis of X-ray diffraction data from single crystals of double helical DNA and RNA fragments reveals that local mobilities of double stranded DNA and RNA are similar to each other and are intrinsic properties of nucleotides. We have determined the directions and magnitudes of translational and rotational local mobility of phosphate, ribose, and base moieties of double stranded nucleic acids. Our primary findings are: (a) the major base pair motions are propeller twisting, rolling (rocking), buckling, and sliding; (b) the mobility of sugar moieties is coupled to their bases; and (c) the local mobilities are partly dependent on base sequences. These local mobilities help us understand intercalation, protein interaction, large scale motion, and other processes involving DNA and RNA.

It is easy to conceptually understand that double stranded DNA and RNA structures are not static but rather dynamic and flexible, fluctuating among many different conformations and perhaps even different helical forms. However, we have very little knowledge about quantitative magnitudes, directions and types of motion of nucleic acids. At the present time, there is no adequate experimental method by which one can directly measure them. However, such quantities can be derived from crystallographic "thermal" parameters (see Fig. 1) which in turn can be obtained by refinement of a model versus single crystal X-ray diffraction data, based on certain assumptions. The first assumption is that each atom in a base, sugar, or phosphate group is neither independent nor free-moving but, rather, constrained as a member of a group, and that the group can be considered the basic unit of motion. This assumption allows one to reduce the number of independent parameters to be refined using X-ray diffraction data. The second assumption is that in a single crystal, the overall molecular mobility or molecular disorder is relatively small compared to the local motion and local disorder of atomic groups in the molecule (see Fig. 1). This assumption is necessary since disorder and motion are indistinguishable from each other by X-ray diffraction.

## METHODS

Details of the methods[1] used to derive the magnitudes and directions

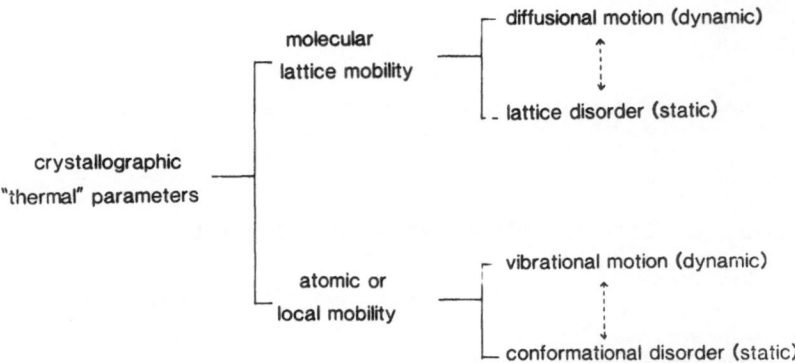

Fig. 1:  A schematic diagram illustrating the elements contributing to the
crystallographic "thermal" parameters.


of local mobility are rather involved and will not be presented here.  The
conceptual background is as follows:

X-ray scattering by a stationary atom ($f_o$) is stronger than that of a
locally moving or disordered atom, f:

$$f = f_o e^{-M}$$

where M represents a 3 x 3 symmetrical matrix containing 6 unique elements:
$U_{11}$, $U_{12}$, $U_{13}$, $U_{22}$, $U_{23}$, $U_{33}$.  These U values are called crystallographic
"thermal" parameters (which is a misnomer), and contain information about
motions and disorders of atoms in a crystal.  Furthermore, where a group of
atoms forms a rigid moiety such as a base, a sugar, or a phosphate, these U
values of the individual atoms can be related to three tensors.  These are
Translation (T), Libration (L), and Screw (S) tensors of the group to which
the atom belongs:

$$U = GL + HS + T,$$

where G and H are tensors calculable from the positions of the atoms in the
group.  Thus, the local mobility of the molecule can be understood if one
can derive the mobility of each individual atom in the molecule from single
crystal X-ray diffraction data.  However, to do so, a very large number of
diffraction data is required.  In general, such large amounts of data are
not available from single crystals of double stranded DNA or RNA fragments.
However, since the atoms in nucleic acids are not all independently free,
but rather constrained as a part of a rigid group (for example, the major
motions of the atoms in a base group are not independent but rather part of
the motion of the base plane), one can drastically reduce the number of
diffraction data required for mobility analysis if one analyzes the mobility
of the group rather than individual atoms.  This method, called the "seg-
mented rigid body", or TLS method[2], allows one to determine direction and
magnitude of the mobility of each group directly without determining the
crystallographic "thermal" parameters of the individual atoms.  This is done
by a least-squares minimization of the difference between the observed diffraction intensities and those calculated from the model while varying the
elements of T, L and S tensors.

SYSTEMS

The rigid body mobility for the phosphate, ribose (or deoxyribose), and base subgroups of the following double stranded DNA and RNA fragments has been studied: the self-complementary RNA dinucleotides ApU and GpC, and the self-complementary DNA fragment CGCGAATTCGCG. All the compounds listed above form double helical segments in the crystal. Three-dimensional structures have been determined by single crystal X-ray diffraction studies of the respective compounds[3,4,5].

REPRESENTATION OF LOCAL MOBILITY

The local mobility of each subgroup has been represented by two types of motion: libration and translation. The libration motion of a group is defined by three principal axes around which the molecule is librating (limited rotation). Similarly, translational motion is also described by defining 3 principal axes along which each group is vibrating. Thus, the direction and magnitude of group mobility can be described by rotation and translation around these principal axes. We calculated all the librational and translational motions for each group, and then superimposed all the nucleotides in DNA or RNA onto a common nucleotide. When this superposition was performed, we found that the librational axes, as well as the translational axes, have a tendency to cluster along particular directions (Fig. 2). This is a strong indication that there are intrinsic local mobilities in nucleic acid constituents.

The average values for the translational and librational mobility of double helical RNA fragment subgroups are listed in Table 1, and equivalent values for the double helical DNA fragment are shown in Table 2. Pictorial

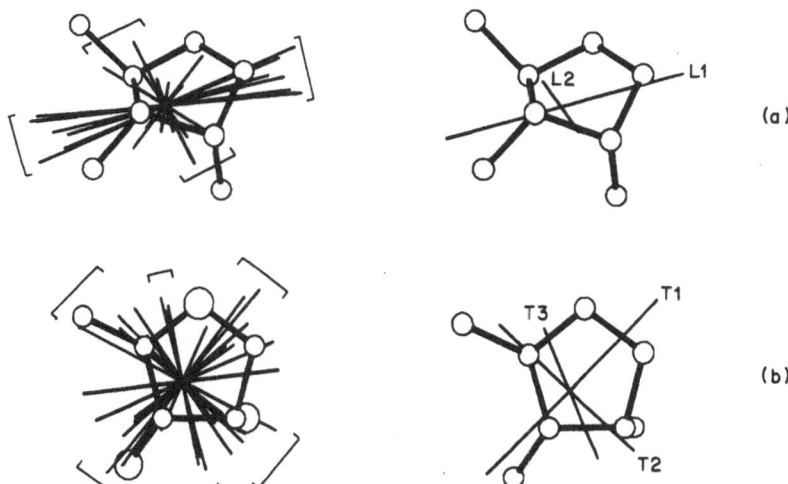

Fig. 2: The librational and translational eigenvectors of all six ribose subgroups of the base paired dinucleoside phosphates ApU and GpC are superimposed onto a common ribose for comparison and clustering. The origin of the eigenvector is at the center of mass and the length is proportional to the associated eigenvalue. The left half shows the superimposed vectors with brackets indicating how the clusters were formed. The right half shows the resultant vectors for each cluster. (a) ribose libration; (b) ribose translation.

17

Table 1: Summary of Average Eigenvalues of Ribooligonucleotide Subgroup
Clusters

| SUBGROUP | MODES[a] | VECTORS/ MODES | RMS DEV.[b] | AVG. MAGNITUDE[c] | VECTOR SUM[d] |
|---|---|---|---|---|---|
| Bases (Libration) | B1 | 6 | 21.7 | 5.56 | 0.862 |
| | B2 | 6 | 22.2 | 4.58 | 0.710 |
| | B3 | 6 | 8.69 | 1.93 | 0.318 |
| (Translation) | B1 | 8 | 37.0 | 0.188 | 0.033 |
| | B2 | 4 | 7.2 | 0.186 | 0.021 |
| | B3 | 3 | 10.1 | 0.206 | 0.017 |
| Riboses (Libration) | R1 | 7 | 26.0 | 5.25 | 0.923 |
| | R2 | 4 | 23.0 | 2.86 | 0.304 |
| (Translation) | R1 | 6 | 24.5 | 0.205 | 0.031 |
| | R2 | 5 | 20.2 | 0.194 | 0.025 |
| | R3 | 5 | 21.5 | 0.185 | 0.024 |
| Phosphate (Libration) | P1 | 2 | 12.6 | 12.63 | 0.689 |
| | P2 | 4 | 40.7 | 6.28 | 0.565 |
| (Translation) | P1 | 3 | 23.7 | 0.209 | 0.016 |
| | P2 | 3 | 18.4 | 0.179 | 0.014 |
| | P3 | 3 | 24.4 | 0.170 | 0.013 |

---------------------------------------------------------------------------

a) Refers to the common modes of libration or translation as shown in
   Figure 3a.

b) The RMS DEV. refers to the root mean square deviation in degrees of the
   vectors comprising that cluster from their mean value.

c) The AVG. MAGNITUDE of a cluster is the sum of the eigenvalues of each
   vector in the cluster divided by the number of vectors in the cluster
   in degrees of libration and angstroms for translation.

d) The VECTOR SUM is obtained by vector addition of the eigenvectors in a
   cluster and normalization (division) by a constant value equal to the
   total number of vectors in the subgroup. Values given are in degrees
   for libration and angstroms for translation.

Table 2:  Summary of Average Eigenvalues of Dodecamer Subgroup Clusters

| SUBGROUP | MODES[a] | VECTORS/ MODES | RMS DEV.[b] | AVG. MAGNITUDE[c] | VECTOR SUM[d] |
|---|---|---|---|---|---|
| Bases (Libration) | B1 | 9 | 14.4 | 15.19 | 1.86 |
| | B2 | 15 | 16.9 | 8.00 | 1.61 |
| | B3 | 7 | 18.4 | 13.26 | 1.22 |
| (Translation) | B1 | 23 | 28.4 | 0.405 | 0.11 |
| | B2 | 8 | 13.9 | 0.690 | 0.07 |
| | B3 | 8 | 13.7 | 0.659 | 0.07 |
| | B4 | 7 | 17.6 | 0.653 | 0.06 |
| Riboses (Libration) | R1 | 17 | 31.7 | 16.97 | 3.59 |
| | R2 | 10 | 21.5 | 17.52 | 2.28 |
| (Translation) | R1 | 14 | 22.2 | 0.755 | 0.14 |
| | R2 | 13 | 27.7 | 0.620 | 0.10 |
| | R3 | 8 | 13.4 | 0.698 | 0.08 |
| | R4 | 7 | 10.4 | 0.767 | 0.07 |
| Phosphate (Libration) | P1 | 12 | 29.0 | 60.77 | 8.89 |
| | P2 | 10 | 20.9 | 65.67 | 8.62 |
| (Translation) | P1 | 17 | 21.6 | 0.634 | 0.14 |
| | P2 | 12 | 29.1 | 0.903 | 0.13 |
| | P3 | 9 | 8.4 | 0.894 | 0.11 |
| | P4 | 9 | 13.8 | 0.849 | 0.10 |
| | P5 | 8 | 21.9 | 0.900 | 0.09 |

---

a) Refers to the common modes of libration or translation as shown in Figure 3b.

b) The RMS DEV. refers to the root mean square deviation in degrees of the vectors comprising that cluster from their mean value.

c) The AVG. MAGNITUDE of a cluster is the sum of the eigenvalues of each vector in the cluster divided by the number of vectors in the cluster in in degrees for libration and angstroms for translation.

d) The VECTOR SUM is obtained by vector addition of the eigenvectors in a cluster and normalization (division) by a constant value equal to the total number of vectors in the subgroup. Values given are in degrees for libration and angstroms for translation.

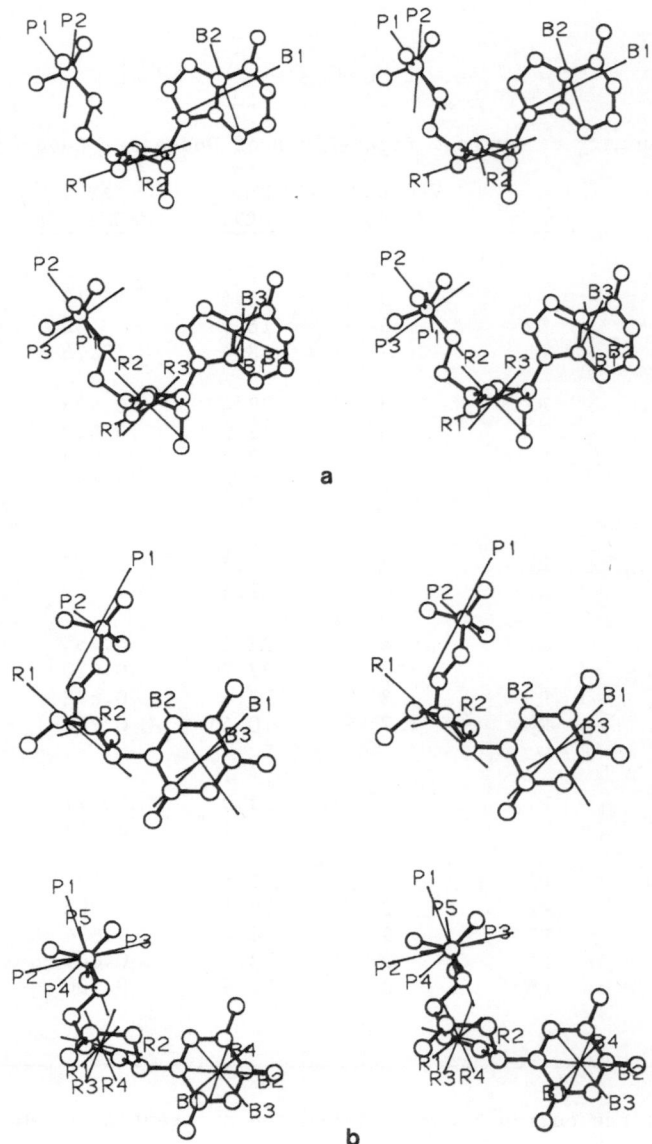

Fig. 3: (a) The common libration and translation axes of each subgroup of
helical RNA fragments ApU and GpC. For illustration, the resultant vectors have been normalized so that the longest vector of each
subgroup is 2.5 Å in length. Vectors within a subgroup may be
compared to each other by their lengths. To compare vectors in
different subgroups, the values of average magnitude or vector sum
given in Table 1 should be used. (Top) libration of the helical
structures; (bottom) translation of the helical structures. (b) The
common libration and and translation axes of the phosphate, ribose,
and base subgroups of the DNA dodecamer. (Top) resultant librational vectors; (bottom) resultant translational vectors. For illustration, the resultant vectors have been normalized so that the
longest vector of each subgroup is 2.5 Å in length. Vectors within
a subgroup may be compared to each other by their lengths. To
compare vectors in different subgroups the values of average magnitude or vector sum given in Table 2 should be used.

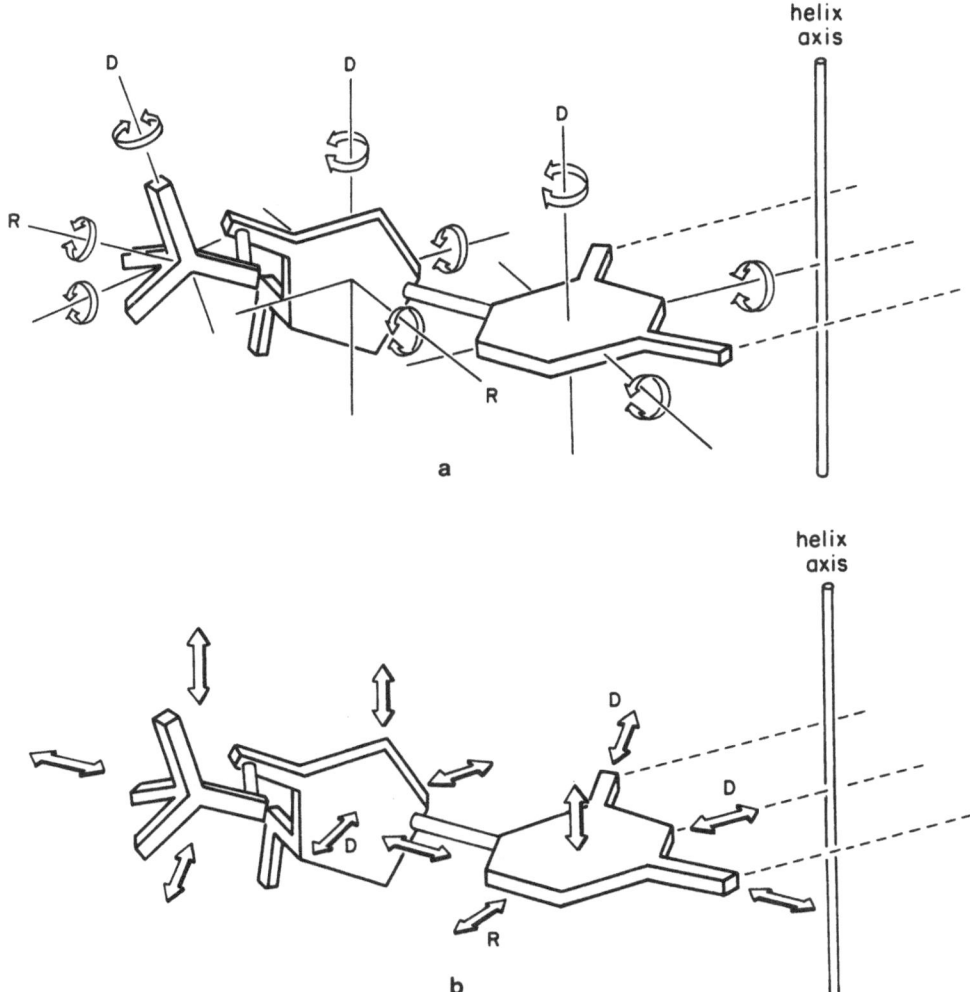

helix
axis

D D D

R

R

a

helix
axis

D

D

D

R

b

Fig. 4: Schematic diagrams summarizing the average rotational (upper) and translational (lower) axes common to helical RNA and DNA as discussed in the text. Straight arrows indicate common translational axes and lines with "circular" arrows around them represent librational axes. The labels "D" and "R" denote axes observed only for DNA or RNA helices respectively. Those without any label are axes common to both DNA and RNA helices. Only one nucleotide is shown for reference.

representations of these two tables are shown in Figure 3. Notice in Table 1 that average translational motions of base, ribose and phosphates are approximately equal and measure about 0.2 angstrom. However, the libration of phosphate is significantly greater than that of ribose or base. This trend is also apparent in the double helical DNA fragment, as shown in Table 2.


RESULTS AND DISCUSSION

An analysis of the average mobility of the nucleotides in double strand-ed DNA and RNA has revealed that many motional directions are similar (see Fig. 4) regardless of crystalline environment or nucleotide sequence. The direction of the motional axes can be associated with a particular physical model as follows:

(a) In most cases, base and sugar appear to move as a unit. This is manifested by the similarity in direction between libration vectors of the base and those of the sugar moieties of DNA and RNA (see Fig. 3). Complex motion of this kind was suggested by carbon-13 NMR experiments[6].

(b) Three primary motions of the base-ribose coupled unit are propeller twisting (Fig. 5a), base pair rocking or rolling (Fig. 5b), and base pair buckling (Fig. 5c).

(c) In the case of DNA, there is one additional major motion, a spinning motion, of the base pair (Fig. 5e).

(d) It appears that there is very little, if any, base pair tilting motion (Fig. 5d) present either in the DNA or in RNA double Some of these mobilities have been proposed by others[7,8] as ways in which nucleic acids use their flecibility to relieve cross strand contacts while maintaining maximum stacking.

The traditional motions are rather uniformly divided among various different directions, except in the case of DNA where there is a clear preference for base pair sliding along the long axis of the base pair, as shown in Figure 5f.

The translational motions are rather uniformly divided among various into 3 categories: (a) parallel to helical axis; (b) tangential to the cylinder which enclosed the double helical nucleic acids; and (c) radial to the helical axis. The radial translational motion probably reflects the breathing motion of the double strands, and the tangential motion probably reflects the partial winding and unwinding of the double stranded nucleic acid. This motion is more predominant for the residues at the end of the double helix than for the middle residues. Finally, the translational motion parallel to the helical axis can cause bending of the helix as well as fluctuation of the groove size, depending on whether or not the motion is synchronized between the two strands.

In summary, we have derived the magnitudes and directions of the local mobility of phosphate, sugar, and base groups in double stranded DNA and RNA based on single crystal X-ray diffraction data. An analysis of these quantities suggests an immediate interpretation of the physical mobility of these groups, thus providing insight into the detailed models of motion of DNA and RNA, the possible mechanism of intercalation of aromatic groups into double stranded nucleic acids, and interaction between nucleic acids and proteins. Furthermore, they show us the motional elements which help us to understand the stability as well as the motion of nucleic acids on a larger scale.

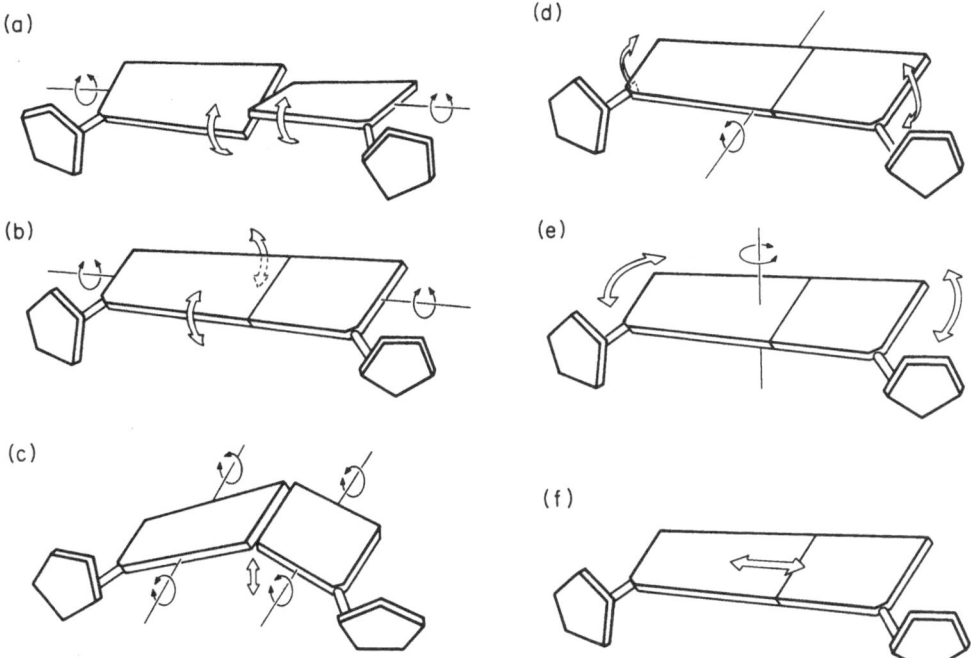

Fig. 5:  Schematic diagrams illustrating the qualitative descriptions of
various nucleoside motions.  The motions illustrated are:  (a)
propeller twisting; (b) base pair rolling; (c) buckling; (d) base
pair tilting; (e) helical turning; (f) base pair sliding; (g)
glycosyl bond rotation.

ACKNOWLEDGEMENTS

We would like to acknowledge Professor Charles Strouse for supplying
us with the computer code for calculating the TLS derivatives which we incorporated in our macromolecular structure factor least squares program,
and Professor Kenneth Trueblood for his program for analysis of the TLS
tensors.  We are also grateful to Professor Richard Dickerson and Dr. Horace
Drew for providing us with the structure factor data and atomic positional
parameters for the dodecanucleotide and for helpful discussions concerning
their previous work.

This research was supported by grants from the National Institutes of
Health (GM29287), the National Science Foundation (PCM-8019468), and the
Department of Energy.

REFERENCES

1. S. R. Holbrook and S.-H. Kim, Local mobility of nucleic acids as
   determined from crystallographic data. I. RNA and B form DNA,
   J. Mol. Biol. 173:361-388 (1984).

2. V. Schomaker and K. N. Trueblood, On the rigid body motion of molecules
   in crystals, Acta Cryst. B24:63 (1968).

3. N. C. Seeman, J. M. Rosenberg, F. L. Suddath, J. J. P. Kim, and A.
   Rich, RNA double-helical fragments at atomic resolution: I. The
   crystal and molecular structure of sodium adenylyl-3',5'-uridine
   hexahydrate, J. Mol. Biol. 104:109 (1976).

4. J. M. Rosenberg, N. C. Seeman, R. O. Day, and A. Rich, RNA double-
   helical fragments at atomic resolution: II. The crystal structure
   of sodium guanylyl-3',5'-cytidine nonahydrate, J. Mol. Biol. 104:
   145 (1976).

5. R. Wing, H. Drew, T. Takano, C. Broka, S. Tanaka, K. Itakura, and
   R. E. Dickerson, Crystal structure analysis of a complete turn of
   B-DNA, Nature 287:755 (1980).

6. R. L. Rill, P. R. Hilliard, L. F. Levy, and G. C. Levy, Natural
   Abundance carbon-13 NMR spectroscopic studies of native and de-
   natured DNA, in: "Biomolecular Stereodynamics", Vol. 1, R.H.
   Sarma, ed., Adenine Press, New York (1981).

7. C. R. Calladine, Mechanics of sequence-dependent stacking of bases in
   B-DNA, J. Mol. Biol. 161:343 (1982).

8. R. E. Dickerson, M. L. Kopka, and H. R. Drew, Structural correlations
   in B-DNA, in: "Structure and Dynamics: Nucleic Acids and Proteins,"
   E. Clementi and R. H. Sarma, eds., Adenine Press, New York (1983).

CONFORMATIONAL CHANGE OF DNA IN SPECIFIC RECOGNITION COMPLEXES BETWEEN

DNA AND PROTEIN

Rosalind Kim[1] and Sung-Hou Kim

Department of Chemistry and
[1]Melvin Calvin Laboratory
University of California
Berkeley, California 94720

ABSTRACT

Specific recognition between protein and DNA is one of the most fundamental interactions in the cell. Many experiments suggest that in such
recognition systems, a protein binds to DNA "non-specifically" first, then
searches for the cognate DNA sequence by sliding, short hopping and/or
inter-strand jumping. When it finds the target site, it may "passively"
stop, or "interactively" binds to DNA, resulting in conformational changes
of DNA and/or protein in forming the complex. Our study with two "specific
recognition" systems shows that DNA in the specific complexes is bent and/
or unwound, but no measurable DNA distortion is revealed in non-specific
interaction.

The small magnitude of the DNA distortion suggests a mechanism of the
active recognition, whereby a population of thermally fluctuating DNA
structures (compatible to formation of a specific recognition complex) is
"captured", thus freezing the distorted DNA structure in the complex, rather
than the protein twisting DNA into a structure normally absent in a free
state. This mechanism also provides an explanation for the effect of the
flanking sequence around the recognition site on DNA because the flexibility
of DNA is likely to be a function of the DNA sequence on and around the
recognized sequence.

INTRODUCTION

Interaction between DNA and protein, which plays an important role in
all living cells, can be divided into two categories. In specific recognition, a protein recognizes a particular DNA sequence a few orders of magnitude tighter than in non-specific recognition, where the protein recognizes
primarily the general features of DNA regardless of the base sequences.
Examples include interaction between restriction enzyme and DNA[1] and between
lactose repressor and DNA[2].

In specific recognition, the mechanism of how a protein finds a particu-
sequence of DNA is under intense study. The current view is that, initially,
a protein binds to DNA non-specifically and then finds a cognate DNA sequence by sliding, short hopping and/or inter-strand jumping[3,4,5].

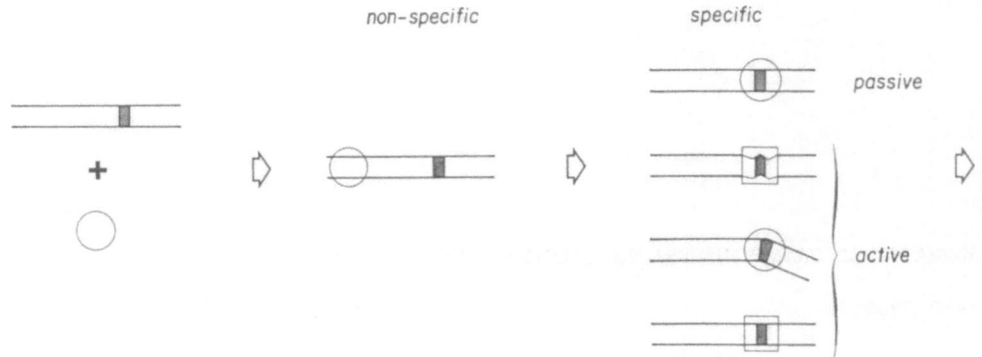

Fig. 1:  Schematic drawing to show the distinction between "passive" and
         "active" recognition.  Initially, a protein is assumed to bind to
         DNA non-specifically without any conformational changes on DNA or
         protein.  The protein then slides or short-hops along DNA and finds
         a cognate DNA sequence.  In passive recognition, the protein simply
         stops at the cognate site in the average conformation of free DNA.
         In active recognition, the conformation of DNA and/or protein in
         the recognition complex is different from the average conformation
         of free DNA and/or protein.

The question we would like to address is what happens to DNA after a protein
binds to its cognate DNA sequence?  Two consequences can arise.  In one, the
protein may simply stop at the cognate sequence (we'll call this "passive
recognition"), and in the other, there may be an active process of recognition between protein and DNA after the protein finds its cognate sequence,
resulting in conformational changes of DNA and/or protein ("interactive
recognition").  These two processes are schematically shown in Figure 1.
The same questiona can be asked for non-specific interaction.  Depending
on the function of protein subsequent to the recognition step, additional
conformational changes of DNA and/or protein may occur.

     In the initial recognition step, the magnitude of the conformational
changes, if any, is likely to be small.  For experimental detection of small
conformational changes, one needs a very sensitive technique to detect small
conformational changes, or to construct a system so that small signals can
be amplified.  We have taken the second route to study conformational changes
of DNA in two specific recognition systems:  lac operator-repressor recognition, and restriction enzyme-restriction site recognition of EcoRI.  The
quantity determined as a measure of conformational change on DNA is the
angle of topological unwinding (or winding) of circular DNA by electrophoresis on agarose gel, according to the methods developed by Keller and
Wandell[6] and exploited so well by various investigators[7,8].

AMPLIFICATION OF SMALL DISTORTION

     To amplify the signal from small topological winding/unwinding of DNA
and to distinguish between duplex twisting and supercoiling, we have constructed three plasmids, pRK112-8, pRK112, and pRK3.  The first contains
15 lac operators and 19 EcoRI restriction sites; the second has 10 lac
operators and 13 EcoRI sites; and the third has 5 lac operators and 7 EcoRI
sites (see Fig. 2).  Plasmids containing multicopies of an insert are often
unstable.  To overcome this instability, we introduced a "spacer sequence"
between inserts.  The insert is 1050 bp long and contains five copies of
lac operator separated by EcoRI sequences (see Fig. 2).  For our purposes,

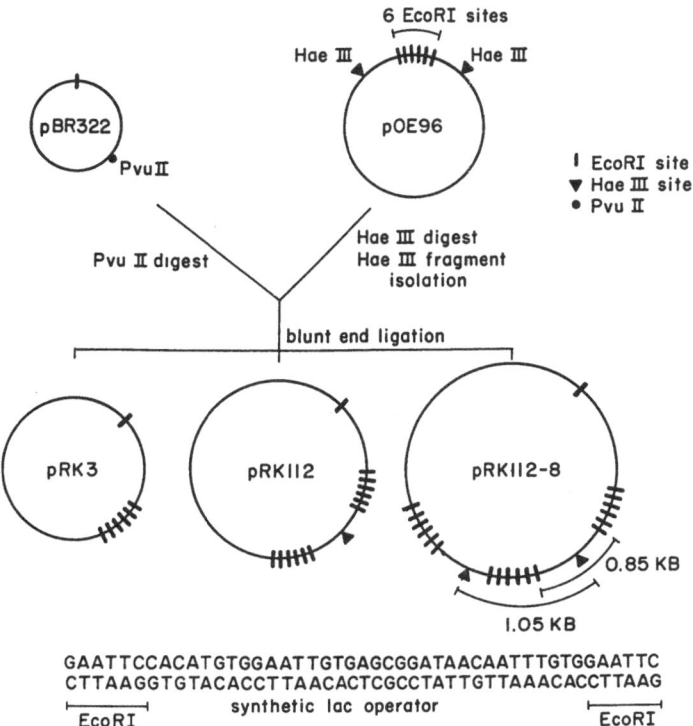

GAATTCCACATGTGGAATTGTGAGCGGATAACAATTTGTGGAATTC
CTTAAGGTGTACACCTTAACACTCGCCTATTGTTAAACACCTTAAG
|——————|      synthetic lac operator       |——————|
  EcoRI                                                EcoRI

Fig. 2:   Construction of pRK3, pRK112, and pRK 112-8. The plasmid pOE96
which contains a cluster of 6 EcoRI sites was digested with HaeIII
restriction enzyme. This fragment is blunt-end ligated into a
PvuII site of pBR 322, which already has one EcoRI site. Three
plasmids were isolated pRK3, pRK112, and pRK112-8, each containing 7, 13, and 19 EcoRI sites, respectively. Any two adjacent
EcoRI sites within the cluster are separated by a 34-base pair long
synthetic lac operator shown at the bottom of the figure.

the relative orientation of each insert with respect to each other in the
plasmid is not important since the <u>handedness</u> of winding or unwinding of DNA
is independent of the orientation of the inserts.

## CONFORMATIONAL CHANGES OF DNA

Our earliest experiment using pRK112-8[10], which has 15 lac operators,
showed that small unwinding per operator-repressor binding is amplified
sufficiently to produce clearly recognizable band pattern shift as shown in
Figure 3a, and that, at saturating conditions, lac repressor binding unwinds
pRK112-8 by 2.27 topological turns (see Fig. 3b). However, non-specific
binding to the same plasmid in the presence of an inducer, or to a plasmid
lacking the lac operator sequence, showed no detectable unwinding or winding.
The 2.27 turn per plasmid corresponds to an average of 55° topological unwinding per lac repressor binding and agrees well with the 35° estimate
based on filter binding method[11]. This small unwinding angle was the basis
for rejecting a cruciform model[12,13] as the structure of lac operator DNA
in the operator-repressor complex.

Using the same plasmid, pRK112-8, which has 19 EcoRI sites, we have now
determined that the EcoRI restriction enzyme at a saturating amount also

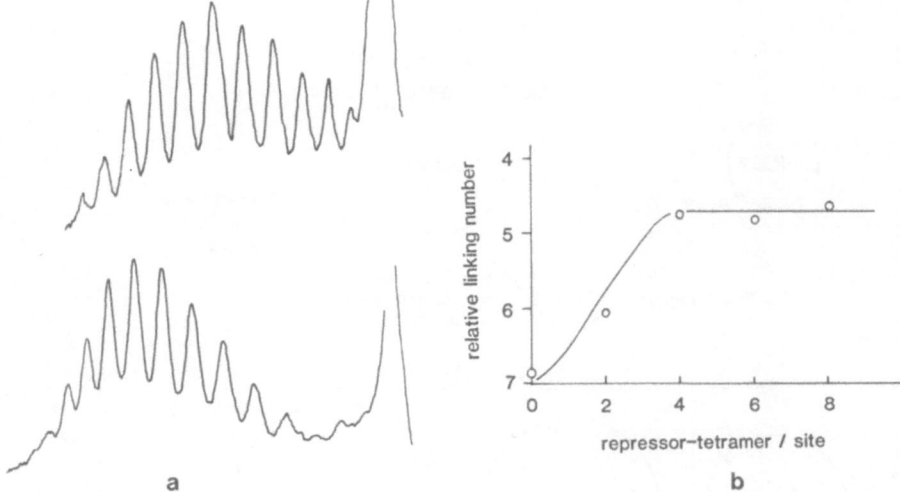

relative linking number

repressor-tetramer / site

a        b

Fig. 3: (a) Densitometer tracing of a band pattern shift.  Bottom:
Control:  pRK112-8, nicked and closed in the absence of lac repressor; Top:  pRK112-8, nicked and closed in the presence of 4
lac repressor tetramers per lac operator.  (b) Unwinding as a
function of lac repressor/operator ratio.  Each of five points in
this figure represents the center of the Gaussian distribution of
pRK112-8 topoisomers from enzymatically relaxed complexes formed
at a lac repressor tetramer concentration of 0.0 M, $1.2 \times 10^{-7}$M,
$2.4 \times 10^{-7}$M, $3.6 \times 10^{-7}$M, and $4.8 \times 10^{-7}$M corresponding to a re-
pressor-tetramer/operator ratio of 0, 2, 4, 6 and 8, respectively.

unwinds the plasmid by 1.31 topological turns corresponding to an average
of 25° topological unwinding per restriction enzyme binding.  This small
unwinding rules out a "cage" model[14],[15] proposed for the restriction enzyme-
DNA recognition, in which six base-pairs of the restriction sequence form
a four-stranded "cage", and where there is a net increase of total hydrogen
bonds (see Fig. 4) and its precursor model of cruciform structure[12],[13].
Such cage or cruciform structure (Fig. 4) should produce unwinding of near
180°, far too large compared to the observed 25°.

These experiments clearly show that there is altered DNA conformation
in both the specific complexes.

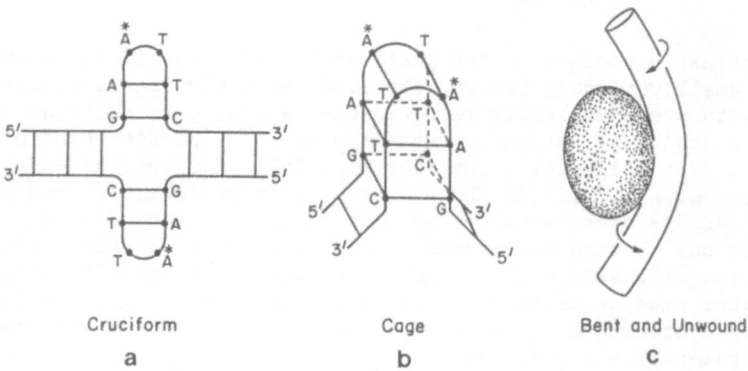

Cruciform    Cage    Bent and Unwound

a      b      c

Fig. 4: Models for DNA conform in EcoRI restriction enzyme-DNA complex.
(a) Cruciform. (b) Cage model. (c) Bent and unwound model.

MEASUREMENT OF THE UNWINDING ANGLE

The experimental details involving EcoRI restriction enzyme are as follows (those for lac repressor have been published[10]). All the plasmid DNA is prepared by buoyant density methods[16]. To test for topological changes induced by EcoRI restriction enzyme, 0.3 μg of supercoiled or pre-relaxed plasmid DNA was mixed with various concentrations of the enzyme (prepared according to Modrich and Zabel[17]) in 15 μl of Buffer A (100mM Tris-HCL pH7.4, 80mM NaCl, 2mM DTT, and 100 μg/ml bovine serum albumin) and incubated at 37°C for 30 minutes. In the absence of Mg ions, the enzyme binds the cognate DNA sequence specifically without cleaving it[17]. The sample was then transferred to a 4°C bath and one unit (the amount of nick and closing enzyme required to totally relax one μg of supercoiled DNA at 4°C in 1 hour in buffer A) of HeLa nick and closing enzyme, topoisomerase I (gift of Dr. H. Gamper, of UC, Berkeley), was added and incubated for 2 hours. One more unit of HeLa nick and closing enzyme was added to make sure relaxation was complete, and was incubated for one more hour. The reaction was terminated by bringing the solution to 20mM EDTA, 24% sucrose, 5% sodium dodecyl sulfate, and 0.075% bromophenol blue. The DNA was subjected to electrophoresis at 37° for 20 hours in an 0.8% agarose gel in 40mM Tris-HCl (pH7.9), 20mM sodium acetate, 1mM EDTA. The voltage gradient was 1.5V/cm. The gels were stained in a 2 μg/ml ethidium bromide solution, illuminated with a short-wave ultraviolet light and photographed on Polaroid Type 665 positive-negative film. The negatives were traced on a Joyce Loebl microdensitometer.

With pRK112-8, the enzyme binding induced a significant shift in band pattern, indicating unwinding of the DNA (Fig. 5a, lanes 2-5). The same results were obtained when pRK112-8 was pre-relaxed prior to the addition of EcoRI restricted enzyme and the subsequent treatments with the HeLa topoisomerase I (Fig. 5a, lanes 6-9). This indicates that the band shift pattern observed is due to EcoRI restriction enzyme binding and not to inhibition of the HeLa topoisomerase I by EcoRI restriction enzyme nor to the supercoil state of the DNA. With pBR322, which contains one EcoRI site, there was no detectable shift induced in the band pattern (results not shown). Furthermore, when the DNA was methylated by EcoRI methylase (a gift of Dr. Paul Modrich), there was also no detectable band shift (Fig. 5b, lanes 7-10) consistent with the observation that EcoRI restriction enzyme does not actively recognize the restriction site that is methylated by the cognate methylase enzyme[1].

An average of eight experiments showed that there is DNA unwinding of 1.31 topological turns per plasmid at a saturating amount of the restriction enzyme. This corresponds to an average DNA unwinding of 25° per EcoRI restriction site, with a standard deviation of 5°. Examples of the titration curve and the densitometer scan of a gel are shown in Figure 6.

NUMBER OF AVAILABLE SITES FOR SIMULTANEOUS BINDING

In order to determine the number of EcoRI restriction enzyme molecules that can bind simultaneously to their specific sites in the plasmid pRK112-8, we used a method described by Fried and Crothers[18]. For this purpose a 1.05 KB HaeIII fragment containing six EcoRI restriction sites and an 0.85 KB spacer fragment (EcoRI fragment from pRK112-8) were used. The 0.85 KB fragment has the same sequence as the 1.05 KB fragment but lacks the EcoRI restriction sites (see Fig. 2). As shown in Figure 7, upon addition of increasing amounts of EcoRI restriction enzyme to the 1.05 KB fragment, six discrete bands can be resolved that migrate slower than the starting DNA fragment, indicating six different DNA-protein complexes, each differing by one protein. On the other hand, with the 0.85 KB fragment no

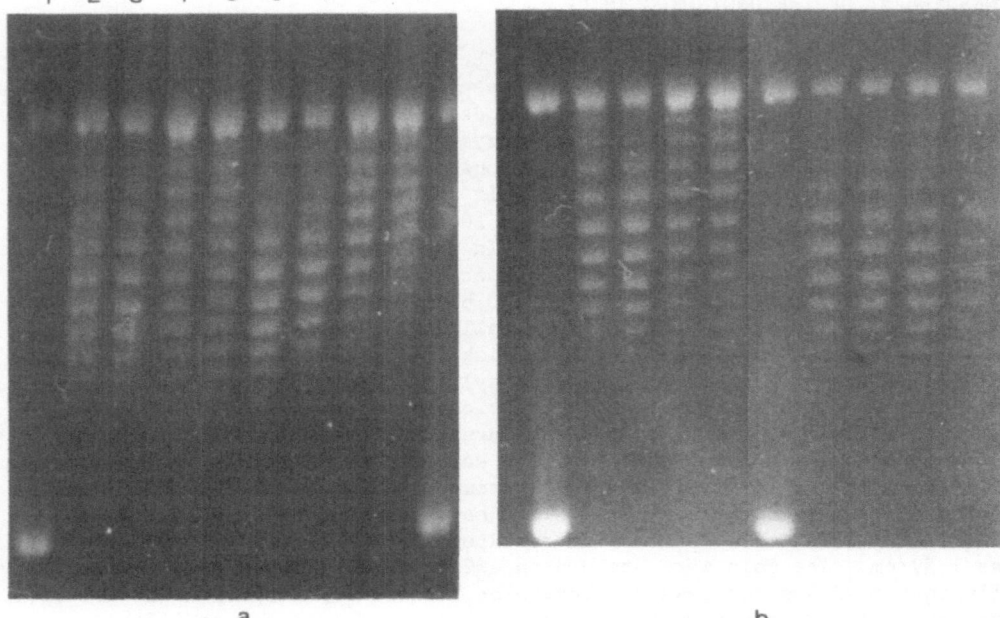

Fig. 5: (a) Lanes 1 and 10 contain supercoiled (bottom band) and nicked (top band) pRK112-8. Lanes 2-5 are pre-relaxed pRK112-8 DNAs nicked and closed in the presence of 0, 0, 7, and 10 molar equivalents of EcoRI restriction enzyme dimers per site. Lanes 6-9 are the same as lanes 2-5 except that the starting DNAs are supercoiled pRK112-8. (b) Lanes 1 and 6 contain supercoiled (bottom band) and nicked (top band) pRK112-8. Lanes 2-5 are supercoiled pRK112-8 DNAs that are nicked and closed in the presence of 0, 0, 7 and 10 molar equivalents of EcoRI restriction enzyme dimer per restriction site. Lanes 7-10 are the same as lanes 2-5 except that the DNAs were methylated by EcoRI methylase.

such discrete bands are observed. Instead only smeared bands due to non-specific binding could be detected (results not shown). Experimental details are as follows: To 0.1 µg of DNA in buffer A were added EcoRI restriction enzymes at two different concentrations (0.285 µM and 0.65 µM), which are equivalent to four and ten EcoRI restriction enzyme dimers per EcoRI restriction site. The samples were very gently mixed by hand and incubated at 37° for one hour. 2.5 µl of a 10 µg/ml xylene cyanol FF solution in 5% glycerol was added to the sample and loaded immediately on a 1% TBE (45mM Tris HCl, pH8.3, 45mM boric acid, 1.25mM EDTA) agarose gel. Electrophoresis was run at 5V/cm for 10 hours.

CONFORMATIONAL CHANGE OF DNA IN COMPLEX

In the two systems of DNA-protein interaction we have studied, it is clear that there is a significant change of DNA conformation in the specific complexes, but no measurable changes in the non-specific interaction. Our preliminary results, using the plasmids with a different number of recognition sites (pRK3 and pRK112) suggest that the DNA in the specific recognition complexes is bent and slightly unwound. Although the physical magnitudes of the bending and unwinding are not measurable at the present time, the topological magnitudes of distortion in the specific recognition

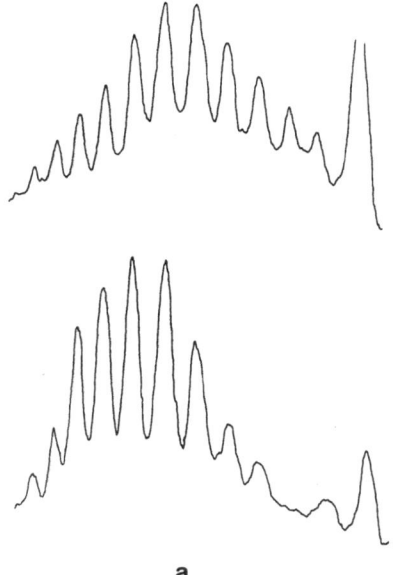

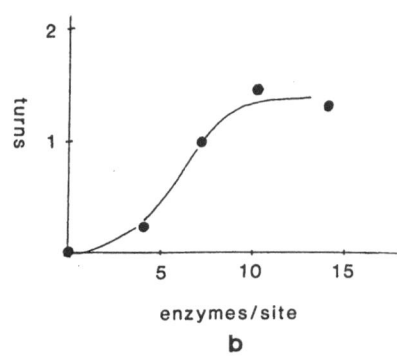

a                                                    b

Fig. 6:    (a) Under our experimental conditions, addition of the EcoRI
           restriction enzyme at the molar ratio of about 8 dimers per site
           in solution saturates all the EcoRI sites on DNA.  Further addi-
           tion of the restriction enzyme does not shift the band pattern
           until the point where the topoisomerase I activity is inhibited.
           At the saturation condition, an average band pattern shift of
           eight experiments is 1.32 topological turn of unwinding.  (b) An
           example of microdensitometer tracing of pRK112-8 DNAs that were
           nicked and closed in the presence of 0 (bottom) and 10 (top) molar
           equivalents of the restriction enzyme dimer per site.

complexes (-55° per lac operator-repressor binding and -25° per EcoRI-DNA
binding) are clearly measurable once the signal is amplified, as we have
done here.  This type of DNA conformational change may be important for
the function of proteins in some of the specific recognition systems.


"CAPTURE" MECHANISM

     The free energy change to induce such topological unwinding of free
and relaxed circular DNA in the absence of interacting protein is small
and positive.  Using the expression of supercoil energy, $\Delta G = 10.0 \times RTN\sigma^2$[19,20] (where R, T, N, $\sigma$ are gas constant, absolute temperate, number
of duplex twists and supercoil density, respectively))total $\Delta G$ is 415 cal/
mol-plasmid and 140 cal/mol-plasmid to induce the extent of unwinding
observed in lac-repressor binding and EcoRI restriction enzyme binding to
the plasmid pRK112-8, respectively.  Although these values represent the
lower limits of distortion free energy, it suggests that the extent of DNA
conformational change is small.  Furthermore, 55° and 25° of unwinding per
lac operator and EcoRI site, respectively, correspond to an average of
3°-4° unwinding per base pair.  This small unwinding is well within the
mobility range of base pairs of DNA fragments even in a crystalline
state[21,22].  Therefore, it is entirely possible that the conformation(s)
recognized by the protein may be present among the molecular population of

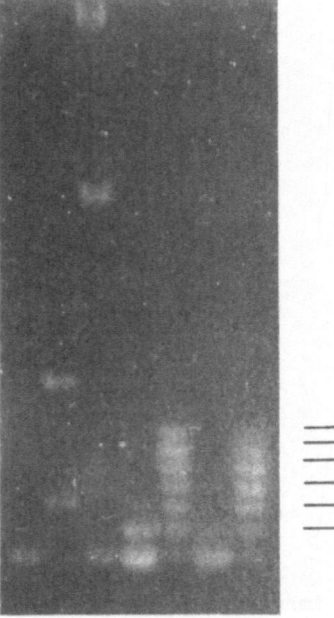

Fig. 7: Binding of EcoRI restriction enzyme to a 1.05 KB fragment containing
6 EcoRI sites. Lanes 1, 4, and 5 are 1.05 KB fragments with 0, 4,
and 10 molar equivalents of EcoRI enzyme dimers per site. Lanes 6
and 7 are the same as 4 and 5, with reduced amount of DNA. Lanes 2
and 3 are DNA size markers. Lanes 5 and 7 show discrete bands in
addition to 1.05 KB band. They are arranged in a logarithmic
fashion.

free DNA in thermal fluctuation. We propose that those conformations compatible to the protein binding then are selectively stabilized by the protei
protein, thus freezing "distorted" DNA conformation.

This line of consideration makes a specific prediction that the flexibility of DNA to generate a large conformational population is important for
the kinetics of specific recognition, and that changes in the flexibility of
the cognate DNA or its flanking regions may change the binding properties.
Such changes can arise due to structural constraints resulting from supercoiling, binding of other proteins (or ligands) proximal to the specific
binding sites, and changes in DNA sequence flanking the binding site. Thus,
specific recognition depends not only on the presence of the cognate DNA
sequence, but also on the flexibility of the DNA region recognized.

ACKNOWLEDGMENTS

The work reported here has been supported by grants from the National Institute of Health (GM 31616, GM 29287), the National Science Foundation (PCM 80 19468), and the Department of Energy. We thank Drs. Jack Sadler (deceased) and Joan Baetz for the plasmid pOE96, which we used as a starting material; and Drs. Paul Modrich and Howard Gamper for the EcoRI methylase and HeLa topoisomerase I, respectively.

REFERENCES

1.  P. Modrich, Studies on sequence recognition by type II restriction and modification enzymes, CRC Critical Reviews in Biochemistry 13: 287 (1982).

2.  S. Bourgeois and M. Pfahl, Repressors, Adv. Protein Chem. 30:1 (1976).

3.  O. G. Berg, R. B. Winter, and P. H. von Hippel, Biochemistry 20:6929 (1981).

4.  J. L. Bresloff and D. M. Crothers, DNA-ethidium reaction kinetics: Demonstration of direct ligand transfer between DNA binding sites, J. Mol. Biol. 95:103 (1975).

5.  P. H. von Hippel, A. Revzin, C. A. Gross, and A. C. Wang, Protein-ligand interactions, in: "Protein-ligand Interactions", H. Sund and G. Blauer, eds., Walter de Gruyter, Berlin (1975).

6.  W. Keller and I. Wendell, Stepwise relaxation of supercoiled SV40 DNA, Cold Spring Harbor Symp. Quant. Biol. 39:199 (1983).

7.  W. Bauer, F. H. C. Crick, and H. White, Supercoiled DNA, Scientific American 118 (1980).

8.  J. C. Wang, L. J. Peck, and K. Becherer, DNA supercoiling and its effects on DNA structure and function, Cold Spring Harbor Symp. Quant. Biol. 47:85 (1983).

9.  J. R. Sadler, M. Tecklenburg, and L. L. Betz, Plasmids containing many tandem copies of a synthetic lactose operator, Gene 8:279 (1980).

10. R. Kim and S.-H. Kim, Direct measurement of DNA unwinding angle in specific interaction between lac operator and repressor, Cold Spring Harbor Symp. Quant. Biol. 47:451 (1983).

11. J. C. Wang, M. D. Barkely, and S . Bourgeois, Measurements of unwinding of lac operator by repressor, Nature 251:247 (1974).

12. A. Gierer, Model for DNA and protein interactions and the function of the operator, Nature 212:1480 (1966).

13. H. M. Sobell, Molecular mechanism for genetic recombination, Proc. Natl. Acad. Sci. USA 69:2483 (1972).

14.  V. I. Lim and A. L. Mazanov, Tertiary structure for palindromic regions of DNA, <u>FEBS Lett</u>. 88:118 (1978).

15.  A. Stasiak and T. Klopotowski, Four-stranded DNA structure and DNA base methylation in the mechanism of action of restriction endonucleases, <u>J. Theor. Biol</u>. 80:65 (1978).

16.  D. B. Clewell, Nature of ColE: Plasmid replication in <u>Escherichia coli</u> in the presence of chloramphenicol, <u>J. Bacteriol</u>. 110: 667 (1972).

17.  P. Modrich and D. Zabel, EcoRI endonuclease: Physical and catalytic properties of the homogeneous enzyme, <u>J. Biol. Chem</u>. 251:5866 (1976).

18.  M. Fried and D. Crothers, Equilibria and kinetics of the repressor-operator interactions by polyacrylamide gel electrophoresis, <u>Nucl. Acids Res</u>. 9:6505 (1982).

19.  D. F. Pulleyblank, M. Shure, D. Tang, J. Vinograd, and H.-P. Vosberg, Action of nicking-closing enzyme on supercoiled and nonsupercoiled closed circular DNA: Formation of a Boltzmann distribution of topological isomers, <u>Proc. Natl. Acad. Sci. USA</u> 72:4280 (1975).

20.  R. Depew and J. C. Wang, Conformational fluctuations of DNA helix, <u>Proc. Natl. Acad. Sci. USA</u> 72:4275 (1975).

21.  H. R. Drew, S. Samson, and R. E. Dickerson, Structure of a B-DNA dodecamer at 16 K°, <u>Proc. Natl. Acad. Sci. USA</u> 79:4040 (1982).

22.  S. R. Holbrook and S.-H. Kim, The local mobility of nucleic acids as determined from crystallographic data. I. RNA and B-form DNA, <u>J. Mol. Biol.</u> 173:361 (1984).

# NUCLEOSOME MOTION:  EVIDENCE AND MODELS

K. E. van Holde and Thomas D. Yager

Department of Biochemistry and Biophysics
Oregon State University
Corvallis, Oregon 97331

## INTRODUCTION:  PUBLISHED EVIDENCE FOR NUCLEOSOME SLIDING IN CHROMATIN

Much of the voluminous literature concerning nucleosome arrangement in chromatin has implicitly assumed this to be a static structure, with the histone cores fixed in place upon the DNA.  There exists, however, a growing body of evidence to indicate that under certain circumstances the cores can migrate along the DNA, both in vitro and in vivo.  The first suggestion of such migration came from observations[1-4] of anomalously close spacing of some histone cores in chromatin that had been depleted of the very lysine-rich histones.  The presence of these "compact oligomers" was observed in the specific cases in which the very lysine-rich histones had been removed by extraction of the chromatin with salt solutions in the concentration range 0.5-0.65 M.  This suggested that such structures might be generated under such conditions.  This postulate was elegantly confirmed by Weischet[5], who showed that nuclei depleted of H1 by a low pH, low salt extraction did not yield compact oligonucleosomes upon nuclease digestion, but that such structures could be found after the nuclei were incubated in salt concentrations greater than 0.3 M.  That sliding, rather than nucleosome displacement and reassociation must be involved was indicated by the earlier studies of Germond et al.[6], who had shown that histone cores could only be displaced from chromatin by salt concentrations in excess of 0.8 M.

The most direct demonstration of nucleosome sliding, however, comes from the work of Beard[7].  In these experiments, DNA was ligated onto linearized SV-40 minichromosomes, and migration onto the added DNA demonstrated by a variety of techniques.  It is notable that Beard's experiments were performed at 0.15 M NaCl, showing that migration could occur, albeit slowly, under physiological salt concentrations.  The possibility of dissociation and reassociation was rigorously excluded by control experiments in which the foreign DNA was added, but not ligated.  No transfer was seen under these conditions.

Further in vitro studies have been carried out by Spadafora et al.[8] and Glotov et al.[9].  The latter workers made the interesting observation that sliding on SV-40 minichromosomes could occur only if a double-strand break were introduced into the closed circular DNA.

All of the experiments mentioned above pertain to sliding in vitro, most often at salt concentrations markedly higher than would be encountered

in cell nuclei.  Is there, then, any evidence that sliding occurs in vivo?
There is, in fact, such evidence.  The most positive indication for in vivo
sliding comes from studies of chromatin replication.  Two laboratories[10-12]
have observed that nucleosomes are first laid down on newly synthesized DNA
in a tightly packed structure.  Within a few minutes, the correct spacing
has been established, presumably by nucleosome sliding.  Similar evidence
has been presented for nucleosome sliding during chromatin repair[13,14].
Thus, it appears likely that motion of the histone cores along DNA can occur
under physiological conditions, and may play a significant role in certain
nuclear processes.

Direct measures of the kinetics of nucleosome sliding on long chromatin
are difficult.  However, there is a closely related process which is much
more amenable to experimental study.  A number of researchers have presented
evidence that mononucleosomes can undergo dissociation into free DNA and the
constituent histone complexes[15-22].  The process is most easily studied at
salt concentrations comparable to those used in most in vitro sliding experiments, but can be observed even at low salt concentrations if the
nucleosome concentration is sufficiently low.  Like sliding, dissociation
occurs only in the absence of the H1 class of histones.  As we shall suggest
in this chapter, dissociation may involve a sliding of the histone core
relative to the DNA.

EXPERIMENTAL STUDIES OF NUCLEOSOME DISSOCIATION:  EVIDENCE FOR A SLIDING
MECHANISM

To investigate nucleosome dissociation, we have prepared two kinds of
nucleosomal particles from chicken erythrocyte nuclei.  Core particles
(which shall herein be referred to as "C-nucleosomes") were obtained by the
technique described by Paton, et al.[23].  As observed in many experiments in
many laboratories, these were characterized by a very narrow DNA size distribution centered on 145 bp, and by presence of only the four core
histones, H2A, H2B, H3 and H4.  For comparison, we also wished to have
nucleosomes with the same histone composition, but containing longer DNA;
these we shall call "L-nucleosomes".  They were prepared by first isolating
H1/H5-containing nucleosomes by KCl precipitation of chromatin from a
nuclear digest, and then removing the H1 and H5 by a low-salt procedure[24];
details are given elsewhere[25].  That the L-nucleosomes contain only the core
histones is shown in Figure 1.  Figure 2 depicts the distribution of DNA
sizes present in these particles.  Although the size distribution is quite
broad, it differs fundamentally from that of the C-nucleosomes in that no
DNA of core size or smaller is present.  We aimed for such a distribution
because it has been suggested that nucleosomes containing DNA lengths even
slightly smaller than 145 bp behave anomalously in dissociation[22].

All nucleosomes were finally purified by sucrose gradient sedimentation.  In the course of these experiments, we have observed that unless
certain precautions are taken, such nucleosome preparations are likely to be
contaminated with small amounts of free DNA.  We find that even modest concentrations of salt, often added to enhance resolution in sucrose gradients,
must be avoided.  In particular, preparative sucrose gradient sedimentation
in salt concentrations as low as 50 mM will produce this artifact.  Use of
10 mM Tris, 0.25 mM EDTA, pH 7.4, without added salt in the preparative centrifugation results in "clean" mononucleosomes.  However, long storage of
mononucleosomes in buffers containing as little as 10 mM NaCl can result in
some dissociation, and should be avoided.  The histones released from the
dissociated nucleosomes during a sucrose gradient separation are lost from
the nucleosome fraction, and will not be available for reassociation even
if that fraction is reconcentrated.  We believe this to be a probable explanation for reports of a "non-equilibrating" fraction of DNA in nucleosome
preparations[16,21].

36

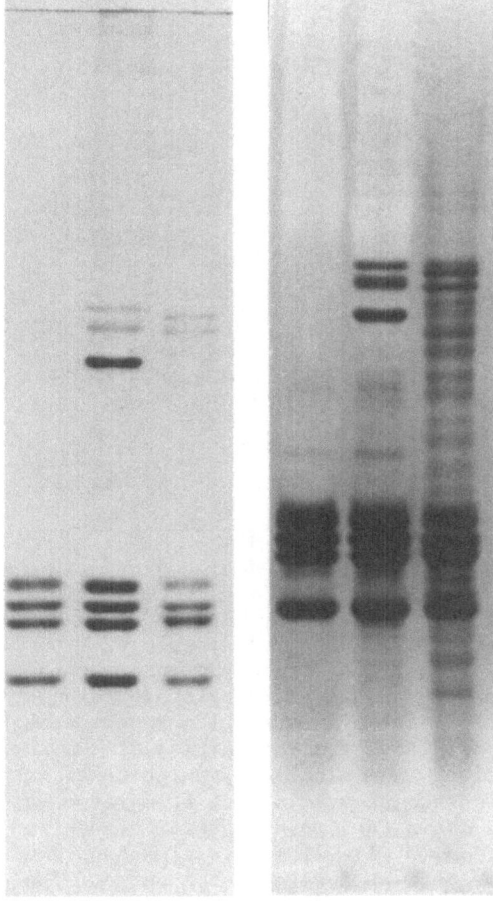

a                    b

Fig. 1: Removal of Non-Core Proteins in the Preparation of L-Nucleosomes.
After precipitation with KCl, but before fractionation on sucrose
gradients, a mixture of mono, oligo, and polynucleosomes were
exposed to a 50 mM NaCl + 30 mg/ml Carboxymethyl/Sephadex. In
Figure 1A, lanes 2 and 1 depict the proteins present before and
after this step, respectively, as revealed by Coomassie Blue
staining of an SDS gel. Lane 3 is a set of calf thymus histones,
as a standard. Lane 1 indicates that virtually all proteins other
than the core histones have been removed, but to provide a more
stringent test, the gel was restained with silver. Figure 1B
shows the result: only traces of other proteins remain, and the
lysine-rich histones have been quantitatively removed.


    We present here only an abbreviated description of our dissociation ex-
periments; details are given elsewhere[25]. C-nucleosomes and L-nucleosomes
were incubated in varying NaCl concentrations (in a buffer containing 10 mM
Tris, 0.25 mM EDTA, pH 7.4) for varying periods of time. With both types of
nucleosomes, a more slowly sedimenting component ($\sim$5S) was observed to be
formed in addition to the remaining nucleosomes. We have demonstrated by
several methods (particle gel electrophoresis, and sucrose gradient sedimentation with analysis of the fractions for DNA and histones) that the
slowly sedimenting component is in fact DNA, and not an unfolded nucleo-

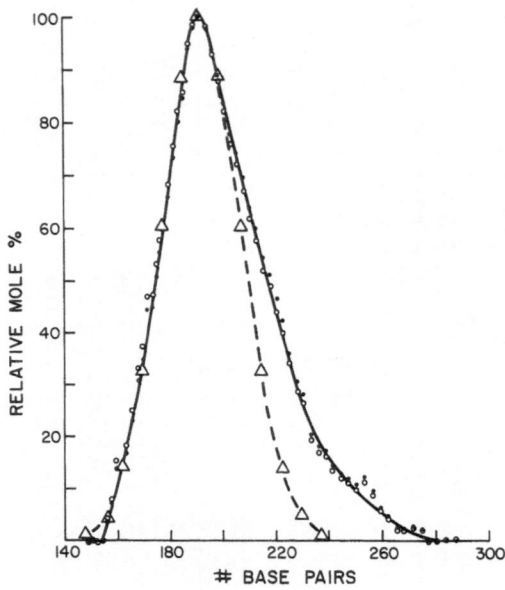

Fig. 2:  Distribution of DNA Sizes in the L-Nucleosomes.
DNA was prepared from a typical sample of L-nucleosomes. In order
to determine the size distribution, photographic negatives of
ethidium bromide-stained polyacrylamide gels were scanned. The
gels contained a set of restriction fragment markers at equal molar
concentrations. From the intensities of the marker bands, a "response function" was calculated, which takes into account relative
staining, fluorescence yield, and film response. The resulting distribution is shown for two different methods for fitting the response function (O, ●). The triangles show a Gaussian distribution
fitted to the left hand side of the curve. The critical point to
note is that these nucleosomes contain no DNA smaller than core
size.

somal structure. This conclusion is supported by the observation that
crosslinking of the histone cores by dimethyl suberimidate does not prevent
the formation of the slow boundary. In fact, crosslinking by this reagent
was found to allow more extensive dissociation at low salt concentration.
A similar effect has been reported in LiCl solutions[20].

The principal results are typified by Figure 3, which depicts the
analysis of a set of analytical ultracentrifuge experiments with C-nucleosomes incubated at varying salt concentrations at 20°C. The amount of the
slow boundary increases with time, reaching, under these conditions, plateau
values in about 200 min. The plateau dissociation is strongly dependent
upon salt concentration, but reaches detectable levels even at 100 mM NaCl.
A closer analysis of this time-dependent dissociation is seen in Figure 4,
which depicts scanner traces for the same sample from centrifuge runs
started 44 min and 424 min after addition of salt to 0.75 M. Figure 5 shows
sedimentation coefficient distributions calculated from these two experiments, using the method of van Holde and Weischet[26]. These are compared
with the distribution obtained for the same nucleosomes prior to salt addition. The amount of slowly sedimenting material at each time is roughly
the same as that estimated directly from the scanner traces (arrows,
Figure 5).

Figure 5 also illustrates the second major observation in these

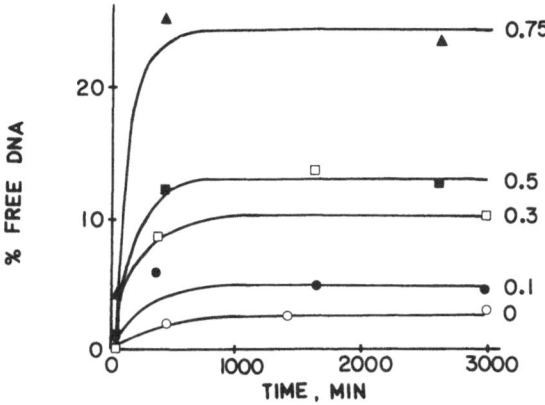

Fig. 3: Dissociation of C-Nucleosomes as a Function of Time.
Sedimentation velocity experiments were started at various times
after mixing a C-nucleosome solution (initially in 10 mM Tris,
0.25 mM EDTA, pH 7.4) with a concentrated NaCl solution to give
the desired final concentration of salt. In each run, several
boundaries (as in Fig. 4) were analyzed for the percent dissociation. The results were corrected for radial dilution and averaged.
Note that the time dependence of the process is clearly shown in
0.75 M, 0.5 M, and 0.3 M NaCl. Solutions were maintained at 20°C
through the experiment.

experiments. The sedimentation coefficient of the fast boundary (residual
nucleosomes) is decreased about 14% from that of the original particles.
Figure 6 shows values of $S_{20,W}$ for the nucleosome boundary immediately after
the salt jump, and at dissociation equilibrium, as a function of salt concentration. It is clear that S is decreased at all salt concentrations
above 0.3 M, and that the change in S is rapid, being observable even before
dissociation can be detected (see also Figures 3 and 5). Thus, the response
of nucleosomes to elevated salt concentration must be considered a two stage
process: a rapid change in conformation is followed by a slow dissociation.

Figure 3 indicates that the dissociation approaches limiting values at
each salt concentration. That this at least approximates a true equilibrium
between dissociation and reassociation is indicated by the experiment shown
in Figure 7. A solution of L-nucleosomes in 10 mM Tris, 0.25 mM EDTA, pH
7.4 (0 M NaCl) was divided into two portions. One part was incubated at
0.75 M NaCl for 30 hr, the other held at zero salt; both were at 20°C, and
at equal nucleosome concentrations. Both solutions were then adjusted to

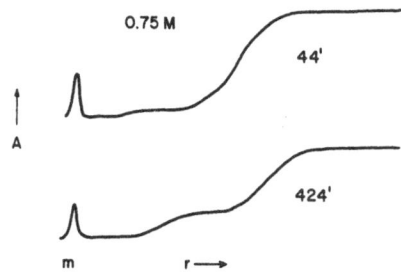

Fig. 4: Scanner Traces of C-Nucleosome Sedimentation in 0.75 M Salt.
Traces were made for runs which had reached speed (44,000 RPM)
44' and 424' after mixing.

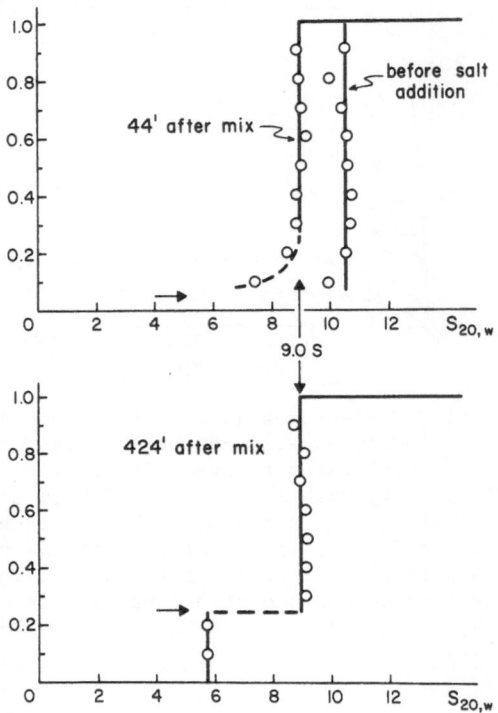

Fig. 5:  Integral Distributions of Sedimentation Coefficient for the Ex-
         periments Shown in Figure 4.
         The method of van Holde and Weischet[26] was used to calculate sedi-
         mentation coefficient distributions from a number of scans (6-8)
         in each run.  NaCl concentration = 0.75 M.  The top panel shows
         that a run started 44 min after mixing exhibits minor dissociation,
         and also a decrease of 14% in the $S_{20,W}$ of the fast (nucleosome)
         boundary.  After 424 min, about 25% of free DNA (5.7 S) has accu-
         mulated.  The sedimentation coefficient of the fact boundary shows
         no further change.

0.5 M NaCl, again at the same final nucleosome concentration.  As Figure 7
shows, the two solutions approach, from opposite directions, approximately
the same percent dissociation.  We believe that the small difference in the
final values is probably attributable to irreversible loss of histones (by
absorption to container walls, for example) in these long experiments.  We
have also demonstrated that the dissociation equilibrium of nucleosomes
is concentration dependent, as would be expected (not shown in Figure 7; see
Yager and van Holde[25]).  Despite the fact that we believe the system to approach thermodynamic equilibrium, we cannot calculate meaningful equilibrium
constants from our data.  This is because the histone octamer, when released,
will at least partially dissociate into $(H3 \cdot H4)_2$ tetramers and $H2A \cdot H2B$ dimers
under these conditions[27].

    Both the L- and C-nucleosomes exhibit the same kind of two-step dis-
sociation process.  The principal difference we have been able to identify
lies in the fact that the dissociation phase is much slower, under comparable conditions, for the L-nucleosomes.

    From the above, the response of nucleosomes to high salt involves both
a slow and a fast component.  We have identified the slow component as a
dissociation process.  What is the nature of the fast component?  We note

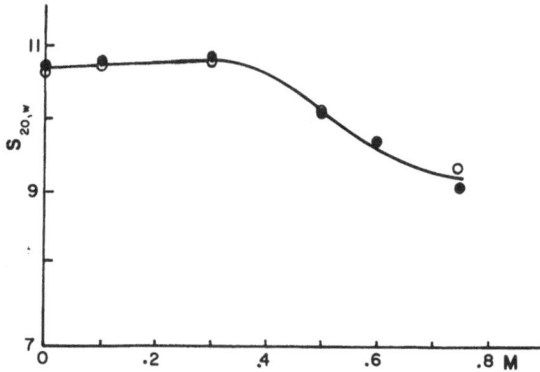

Fig. 6: The Effect of Salt Concentration on the Sedimentation Coefficient
of the Nucleosome Boundary.
Samples were "jumped" to various NaCl concentrations (abscissa)
and the sedimentation coefficient measured as soon as possible
(30-50 min) after mixing (open circles). The sedimentation coefficient of the nucleosome boundary was then redetermined (filled
circles) after dissociation equilibrium had been attained (e.g.
after several thousand minutes; see Figure 3).


that the fast step, as observed by ourselves and others[18,21,28,29], corresponds to a maximal decrease of about 15% in $S_{20,W}$. Two kinds of events
might be postulated to explain this decrease in sedimentation coefficient:
the loss of one or more histones, or a conformational change. The first
is excluded by experiments in which L-nucleosomes were sedimented through
sucrose gradients containing 0.6 M NaCl[25]. Gel electrophoresis of fractions
showed that the rapidly sedimenting boundary contained all four histones,
in the correct proportion. Excluding the possibility that a whole heterogeneous tetramer was lost - a hypothesis inconsistent with the small change

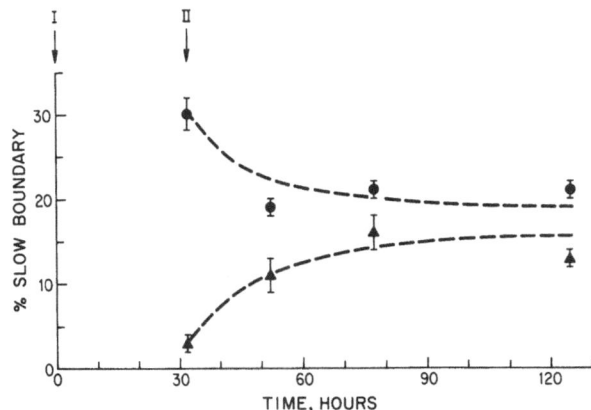

Fig. 7: The Approach to Dissociation Equilibrium for L-Nucleosomes.
A solution of L-nucleosomes initially in 10 mM Tris, 0.25 mM EDTA,
pH 7.4, was divided into two portions. One part was increased in
salt concentration to 0.75 M, the other left in low salt. Both
were incubated at equal nucleosome concentrations for 30 hr at
20°C, and then readjusted to be at 0.5 M salt, again at equal
nucleosome concentrations. Sedimentation experiments were then
performed over an additional 90 hr to follow the re-equilibration.

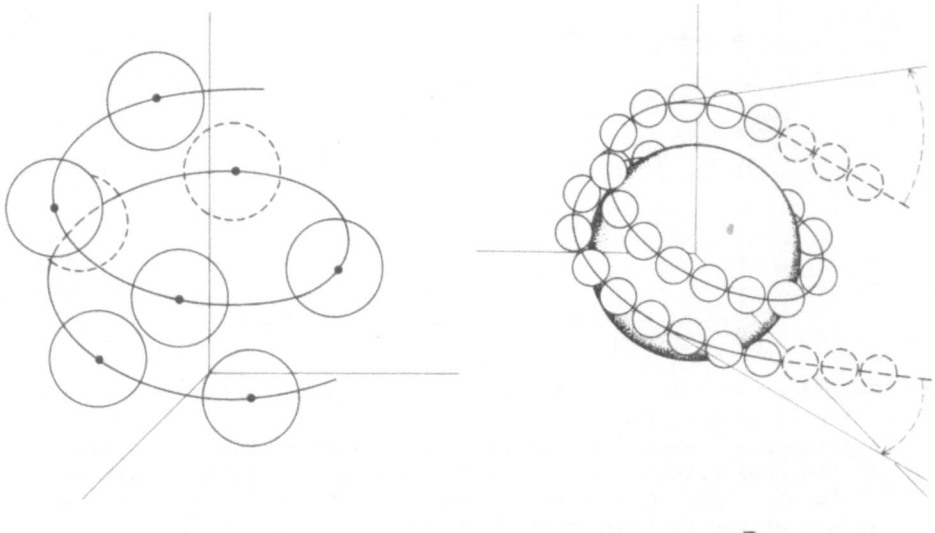

A                       B

Fig. 8:  Models used for the Estimation of the Effect of Conformational
Changes on the Sedimentation Coefficient.
A. Model for nucleosome expansion: the C-nucleosome is represented
as 8 nucleoprotein beads, each corresponding to 1/8 of the total
nucleic acid and protein in the core particle. Broken circles
represent beads in background. Either the number of superhelical
turns, or the distance between the first and eighth beads were
varied. B. Model for DNA unwrapping: the histone core was represented as one large bead, surrounded by a helical chain of
smaller beads depicting the DNA. Either the core particle or an
L-nucleosome can be depicted, by adding extra small beads in the
latter case (broken circles). In both models, the relative contribution to S of hydration was assumed to not vary as the conformation changed. Thus the effects of hydration were cancelled
out of the ratio $S/S_o$.

in S - this means that <u>no</u> histones were lost.

If the fast change is conformational, then three possibilities can be
suggested from other studies of nucleosomal conformation changes: (1) a
general loosening and expansion of the whole nucleosomal structure; (2)
an unwrapping of a portion of the DNA from the histone core; or (3) release
of histone tails. In an attempt to estimate how large such changes would
have to be to account for the observed decrease in $S_{20,w}$, we have employed
the Kirkwood algorithm[30,31] for the calculation of the frictional coefficients of complex objects. The models chosen for hypotheses (1) and (2)
are shown in Figure 8 and the results of such calculations depicted in
Figure 9. The major conclusion to be drawn from these calculations is that
the conformational change cannot be large. Either a small expansion of the
core, or the unwrapping of 20-30 bp of DNA from either end will suffice.
The calculations do seem, however, to exclude the drastic conformational
change that Dieterich et al.[32] have proposed to occur in high salt. A possible explanation lies in the fact that the experiments of Dieterich et al.
utilized nucleosomes that had been reconstituted after the addition of
rather bulky dye ligands to each of the H3 sulfhydryl groups. Since the
sulfhydryl groups can easily be oxidatively crosslinked, they must lie close
to one another in the histone core. Modifications at such sites could well
be expected to destabilize the nucleosomes.

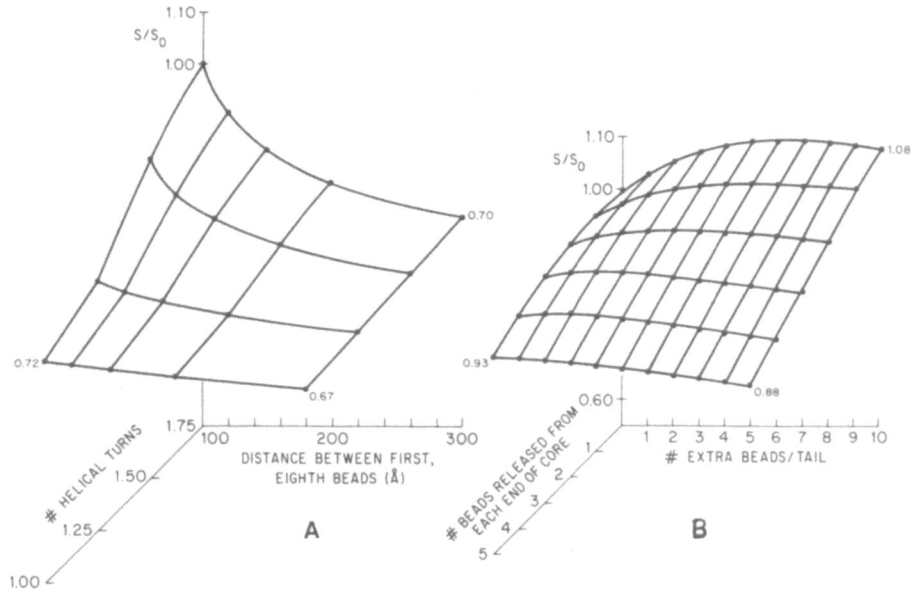

Fig. 9: The Predicted Effect of Conformational Changes on the Sedimentation
Coefficient of Nucleosomes.
Using the models shown in Figure 8, the effects of nucleosomes
expansion (A) or partial DNA unwrapping (B) were calculated, as
described in the text.

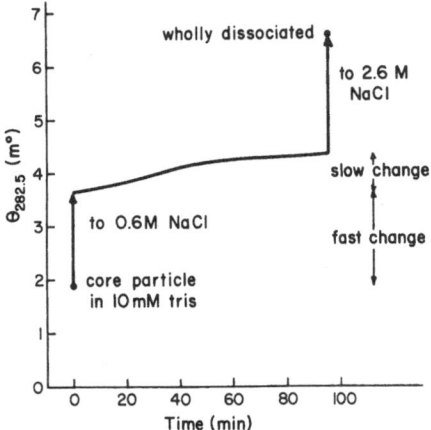

Fig. 10: A Schematic Representation of the Results of a "Salt Jump"
Circular Dichroism Experiment.
A solution of C-nucleosomes in 10 mM Tris, 1mM EDTA, pH 7.5
($A_{260} \cong 0.1$) was placed in a 10 cm pathlength cell in a Jasco
J-40 circular dichroism apparatus. The cell was thermostatted
at 33.5°C. The ellipticity was recorded at 282.5 nm, and 5 M
NaCl was added with rapid stirring to bring the concentration to
0.6 M. After the slow change had apparently ceased, solid NaCl
was added to completely dissociate the nucleosomes.

In any event, we favor the unwrapping of DNA ends or histone tails as an explanation for the change in sedimentation coefficient. The change in S is about the same as that observed by Simpson[33] in the first stage of thermal denaturation of core particles, which has been shown to correspond to an unwrapping of about 20 base pairs at either end of the core DNA[34]. Furthermore, calculations of the electrostatic binding of these end domains to the histone core[35] indicate that at high salt these should be destabilized.

To provide more definite information concerning the fast and slow changes, we have turned to circular dichroism measurements. The rationale for such experiments is based on the observation that the CD of nucleosomes (at about 280 nm) is much lower than that of free DNA, and that, for core particles, partial release and straightening of the two end segments of the DNA causes a proportional increase in the CD signal[33]. Figure 10 diagrams the kind of experiment we have performed. The CD spectrum of a nucleosome preparation in 0 M salt was recorded, and the monochrometer then fixed at 282.5 nm. Concentrated (5 M) salt was then slowly added, with vigorous mixing, and the change in CD noted. There was a rapid (<5 min) increase in CD, followed by a much slower, small further increase. After this reached a plateau, more salt was added to yield a final concentration of 2.6 M, which resulted in a large additional CD increase. Analysis of the data requires correction for the dilution at each step, as well as the fact that free B-form DNA exhibits somewhat different CD intensity at the different salt concentrations[36]. Details are given elsewhere; it suffices to say at this point that the data support the hypothesis that the rapid step involves an unwrapping of about 20 bp of DNA from each end of the core particle, as in the thermal denaturation. In the example shown (Figure 10) the fast change corresponds to the transformation of 40 bp of DNA from a nucleosome-like conformation to a B-form DNA conformation. The total magnitude of the slow CD change is consistent with 11% of these particles becoming wholly unwrapped, a value in reasonable agreement with the result ($\sim$ 15%) observed by sedimentation under these circumstances.

An alternative explanation, which cannot be ruled out at this point, is that histone tail release "relaxes" constraints on the DNA, allowing a change in twist of all or a portion of the core DNA. This could have a comparable effect on the CD.

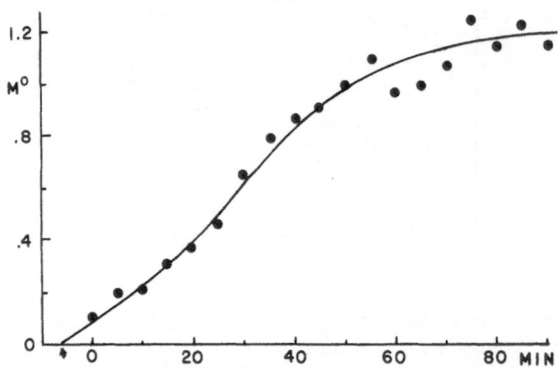

Fig. 11:  The Slow Change in Ellipticity for the Experiment Diagrammed in Figure 10.
The ellipticity in millidegrees is graphed versus time. The arrow shows the point at which the NaCl concentration was made 0.6 M; data recording was resumed at t = 0.

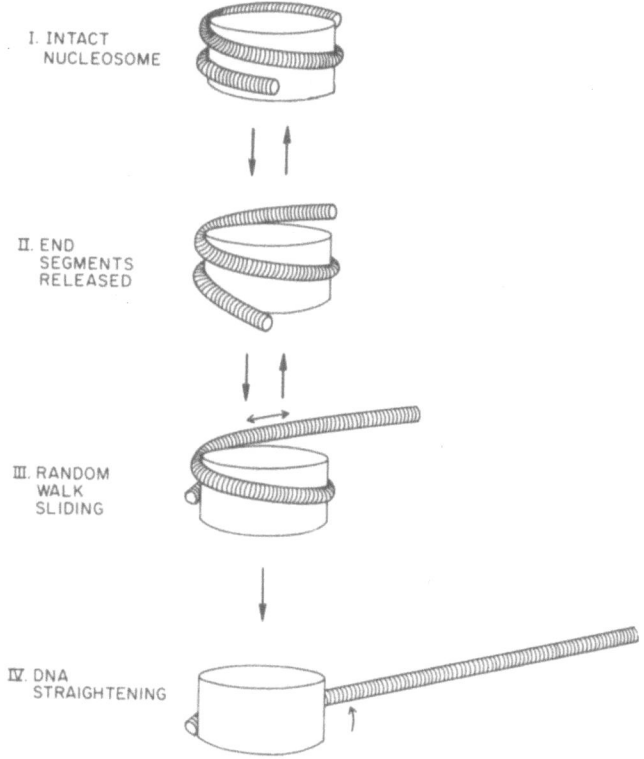

Fig. 12:  A Model for Nucleosome Dissociation.
We assume that the "fast change" corresponds to a relaxation of
DNA from the ends of the nucleosome.  This could be an unwrapping,
as depicted, or simply a release of local constraints.  This
allows sliding, which proceeds by a random walk process until one
end reaches a point at which it becomes bound to the core.  Beyond
this point sliding will be mainly undirectional, since it is
favored by straightening of the DNA at the other end.


It is difficult to follow the kinetics of the slow change with precision, but the data (Figure 11) suggest a sigmoidal curve.  They definitely
do not indicate a first-order process, as would be expected if the DNA
simply "fell off" the histone core.  The very existence of a slow process
suggested to us that a sliding mechanism might explain the dissociation.
Our present hypothesis is this:  high salt concentrations induce the release of the terminal portions of the DNA from the histone core.  Such
"opened" nucleosomes are then susceptible to core-sliding along the DNA.
The sliding is initially a random-walk process, but when a critical point
is reached, straightening of the DNA provides a driving force for release
(see Figure 12).  We then ask:  is there a reasonable mechanism for nucleosome sliding which is capable of explaining, even semi-quantitatively, the
observed dissociation data?


A MODEL FOR NUCLEOSOME SLIDING

Mirzabekov et al.[37] have shown that, for the central 100 bp of DNA in
a core particle, a DNA-histone "interaction" occurs about once every five
base pairs.  What is the nature of this interaction?  We know that the
histone core does not display a strong preference for binding to particular

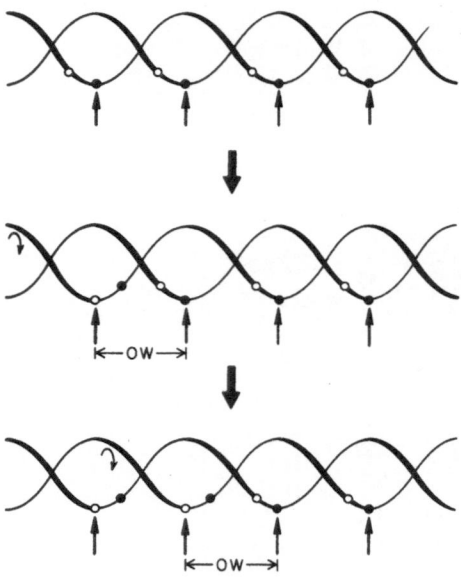

Fig. 13:   The Mechanism Proposed for DNA Sliding on the Histone Core.
It is assumed that DNA phosphate residues at the core surface
make ionic bonds to positively charged residues. Occasionally,
twisting motions in the free DNA ends will produce a one-phosphate
displacement, with consequent over- or under-twisting in the first
"cell".  This twist-defect can then migrate through the lattice of
cells.  It emerges from the other end, the DNA will have moved by
one base pair with respect to the core.

DNA sequences; this suggests that the interactions are relatively non-
specific.  We also know that certain nucleosome instabilities (sliding and
dissociation) are induced by raising the salt concentration. This suggests
that the histone-DNA interactions are electrostatic in nature.  We therefore visualize the interactions as electrostatic bonds between DNA phosphates and arginyl or lysyl side chains on the surface of the histone core.
We schematically depict in Figure 13 (top panel) a segment of DNA interacting with the histone core.

     Now suppose that DNA segments at the ends of partially relaxed core
particle (or core domain in H1-depleted chromatin), are able to undergo
rapid torsional ("twisting") oscillations.  There is both a firm theoretical
basis and fairly direct experimental evidence for such twisting motions in
free DNA:  (1) The analysis from classical mechanics of Barkley and Zimm[38],
which treats a DNA molecule in solution as a semi-rigid rod, predicts both
bending and twisting harmonic motions, of periods on the order of nanosec-
onds.  (2) Miller et al.[39], and Hogan et al.[40] have designed experiments to
measure the fluorescence depolarization of a dye intercalated between the
base pairs of DNA in solution.  Their experiments yield anisotropy decay
curves in quantitative agreement with predictions from the theory of
Barkley and Zimm, assuming the dye follows the twisting motion of the DNA
base pairs.  Wang et al.[41] have gone on to show the same apparent twisting
motion for DNA that is bound up in nucleosome core particles.  (3) Holbrook
and Kim[42] have devised a method of analyzing the thermal noise inherent in
the X-ray diffraction pattern of a single crystal of an arbitrary macromolecule.  They have applied this method to the crystals of DNA dodecamer
studied by Dickerson and coworkers[43].  In their analysis, thermal noise is
resolved into coupled vibrations and translations of the phosphate, sugar

46

and base groups within the DNA. They conclude that twisting of base pairs occurs to an extent (averaged over all base pairs in the dodecamer) of about 13°.

From this discussion, we envision twisting harmonics to occur in the free DNA segments at the ends of the core domain, with periods in the nanosecond range. Occasionally, a twisting motion will be large enough to displace the first binding site on the core by one phosphate (1 bp). If this happens, the DNA between this and the next binding site will become locally overwound or underwound (Figure 13, middle panel). There are two ways of relieving this local strain: (1) the structure can revert to its original form (passing the strain back out to the free DNA); or (2) the next binding phosphate can be displaced. If the latter happens, then the local miswinding will be passed to the next cell; this amounts to a dislocation in the DNA-histone bonding lattice (Figure 13, bottom panel). The dislocation will wander in a random sense until it emerges from the lattice, either at the same end from which it entered, or at the opposite end. If the former occurs, there is no net result. In the latter case, the entire histone core will have moved by one base pair with respect to the DNA.

Such a mechanism for core migration sounds extremely inefficient. However, it should be noted that local DNA oscillations occur on a nanosecond time scale, and our studies of nucleosome dissociation suggest that minutes or hours are required for significant motion. Therefore, a factor of $10^{10}$ to $10^{12}$ is involved.

It is possible to build stochastic models of the diffusion of quanta of "DNA mistwisting" through a network of DNA-histone bonds in a nucleosome. Here we present one such model, and use it to demonstrate that a twist-migration mechanism is efficient enough to account for observed nucleosomal sliding rates.

Imagine a linear array of alternating "cell boundaries" and "cells"; in our terminology, a cell boundary is a DNA-histone bond, and a cell is the relatively mobile segment of DNA between two bonds. Assume there are $(a + 1)$ cells numbered $0, 1, \ldots, a-1$, with cells $(0)$ and $(a)$ having only an interior boundary, and thus being open to the external space. The twist of the DNA in cells $(0)$ and $(a)$ fluctuates rapidly, reflecting the continual torsional oscillations of the (unbound) DNA which is external to the body of the nucleosome. Single bp "quanta" of local DNA mistwisting can spontaneously move from cell $(0)$ to cell $(1)$ or from cell $(a)$ to cell $(a-1)$; the rarity of such movement reflects the activation energy for propagation of a quantum of mistwisting across a cell boundary.

We seek: (1) the probability that a quantum of mistwisting, having entered either cell $(1)$ or cell $(a-1)$, will migrate through the entire lattice of cells and emerge at the other end (consequently displacing the histone core 1 bp along the DNA); and (2) the distribution of waiting times for emergence, in the case of such a successful migration.

Assuming the ease of passage of a quantum of mistwisting to be the same between all cells, the probability of successful migration is $1/a$, and the distribution of waiting times for success is given by[44]:

$$0, \quad n < a-1$$

$$P_n = \frac{1}{a} \sum_{i=1}^{a-1} \cos^{n-i} \frac{i\pi}{a} \cdot \sin \frac{i\pi}{a} \cdot \sin \frac{i\pi(a-1)}{a}, \quad n > a-1, \tag{1}$$

where $P_n$ is the probability that a successful migration takes n barrier crossings, and $\Sigma pn = 1/a$.

From this, a rough estimate of the (macroscopic) nucleosomal sliding rate may be obtained:

(1) Assume that the rate-limiting step in the movement of a quantum of mistwisting between two cells is the transitory breakage of the cells' separating boundary. Both theory[38] experiment[39,40] suggest that DNA twisting motion can propagate over a 20 bp length of _free_ DNA (two cells' width) in about 1-30 ns. For boundary breakage to be rate-limiting, therefore, it must occur no more frequently than about every 100 ns. From the theory of absolute reaction rates:

$$\tau = \frac{kT}{h} e^{-\Delta G^{\neq}/RT}.$$

(2)

A period of $\pi = 100$ ns implies an activation energy for bond rupture of 8 kcal/mol.

(2) From the theory of random walks[44], the expected lifetime of a quantum of mistwisting which has already migrated into cell (1) or cell (a-1) is (a-1) $\tau$. For the purposes of argument we suppose that, on the average, there is always 1 quantum of local over- or undertwisting within the lattice at any time. We therefore set the entrance rate of quanta of mistwisting at $[(a-1)\tau]^{-1}$.

(3) It will take on the average (a) entrance events for there to be one successful propagation of a quantum of mistwisting across the entire cell lattice, and out the other side. Under these conditions, the predicted success rate (i.e., macroscopic core sliding rate) is given by $[a(a-1)\tau]^{-1}$. For $\tau = 100$ ns and a = 25 cells, this equals $\sim 10^4$ bp/sec.

Since the sliding is considered to be a one-dimensional random walk, we can obtain a feeling for the actual displacement to be expected for a nucleosome core by recalling that the root-mean-square displacement $[(\overline{m^2})^{1/2}]$ expected after n steps is given by

$$(\overline{m^2})^{1/2} = n^{1/2}$$

(3)

For the case given above, this corresponds to 100 bp in one second of walk. This is, in fact, considerably more rapid than is usually observed for nucleosome sliding. Thus the proposed mechanism can be, in fact, considerably more efficient than is needed to explain the observed sliding rates. To bring the theory into accord with the order of magnitude or rates observed, we will have to postulate either a higher energy barrier for the entrance of quanta of mistwisting into the lattice, or additional internal energy barriers for their displacement across cell boundaries.

This analysis may be related back to the kinetics of dissociation (Figure 11), through the postulate of a "critical migration distance". Imagine the rate-limiting step in nucleosome dissociation to be the random walk of the histone core to a critical distance. In the theory of random walks, such a movement will be characterized by a "first passage time"[44]. Assuming, from above, one bp of sliding in $10^{-4}$ sec, Figure 14 then gives the cumulative percent of nucleosomes in a population which will have randomly walked the critical distance (a/2) after a certain number of $(10^{-4})$ sec steps[44]. We see that, as the critical distance approaches about 20-25 bp, the distribution curve takes on a sigmoidal character, in qualitative agreement with the dissociation kinetics of Figure 11.

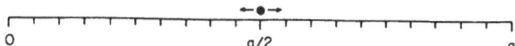

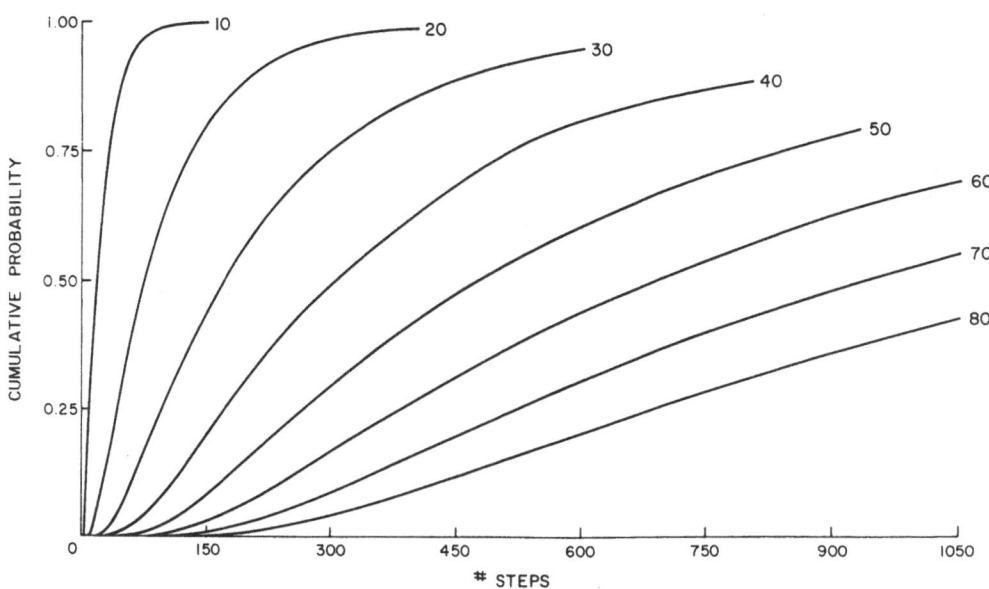

Fig. 14: Theoretical Distribution of First Passage Times, for a Critical-
Distance Random Walk by the Nucleosome Core.
The central base pair (bp) of the DNA in a nucleosome is imagined
to be initially at position (a/2), in a 1-dimensional lattice of
positions 0, 1, 2, . . ., a-1, a. Sliding of the nucleosome core
then proceeds as a random walk having 1 bp "quanta", or "steps"
(abscissa). After a certain number of steps the percent of nucleosome cores which have made the critical excursion of (a/2) bp, to
bring the central bp of the DNA to either end of the lattice, is
graphed (ordinate), for various values of (a). Note the appearance of a clearly sigmoidal character (cf. Figure 11) as (a/2)
increases to 20-25 bp. This theoretical distribution comes from
Lagrange's solution to the problem of a 1-dimensional random
walk[44].

The theory presented here is clearly a first approximation to a complete description of the process. A more sophisticated analysis would take
into account the simultaneous presence of multiple dislocations within the
lattice, with certain complicating consequences: i.e., the possibility of
mutual annihilation of (+) and (-) dislocations. Even more urgently needed
are experimental measurements of sliding rates, and we are endeavoring to
obtain such measurements in experiments currently in progress. What we have
shown here is that a sliding mechanism of this kind can explain, in a
qualitative or semi-quantitative sense, the observations we have made concerning nucleosome dissociation.

ACKNOWLEDGEMENTS:

The major portion of this work was supported by research grants from the American Cancer Society (NP355A) and the Public Health Service (GM22916); support also came from Oregon State University, in the form of President's and Tartar Fellowships to T. D. Y. One of us (K. v. H.) wishes to express appreciation for an American Cancer Society Research Professorship.

Within our research group, we would like to thank A. Paton, C. McMurray and C. Poklemba for preparation of the C-nucleosomes, and G. Riedel for technical help with particle gels and silver staining. We would also like to thank I. Isenberg and T. Tibbits for robust fitting programs, W. Weischet and M. Zehfus for integral distribution-of-S programs, P. Meagher for help implementing our hydrodynamic models on the computer, and Sue Conte and Pat Duckworth for their careful typing of the manuscript.

REFERENCES

1. L. Klevan and D. Crothers, Isolation and characterization of a spaceless dinucleosome from H-1 depleted chromatin, Nucleic Acid Res. 4:4077-4089 (1977).

2. D. Lohr, K. Tatchell, and K. E. van Holde, On the occurrence of nucleosome phasing in chromatin, Cell 12:829-836 (1977).

3. M. Steinmetz, R. E. Streek, and H. Zachau, Closely spaced nucleosome cores in reconstituted histone-DNA complexes and histone H-1 depleted chromatin, Eur. J. Biochem. 83:615-628 (1978).

4. K. Thatchell and K. E. van Holde, Compact oligomers and nucleosome phasing, Proc. Natl. Acad. Sci. USA 75:3583-3587 (1978).

5. W. O. Weischet, On the de novo formation of compact oligonucleosomes at high ionic strength. Evidence for nucleosome sliding at high salt, Nucleic Acids Res. 7:291-304 (1979).

6. J. Germond, M. Bellard, P. Oudet, and P. Chambon, Stabiligy of nucleosomes in native and reconstituted chromatin, Nucleic Acids Res. 3:3173-3192 (1976).

7. P. Beard, Mobility of histones on the chromosome of Simian virus 40, Cell 15:955-967 (1978).

8. C. Spadafora, P. Oudet, and P. Chambon, Rearrangement of chromatin structure induced by increasing ionic strength and temperature, Eur. J. Biochem. 100:225-235 (1979).

9. B. O. Glotov, A. Y. Rudin, and E. S. Severin, Conditions for sliding of nucleosomes along DNA: SV-40 minichromosomes, Biochim. Biophys. Acta 696:275-284 (1982).

10. A. Levy and K. M. Jakob, L. Nascent DNA in nucleosome-like structures from chromatin, Cell 14:259-267 (1978).

11. G. Galili, A. Levy, and K. M. Jakob, Changes in chromatin structure at the replication fork. II. The DNP's containing nascent DNA and a transient chromatin modification detected by DNAse I, Nucleic Acids Res. 9:3991-4005 (1981).

12. A. T. Annunziato and R. L. Seale, Maturation of nucleosomal and non-nucleosomal components of nascent chromatin: differential requirements for concurrent protein synthesis, Biochemistry 21:5431-5438 (1982).

13. M. W. Lieberman, M. J. Smerdon, T. D. Tlsty, and F. B. Oleson, The role of chromatin structure in DNA repair in human cells damaged with chemical carcinogens and ultraviolet radiation, in: "Environmental Carcinogenesis," P. Emmelot and J. Kreid, eds., Biomedical Press, Elsevier North-Holland, Dordrecht, Holland (1979).

14. M. J. Smerdon and M. W. Lieberman, Distribution within chromatin of deoxyribonucleic repair synthesis occurring at different times after ultraviolet radiation, Biochemistry 19:2992-3000 (1980).

15. D. R. Burton, M. J. Butler, J. E. Hyde, D. Phillips, C. J. Skidmore, and I. O. Walker, The interaction of core histones and DNA: Equilibrium binding studies, Nucleic Acids Res. 5:3643-3663 (1978).

16. A. Stein, DNA folding by histones: The kinetics of chromatin core particle reassembly and the interaction of nucleosomes with histones, J. Mol. Biol. 130:103-134 (1979).

17. D. M. J. Lilley, M. F. Jacobs, and M. Houghton, The nature of the interaction of nucleosomes with a eukaryotic RNA polymerase II, Nucleic Acids Res. 7:377-399 (1979).

18. J. Bode and K. G. Wagner, Cooperative exposure of histone H3 thiols in core particles, Int. J. Biol. Macromol. 2:129-136 (1980).

19. R. W. Cotton and B. A. Hamkalo, Nucleosome dissociation at physiological ionic strength, Nucleic Acids Res. 9:445-457 (1981).

20. L. Vassilev, G. Russev, and R. Tsanev, Heterogeneity of nucleosomes upon dissociation with salts, Int. J. Biochem. 13:1247-1255 (1981).

21. H. Eisenberg and G. Felsenfeld, Hydrodynamic studies of the interaction between nucleosome core particles and core histones, J. Mol. Biol. 150-537:555 (1981).

22. M. Erard, J. Pouyet, A. Mazen, M. Champagne, and M. Daune, Core particle stability critically depends upon a small number of terminal nucleotides, Biophys. Chem. 14:123-133 (1981).

23. A. Paton, E. Wilkinson-Singley, and D. E. Olins, Non-histone nuclear high mobility group proteins 14 and 17 stabilize the nucleosome core particle, J. Biol. Chem. 257:13221-13229 (1984).

24. L. J. Libertini, and E. W. Small, Salt induced transition of chromatin core particles studied by tyrosine fluorescence anisotropy, Nucleic Acids Res. 8:3517-3534 (1980).

25. T. D. Yager and K. E. van Holde, Dynamics and equilibria of nucleosomes at elevated ionic strength, J. Biol. Chem. 259:4212-4222 (1984).

26. K. E. van Holde and W. O. Weischet, Boundary analysis of sedimentation velocity experiments with monodisperse and paucidisperse solutes, Biopolymers 17:1387-1403 (1978).

27.  T. H. Eickbush and E. N. Moudrianakis, The histone core complex:  An octamer assembled by two sets of protein-protein interactions, Biochemistry 17:4955-4964 (1978).

28.  M. Zama, P. N. Bryan, R. E. Harrington, A. L. Olins, and D. E. Olins, Conformational states of chromatin, Cold Spring Harbor Symp. Quant. Biol. 42:31-41 (1977).

29.  M. L. Wilhelm and F. X. Wilhelm, Conformation of nucleosome core particles anc chromatin in high salt concentration, Biochemistry 19:4327-4331 (1980).

30.  J. G. Kirkwood, The general theory of irreversible processes in solutions of macromolecules, J. Polymer Sci. 12:1-14 (1954).

31.  V. Bloomfield, W. O. Dalton, and K. E. van Holde, Frictional coefficients of multisubunit structures. I.  Theory, Biopolymers 5:135-148 (1967).

32.  A. E. Dieterich, R. Axel, and C. R. Cantor, Salt-induced structural changes of nucleosome core particles, J. Mol. Biol. 129:587-602 (1979).

33.  R. T. Simpson, Mechanism of a reversible, thermally induced conformational change in chromatin core particles, J. Biol. Chem. 254:10123-10127 (1979).

34.  W. O. Weischet, K. Tatchell, K. E. van Holde, and H. Klump, Thermal denaturation of nucleosomal core particles, Nucleic Acids Res. 5:139-160 (1978).

35.  J. D. McGhee and G. Felsenfeld, The number of charge-charge interactions stabilizing the ends of nucleosomal DNA, Nucleic Acids Res. 8:2751-2769 (1980).

36.  V. I. Ivanov, L. E. Minchenkova, A. K. Schyolkina, and A. I. Poletayev, Different conformations of double-stranded nucleic acid in solution as revealed by circular dichroism, Biopolymers 12:89-110 (1973).

37.  A. D. Mirzabekov, V. V. Shick, A. V. Belyavsky, and S. G. Bavykin, Primary organization of nucleosome core particle of chromatin: Sequence of histone arrangement along DNA, Proc. Natl. Acad. Sci. USA 75:4184-4188 (1978).

38.  M. D. Barkley and B. H. Zimm, Theory of twisting and bending of chain macromolecules; analysis of the fluorescence depolarization of DNA, J. Chem. Phys. 70:2991-3007 (1979).

39.  D. P. Millar, R. J. Robbins, and A. H. Zeward, Direct observation of the torsional dynamics of DNA and RNA by picosecond spectroscopy, Proc. Natl. Acad. Sci. USA 77:5593-5597 (1980).

40.  M. Hogan, J. Wang, R. H. Austin, C. L. Monitto, and S. Hershkowitz, Molecular motion of DNA as measured by triplet anisotropy decay, Proc. Natl. Acad. Sci. USA 79:3518-3522 (1982).

41.  J. Wang, M. Hogan, and R. H. Austin, DNA motions in the nucleosome core particle, Proc. Natl. Acad. Sci. USA 79:5896-5900 (1982).

42. S. R. Holbrook and S.-H. Kim, Local mobility of nucleic acids as determined from crystallographic data. I.  RNA and B form DNA, _J. Mol. Biol_. 173:363-383 (1984).

43. R. Wing, H. Drew, T. Takano, C. Broka, S. Tanaka, K. Itakura, and R. E. Dickerson, Crystal structure analysis of a complete turn of B-DNA, _Nature_ 287:755-758 (1980).

44. W. Feller, "An introduction to probability theory and its applications," Volume I, 2nd edition, J. Wiley and Sons, New York (1957).

# THE STRUCTURE OF SATELLITE-CONTAINING CHROMATIN OF THE RAT

Tibor Igo-Kemenes

Institut für Physiologische Chemie, Physikalische Biochemie
und Zellbiologie der Universität München
Goethestrasse 33, D-8000 München 2
Federal Republic of Germany

## INTRODUCTION

During the last decade the main principles and general features of the chromatin structure have been established. The basic repetitive unit within the hierarchy of chromatin superstructures is the nucleosome, a structure revealed both by nuclease digestion of chromatin[1-3] and by visualization of chromatin in the electron microscope[4]. At a second level of chromatin organization, the polynucleosomal chain (100 Å filament) is condensed into 250-300 Å fibers. Although most of the experimental results suggest that the polynucleosomal chain in these fibers is organized in a continuous helical fashion called a solenoid[5], alternative structures with discontinuous globular particles called superbeads[6,7] or other arrangements involving four interwoven filaments[8] have been proposed. At a third level, the 250-300 Å fibers are folded into loops or domains in both interphase nuclei and metaphase chromosomes[9-11]. While these three levels of condensation may account for the compaction of chromatin in interphase, additional levels of compaction were suggested in metaphase chromosomes[12-13]. (For comprehensive reviews on chromatin structure see references 14, 15).

Despite the rapid accumulation of data on the structure of chromatin in general, little is known about particular chromatin fractions containing specific DNA sequences. Different DNA sequences are packaged in distinct ways in interphase nuclei giving rise to more condensed or less condensed chromatin regions. The more condensed chromatin regions called heterochromatin were defined by cytological criteria as that part of the chromatin that does not decondense during interphase. It has been shown later that highly repetitive satellite DNA is often, if not always, associated with this chromatin fraction[16].

Some early attempts to fractionate chromatin have been made to prepare condensed heterochromatin[17]. Later on, the advent of restriction nucleases has provided a technology to isolate chromatin fractions enriched in highly repeated DNA[18-20]. The aim of the present work is to give an overview on satellite-containing chromatin. Most of the material will deal with the satellite I of the rat, the evolutionary origin of this satellite, its chromatin structure, and possible function in chromosome and species evolution. Some data are discussed in relation to findings on satellites from other species. Emphasis will also be given to the question of nucleosome phasing, a widely discussed problem.

At the time when satellite I was detected and characterized it was not clear if further satellites (II, III, etc.) are present in the rat genome. This now seems to be rather unlikely. Yet, for reasons of consistency with earlier literature, we continue to use the Roman numeral I.


## SUBUNIT STRUCTURE AND NUCLEOTIDE SEQUENCE OF SATELLITE I

Initial attempts to isolate and characterize satellites from rat tissues failed. This was due to the fact that the (G + C) content of rat satellite I is rather similar to that of the bulk DNA precluding fractionation by buoyant density gradients. A new approach was necessary in order to detect and to isolate satellite DNA from rat tissues. Such a new approach will be described below.

### Isolation of Satellite I DNA

If a repetitive DNA component differs from the rest of the DNA by having either a very high or, alternatively, a very low number of sites for a certain restriction nuclease, a purification scheme can be devised based on separation by size. Incubations of rat DNA with Sau3A I (cleavage site GATC) converted about 97% of the DNA to short fragments and left satellite I DNA as a small fraction of high molecular weight (marked by asterisks, Fig. 1B). The total amount of this fraction in the rat genome was estimated to be about 3%[22-23] and the average length to be 10,000 base pairs (bp).

Satellite DNA was purified on a preparative scale by gel filtration of a Sau3A I digest on a Sepharose 2B column (Fig. 1A). Early fractions of the elution diagram of Figure 1 contained satellite I (hatched area) of approximately 60% purity. The satellite DNA content of individual fractions was assayed by Eco RI digestion (Fig. 1C) and quantitative evaluation of the ethidium bromide fluorescence of the resulting satellite bands (asterisks). Pooled fractions of preparations which had been scaled up by a factor of 10 contained 30-40% satellite I. Highly purified satellite I DNA was obtained, however, from partially purified preparations by preparative gel electrophoresis and was estimated to be at least 95% pure.

Although highly repetitive DNA components have usually been called satellite DNAs only when they could be separated by centrifugation techniques, it seems justified to use the designation satellite I for this thoroughly characterized DNA component, which closely resembles other satellite DNAs.

Rat DNA contains several highly repetitive components in addition to satellite I. Sau3A I digests of rat DNA revealed a large number of sharp bands in electropherograms (e.g. tracks h-k in Fig. 1B and 1C) which in blotting experiments did not hybridize with nick-translated cloned satellite I. These bands may correspond to short interspersed repetitive elements called SINES and/or long interspersed repetitive elements called LINES[24].

### Characterization of Satellite I-DNA by Restriction Nuclease Digestion and Sequence Analysis

A characteristic feature of satellite DNAs is the organization of a basic repeat unit into long tandem arrays. This type of arrangement can be most easily revealed by partial digestion of satellites with restriction nucleases and separation of the fragments by gel electrophoresis. Since cloned satellite probes are available, this kind of analysis can even be performed on total DNA without prior purification of satellites. In

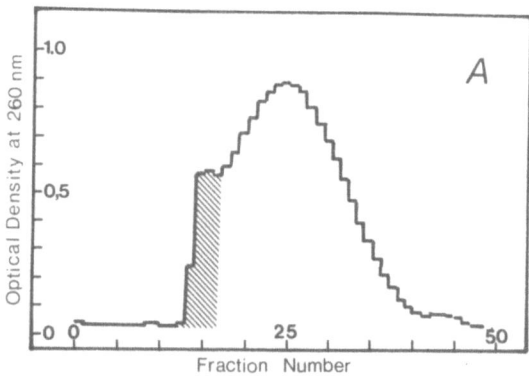

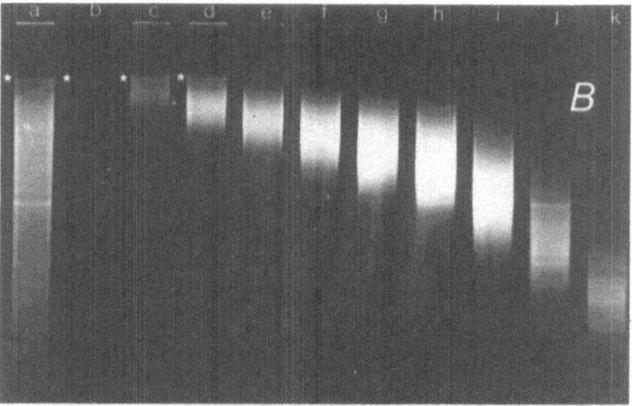

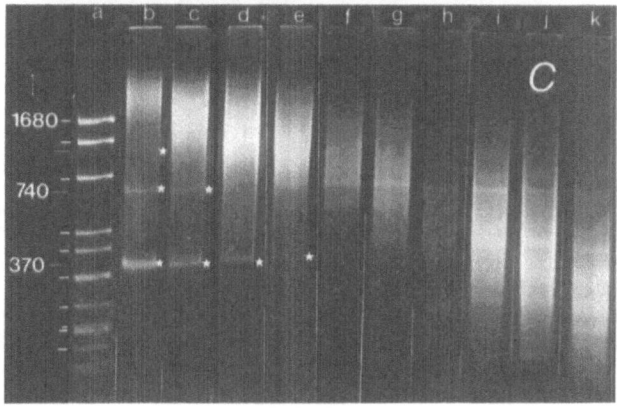

Fig. 1: Isolation of rat satellite I DNA by Sau3A digestion and gel filtration. 5mg of rat DNA, digested with an excess of Sau3A I was
loaded on a 2 x 100 cm column of Sepharose 2B equilibrated with 10
mM Tris-HCl, pH 7.6, 1 mM EDTA, 10 mM NaCl at 4° and eluted with the
same buffer (Fig. 1A). DNA was recovered by ethanol precipitation.
The hatched area of the elution profile represents fractions enriched in satellite I. Aliquots from each fraction were submitted
to electrophoresis on a 0.6% agarose gel (Fig. 1B, tracks b-k) together with DNA prior to fractionation (track a). Satellite I DNA
is visible as the slowest band (asterisk). For a quantitation of
satellite I, aliquots from column fractions were digested with Hae
III and run on a 1.2% agarose gel (Fig. 1C). The monomeric 370 bp
satellite band and multiples of this unit are labeled with asterisks. Repetitive DNA different from satellite I can also be seen
as sharp bands in both gels (e.g. tracks f-k). Track a in Figure
1C contains marker fragments: λdvl DNA digested with Hae III.

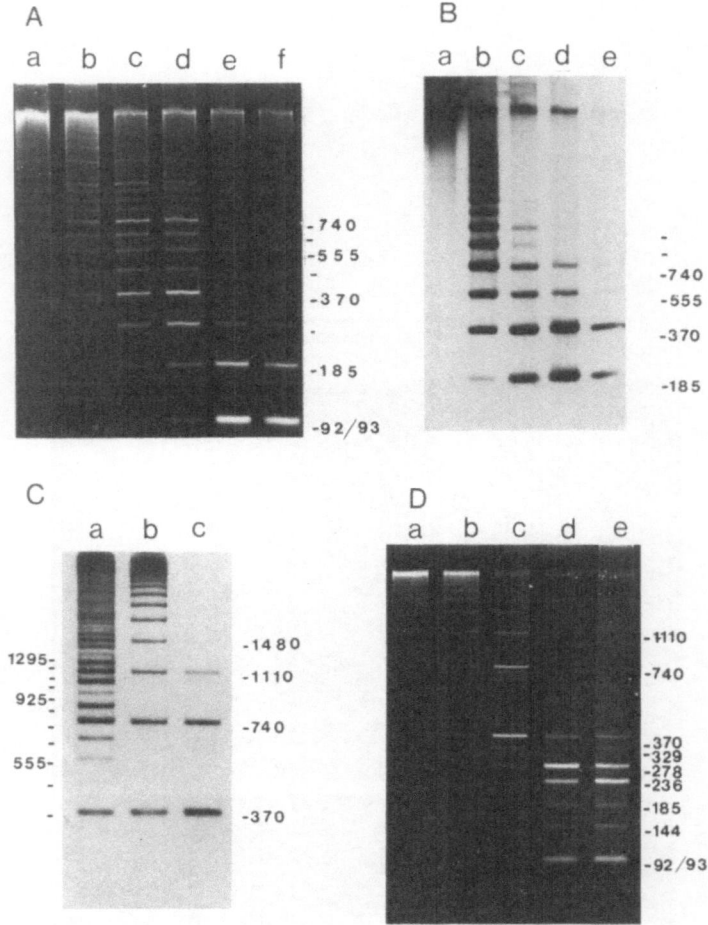

Fig. 2: Course of digestion of satellite I DNA with Eco RI (A), Dde I (B), Hae III (C), and Hinf I (D). About 1.25 μg each of satellite DNA (A, D) or 2.5 μg unfractionated rat DNA (B, C) were digested with increasing amounts of restriction nucleases and subjected to gel electrophoresis. The satellite bands in A and D were revealed by staining the gel with ethidium bromide and in B and C by blotting the DNA to nitrocellulose filters and hybridization with a radio-active satellite probe. Fragment lengths are given in base pairs. In Figure 2C a partial (b) and a limit digest (c) were applied to-gether with an Eco RI digest of rat liver nuclei (a) which displays a 92/93 bp ladder. The first three bands (92/93, 185 and 277/278 bp) run out of the gel.

Figure 2 restriction nuclease digests of purified satellite I DNA are shown (2A, D); alternatively digests of total DNA have been investigated, and the distribution of satellite fragments was displayed by Southern blotting and hybridization with labeled satellite probes (2B, C). By comparing partial digestion products of satellite I DNA with various restriction nucleases, regular "ladders" of bands became visible. The lengths of fragments are integral multiples of basic unit lengths, providing evidence for a tandem arrangement of satellite I.

With Hind III and Hae III, fragments of 370 bp and multiples of this size were obtained, with DdeI fragments of 185 bp and integral multiples of

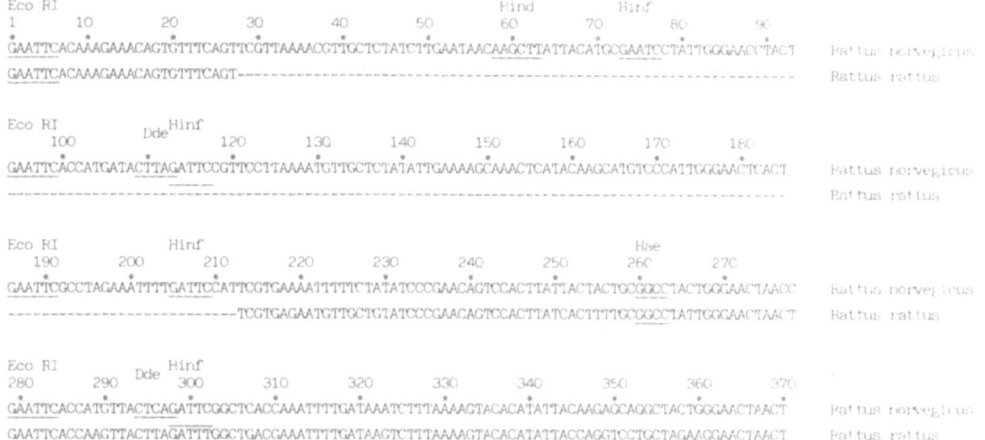

Fig. 3: Homologies between the nucleotide sequence of the 370 bp repeat
unit of satellite I of a laboratory strain rat (R. norvegicus) and
the 185 bp repeat unit of satellite I' (27) from another rat
species (R. rattus). Restriction endonuclease cleavage sites
relevant for this paper are indicated, and the corresponding
sequences are underlined. The R. norvegicus sequence is a con-
sensus sequence derived from 50 clones (see Fig. 9). This con-
sensus sequence differs in 4 positions from the one of Pech et
al.[21]. These differences may be due to the use of rats obtained
from different suppliers. The numbering of the satellite sequence
follows that of Pech et al.[21].

this size were generated. Finally with Eco RI, a 92/93 bp ladder was produced. These findings provided information on the internal subunit structure
of satellite I: the 370 bp unit is composed of four related subunits, 93
and 92 bp in length, respectively. Each of the internal subunits carry
Eco RI sites, but only two of them carry DDE I sites. One of the four 93/92
subunits contains a Hind III site, another one contains a Hae III site
(see Fig. 3).

A somewhat more complex digestion pattern was obtained by digesting
satellite I DNA with Hinf I (Fig. 2D). This complex pattern is due to the
fact that not all four Hinf sites are spaced at equal distances (see Fig. 3)
and those sites which carry a methylated C-residue are cleaved much less
efficiently. Digestion experiments with all kinds of combinations of two
restriction enzymes and analysis of the produced fragments led to the
establishment of a restriction map which fully agrees with the results
from sequence analyses[21,23,25].

Evolution and Species Differences in Satellite I

If one compares satellites from related rodent species like rat and
mouse, the differences in subunit organization and nucleotide sequence are
striking. While the satellite unit of the rat is 370 bp long and is composed of four consecutive 93 and 92 bp subunits, it was shown by sequence
analysis[26] that the unit length of the mouse satellite is 234 bp and is
composed of diverged 9 bp subunits. Apparently, even in related species
considerable differences exist in satellite structures. It is tempting
to speculate that speciation is accompanied by major changes in satellite
structure, or vice versa, although little experimental evidence is
available.

At present the satellites of only two rat species have been thoroughly investigated.  The nucleotide sequence of _Rattus norvegicus_ satellite I was completely determined by Pech et al.[21], and partial sequence analyses were provided by others[23,25].  Witney and Furano[27] cloned and sequenced satellite I' from the Oceanian type black rat _Rattus rattus_.  While the _R. norvegicus_ satellite has a 370 bp repeat unit, the unit of the _R. rattus_ satellite has a length of 185 bp.  The nucleotide sequence of the two satellite repeats are shown in Figure 3.  Both satellites are composed of 93 and 92 bp internal subrepeats.

The subunit architecture of both rat satellites give some insight into the mechanisms by which these DNA sequences may have evolved.  The high degree of sequence homology found in those regions of the satellite which are shared by both species provided evidence for the model proposed by Southern[28].  A process of mutations in one of the subunits was followed by the amplification of a longer segment, for example a diverged dimer.  Such an event occurred once during the development of _R. rattus_ from a hypothetical ancestor, while in _R. norvegicus_ two rounds of mutations and amplifications have to be invoked to explain the present day 370 bp repeat unit.

Extensive investigations on species evolution in the genus _Rattus_ has been carried out by Yosida et al.[29,30].  Karyotype analyses suggest that the long-tailed giant rat, _R. sabanus_, is an ancestral form of the _Rattus_ group.  The Asian type black rat _R. rattus_ evolved from the ancestral form by pericentric inversions of chromosomes 13-18.  About two million years ago[27] _Rattus norvegicus_ diverged from a variant of the Asian type black rat[29] carrying pericentric inversions at chromsomes 1, 9 and 13.  The Oceanian type black rat developed from another variant[30] carrying pericentric inversions at chromosomes 1 and 9, by Robertsonian fusion of the acrocentric pairs 4/7 and 11/12 (Fig. 4).  The schemes for the evolution of rat species are compatible with those for the evolution of satellite structures.  Needless to say, it would be highly interesting to identify possible changes in satellite structures in other well defined and well characterized rat species.

## Location of Satellite I in Metaphase Chromosomes

One of the common characteristics of satellites is their location in heterochromatin, either in pericentric, or telomeric sites of metaphase chromosomes[31].  The chromosomal location of satellite I has been determined by Sealy et al.[23] by _in situ_ hybridization using labeled satellite I probes.  As in the case of satellites in other species, satellite I was found in pericentric and telomeric regions of the chromosomes.  Unfortunately, in their study most of the chromosomes of the rat karyotype could not be identified individually because the _in situ_ hybridization procedure causes some deterioration in chromosome morphology and silver grains often obscure parts of the chromosomes.  Nevertheless, satellite sequences were found in chromosomes of all size classes.  No chromosome in the rat karyotype consistently showed a greater than average label from which it was concluded that neither the X nor the Y chromosome possesses particularly large or extensive blocks of satellite I.  An average of 32 labeled chromosomes per cell could be estimated, suggesting that most, if not all, of the 42 chromosomes do contain satellite I sequences.

## NUCLEOSOME STRUCTURE OF SATELLITE I

### Ultrastructural Studies

On the basis of biochemical experiments[32], it became clear that satellite I is organized in a nucleosome structure.  It was of interest to check

A

R. rattus
(Asian type)

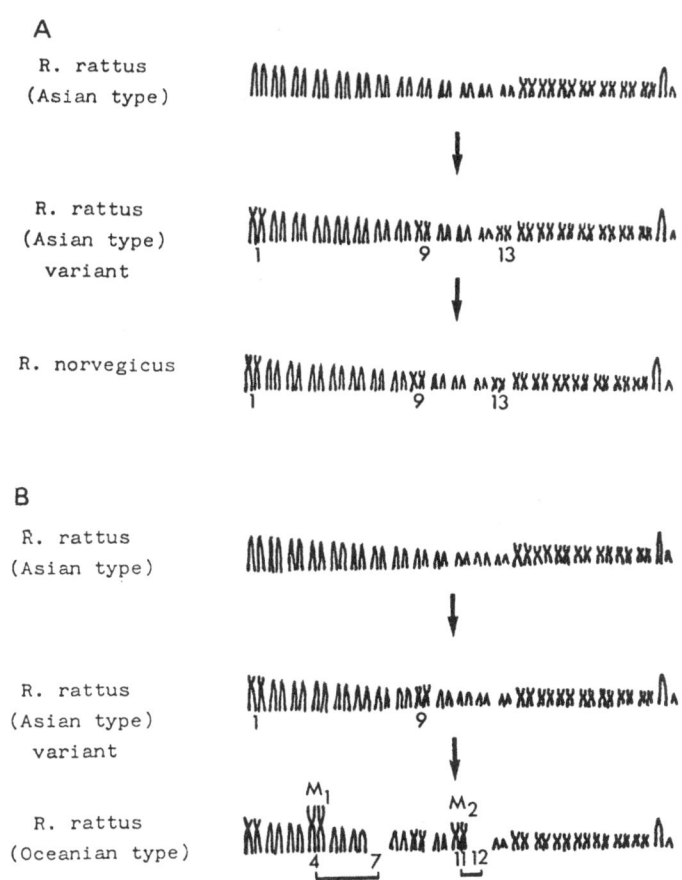

R. rattus
(Asian type)
variant

R. norvegicus

B

R. rattus
(Asian type)

R. rattus
(Asian type)
variant

R. rattus
(Oceanian type)

Fig. 4: Karyotypes of rat species and variants are shown in the idiograms. A possible scheme how R. norvegicus may have evolved from an Asian type R. rattus variant, carrying pericentric inversions at chromosomes 1, 9 and 13, is shown in A. A possible developmental scheme for the evolution of the Oceanian type black rat with 38 chromosomes, from the Asian type black rat with 42 chromosomes, is presented in B. These data were adopted from references 29 and 30.

whether differences can be detected by electron microscopy between chromatin samples containing satellite DNA and non-repetitive DNA. Satellite I-containing chromatin was therefore prepared[33] and investigated by electron microscopy[34]. Due to the purification procedure used, the average size of the satellite-containing chromatin chains was rather small (approximately 8-10 nucleosomes). Nevertheless, the typical beaded structure characteristic of nucleosomes became clearly visible, but at the present level of resolution no differences between these and other chromatin samples could be detected with respect to average internucleosomal distances or to other features.

## Satellite I-containing Chromatin has a Different Nucleosomal Repeat than the Bulk of the Chromatin

Besides electron microscopy and a number of other physical techniques, digestion studies with non-specific nucleases have laid the foundation of our present knowledge of chromatin structure. Digestion experiments with

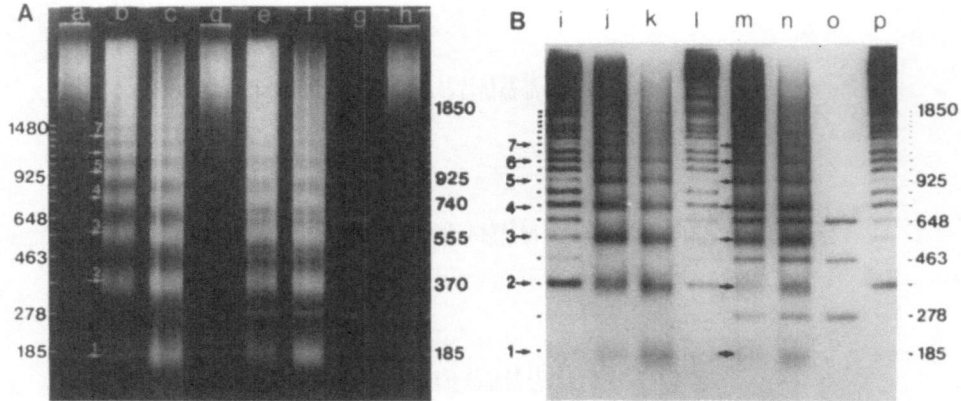

Fig. 5: Analysis of micrococcal nuclease digests of rat liver chromatin
indicates that the repeat length of satellite I-containing chromatin
is shorter than the one of bulk chromatin. Electrophoresis was on
1.8% agarose gels. Ethidium bromide fluorescence patterns (A), and
hybridization patterns (B) with $^{32}$P-labeled satellite I DNA are
shown. A short and a long digest (b, c). The same digests are
shown in tracks e and f, respectively, with added satellite DNA
bands of 278, 463 and 648 bp as chain length markers. Track g,
markers alone. Partial Eco RI digests of enriched satellite DNA
in tracks a, d and h serve as chain length markers (in bp). Tracks
i-p of Fig. 1B correspond to tracks a-h of Fig. 1A. The arrows
point to the positions of mono- and oligonucleosomes, labeled 1-7.
Two gels were run in parallel which were identical except for the
amounts of markers: in (A) amounts detectable by ethidium bromide
staining (which are too high for hybridization) and in (B) amounts
suitable for hybridization were applied. This figure is from
reference 32.

micrococcal nuclease, DNase II, and the $Ca^{2+}/Mg^{2+}$-dependent endogenous
nuclease of rat liver nuclei revealed a difference in the nucleosomal repeat
length between satellite I-containing chromatin and bulk chromatin[32]. These
results suggested that spacing of nucleosomes may be a defined property of
certain regions of the genome. Differences in repeat lengths which have been
found between different species, between different cells of the same organism, and also between a specific gene and the bulk of the chromatin within
the same cell[14,35] are attributed to the linker region of the nucleosomes.
In the following sections, experiments are described that establish the
distinct nucleosome repeat of satellite I-containing chromatin. The role
of histone and nonhistone proteins in spacing was analyzed on purified
satellite I-containing chromatin.

Studies with Micrococcal Nuclease. Brief digestion of rat liver nuclei
with micrococcal nuclease is known to result in the liberation of mono- and
oligonucleosomes from the chromatin fiber. In such a digest the distribution
of satellite I DNA sequences can be analyzed with the blotting technique of
Southern. As a probe, we used highly purified satellite I DNA which had been
labeled by nick-translation. The probe did not contain sizeable amounts of
other rat DNA sequences; at least such sequences, if present at all, did not
contribute significantly to the radioactive signals of our blots under the
hybridization and autoradiography conditions used.

In Figure 5A micrococcal nuclease digestion patterns visualized by
ethidium bromide staining are shown. If the positions of the EcoRI marker

fragments are compared with the positions of nucleosomal fragments a systematic deviation in the relative electrophoretic mobilities becomes
evident. Based on the known repeat length of the satellite fragments
(alternatingly 92 and 93 bp) the evaluation of scans yielded 195 bp as the
bulk nucleosome repeat length in micrococcal digests. Autoradiography of
the Southern blot after hybridization with a satellite probe (Fig. 5B)
revealed that the nucleosomal bands derived from satellite I-containing
chromatin have a different spacing. They comigrate with the bands of the
EcoRI digest of satellite I DNA and therefore are spaced at 185 bp intervals.
The difference in spacing between bulk and satellite I-containing chromatin
is best seen for the higher oligonucleosomes; compare, for instance, the
relative positions of the 925 bp satellite DNA marker fragments in tracks
a and i with pentanucleosome fragments in tracks b and j, respectively.

Because of very weak bands in the hybridization background we cannot
exclude, however, that a small fraction of the satellite DNA is organized
in a 195 bp register.

Control experiments with added markers showed that migration artifacts
of various kinds play a negligible role. The G + C content of rat satellite
I is close to that of bulk DNA. Therefore, base composition dependent
deviations of the electrophoretic mobilities are unlikely.

The intensity distributions of bands in the ethidium bromide stained
gel and in the autoradiogram are rather similar indicating a comparable
susceptibility to micrococcal nucleases of satellite DNA and bulk DNA
containing chromatin.

Studies with a $Ca^{2+}/Mg^{2+}$-dependent Endogenous Nuclease. Autodigestion
of nuclei in the presence of $Ca^{2+}$ and $Mg^{2+}$ led to the known nucleosomal
pattern (Fig. 6A) upon gel electrophoresis. When the bands were blotted
and hybridized with labeled satellite I DNA (Fig. 6B), hybridization was
seen in a 185 bp register, as in the micrococcal nuclease digests. A
nearly perfect coincidence was observed between the radioactive nucleosomal
bands produced by the endogenous nuclease and the marker bands originating
from the digestion of satellite DNA by Eco RI. Artifacts of electrophoresis were excluded by the addition of marker DNA to the autodigested
material.

Analogous results were obtained in DNase II digestion experiments
(not shown). The bands visualized by ethidium bromide staining were spaced
at 195 bp distances in agreement with the 195 bp repeat length of nucleosomes of the bulk of rat liver DNA. After hybridization there was again a
coincidence in the mobilities of DNase II and Eco RI produced satellite
marker fragments indicating a 185 bp rather than a 195 bp repeat length of
the nucleosomes on satellite I DNA.

The Spacing of Nucleosomes in Satellite I-containing Chromatin is
Variable. The simple 1:2 relationship between the nucleosomal repeat
length of satellite I-containing chromatin and the satellite DNA repeat
itself would allow for a direct phase relationship between the two repeats.
An important prerequisite for a perfect phase relationship is that the
spacing of nucleosomes is constant along the chromatin fiber. It was
therefore of interest to investigate possible variations in linker length.
One approach to detect length variations of linker DNA was outlined by
Prunell and Kornberg[36], who used a combination of endo- and exonucleases
for this purpose. A partial micrococcal nuclease digest of chromatin was
prepared and oligonucleosomes were trimmed by the action of exonuclease
III and S1 nuclease.

The result of such an experiment is shown in Figure 7. The action of

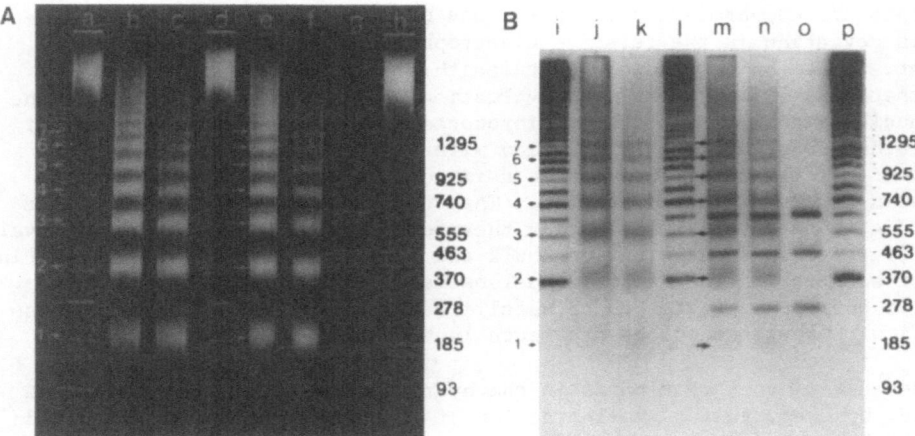

Fig. 6: Digests of rat liver nuclei with the $Ca^{2+}/Mg^{2+}$-dependent endogenous nuclease show that the repeat length of satellite I-containing chromatin is shorter than the one of bulk chromatin. Electrophoresis was on 1.8% agarose gels. Ethidium bromide fluorescence
patterns (A), and hybridization patterns (B) with $^{32}P$-labeled
satellite I DNA are shown The 90 min and 2 h digests (b,c). The
same digests are shown in tracks e and f, respectively, with
added satellite DNA bands of 278, 463 and 648 bp as chain length
markers. Track g, markers alone. Partial Eco RI digest of enriched satellite I DNA in tracks a, d and h serve as chain length
markers (in bp). Tracks i-p of Fig. 6B correspond to tracks a-h
of Fig. 6A. The arrows point to the positions of mono- and
oligonucleosomes, labeled 1-7. Two gels were run in parallel
which were identical except for the amounts of markers: in (A)
amounts detectable by ethidium staining (which are too high for
hybridization) and in (B) amounts suitable for hybridization
were applied. This figure is from reference 32.

exonuclease III and S1 nuclease led to increased mobilities of the nucleosomal DNA fragments. The mononucleosome (185 bp) was trimmed to a sharp 145
bp fragment, corresponding to the size of the core DNA. The dinucleosomal
DNA was clearly shortened, but the width of the band was virtually unchanged,
meaning that linkers between nucleosomes must be of variable size. In
higher oligonucleosomes, the resolution of the gel was not sufficient to
allow a clear interpretation. In control incubations in which either exonuclease III or S1 or both nucleases were omitted, no change in mobility or
width of the mono- or dinucleosomal bands was detected.

These findings clearly showed that there is a variation of linker-
lengths in satellite I-containing chromatin. As a consequence, a perfect
and simple phase relationship between the nucleosome and the satellite I
DNA periodicities over a long range has been excluded. However, the
findings do not allow the conclusion that the nucleosomes are randomly
distributed on the satellite I DNA. In fact we found a more complex, but
still specific arrangement of nucleosomes (see below).

## Protein Composition of Purified Satellite I-containing Chromatin

The molecular basis for the shorter repeat length of satellite-I containing chromatin as well as the higher degree of condensation may be
related to variations in H1 and/or nonhistone protein composition. It was
reported that in the α-satellite of African Green Monkey cells, histone H1

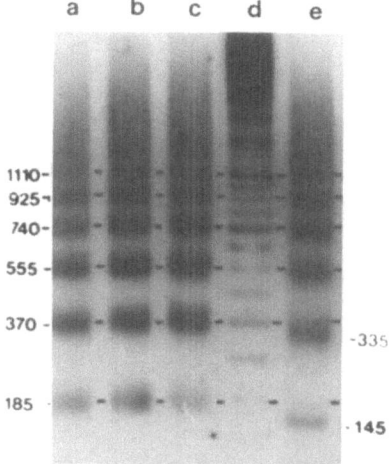

Fig. 7: Demonstration of length heterogeneity of nucleosome spacing in
satellite I-containing chromatin. Chromatin fragments generated
by micrococcal nuclease digestion of nuclei were trimmed with
exonuclease III and S1 nuclease and the DNA subjected to gel
electrophoresis on a 1.5% agarose slab gel, track e. A partial
EcoRI digest of enriched satellite I DNA is shown in track d for
chain length markers. The wells a-c were loaded with DNA from
control samples where S1 nuclease (c), exonuclease III (b), or
both nucleases (a) were omitted from the incubation mixture.
Hybridization patterns with [32]P-labeled satellite I DNA are shown.
This figure is from reference 32.

is replaced by a set of nonhistone proteins[19]; a loss of H1 from the
fraction by arrangement or degradation was not excluded, however. In
Drosophila egg extracts, a protein has been discovered that binds tightly
and with high specificity to a Drosophila satellite[38]. Other nonhistone
proteins claimed to be specific for Drosophila satellites have been
described recently[39,40].

The availability of purified satellite DNA-containing chromatin
fractions has allowed a search for proteins unique to this chromatin. For
the isolation of purified satellite I-containing chromatin the following
approach was used utilizing the specific mode of cleavage of restriction
nucleases. Eco RI restriction endonuclease cleaves the 370 bp satellite
unit at four positions. Since this sequence is repeated very frequently
within the genome, it follows that this region of the chromatin will be
cut into much smaller fragments than the bulk of the chromatin. Chromatin
was extracted from Eco RI digested rat liver nuclei and satellite I-containing chromatin which is enriched in such an extract, was further purified
by sucrose gradient centrifugation[33]. DNA and protein from five gradient
fractions were analyzed on agarose and SDS polyacrylamide gels, respectively, (Fig. 8). The high molecular weight region on the gradient (fraction
4, 5) contained bulk chromatin which according to Eco RI digestions of the
deproteinized DNA had less than 10% satellite I DNA. The low molecular
weight region consisted of practically pure satellite I-containing chromatin
(fraction 2). Free protein together with mono- and dinucleosomes from
satellite I-containing chromatin were seen in the slowest sedimenting region
(fraction 1).

In fraction 2-5 the proportions of H2A, H2B, H3 and H4 histones were
virtually the same as well as the proportions of the H1 subspecies. The

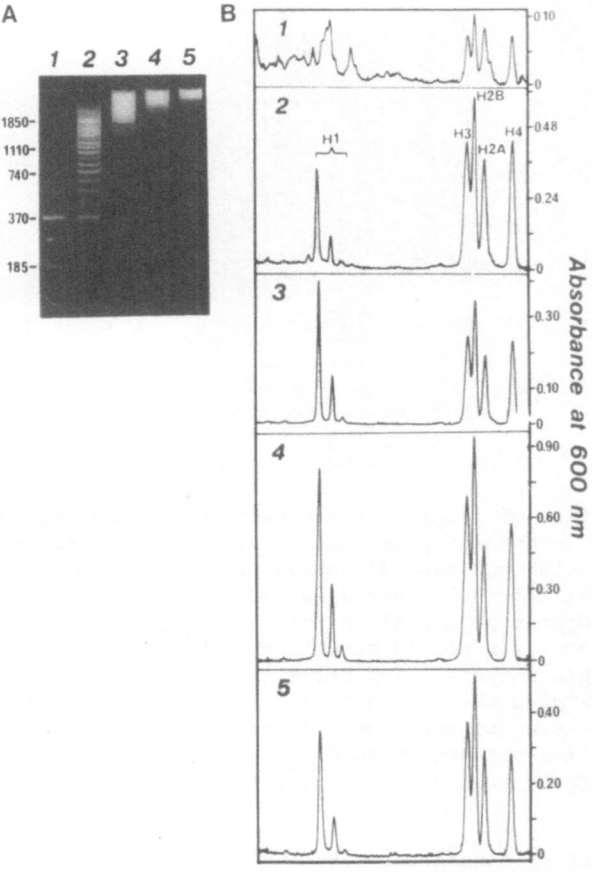

Fig. 8: The histone composition is similar in bulk chromatin and in
satellite I-containing chromatin. Soluble chromatin was prepared
by digestion of rat liver nuclei with Eco RI[33]. 2.5 $A_{260}$ units
each of the digest were layered on 10-30% isokinetic sucrose
gradient and centrifuged in a SW41 rotor of a Beckman Spinco
ultracentrifuge at 4° for 16 h at 22,500 rpm. Under these conditions approximately 80% of the chromatin material was pelleted.
Corresponding fractions from 5 tubes were pooled. The numbers denote the fractions, 1 being the slowest and 5 the fastest sedimenting fraction. DNA and protein were separated and analyzed on
a 1.5% agarose gel (A) and a 12% polyacrylamide gel (B), respectively. Approximately 2 μg of DNA and 50 μg of protein were
applied per track. This figure is from reference 32.

amount of histone H1, however, was reduced to about half in satellite I-
containing chromatin (fraction 2) compared to bulk chromatin (fractions
4, 5) when it was measured in relation to histone H4 and the other histones.
The H1 deficiency may be a true property of satellite I-containing chromatin.
It is a general observation, however, that the mono- and small oligonucleosomes are H1 deficient. We therefore believe that at least part of the H1
has been lost during preparation of the satellite I-containing chromatin due
to its small size.

Most of the nonhistone proteins sedimented near the top of the gradient
(fraction 1) and therefore represent free protein. In agreement with
previous results[41], chromatin-bound nonhistone proteins were detected only

66

in low amounts (fractions 2-5), which made quantitation difficult. We estimate that in those fractions the amounts of individual non-histone proteins did not exceed 1 molecule per 10-20 nucleosomes.

Similar results were obtained in histone and non-histone protein analyses of satellite DNA containing chromatin which was prepared by gel filtration[34] instead of sucrose gradient centrifugation. These results suggested that no satellite I specific nonhistone protein is present in rat satellite I in amounts similar to histone H1 or other histones, although the loss of such a protein during our chromatin preparations cannot be excluded completely. This result is in disagreement with findings of others[19,39,40]. We believe that it is not a nonhistone protein that causes the different nucleosomal repeat length in satellite I-containing chromatin. This property may be due to the specificity of the interaction between the nucleotide sequence of the satellite and histone octamers.

PHASING IN SATELLITE I-CONTAINING CHROMATIN

How nucleosomes are arranged relative to the DNA sequence has recently received much attention (for reviews see: 14, 42, 43). One possibility is that they are arranged randomly. Alternatively they may either be located in unique positions that are identical in a population of cells of the same kind; or they may occupy a small number of distinct preferred positions. Such arrangements have been termed phasing. Interest in phasing stems from the idea that preferential or specific nucleosome locations may be important in chromosome mechanics and could be one means of controlling gene expression and/or replication. While the issue was controversial a few years ago, more recent reports agree that, in the systems investigated, there exists a preference of the nucleosomes for certain positions.

Mapping of Nucleosome Positions by Cloning and Sequence Analysis of Nucleosome Core DNA

Determination of the sequence of core DNA permits conclusions to be reached concerning the location of histone octamers on the DNA. One obvious problem concerning this approach is that any DNA sequence in the core preparation, even highly abundant repetitive DNA sequences, comprises only a small proportion of the total population of DNA sequences. It is impossible to perform sequence analysis with a mixture of fragments. This problem was overcome by the application of commonly used methods of gene technology. Cloning linkers were attached by blunt end ligation to the ends of the core DNA fragments and cloned in E. coli cells using pBR322 plasmid DNA as a vector. By the use of colony hybridization techniques, a number of clones could be easily identified which contained satellite I core DNA. Approximately 50 of the isolated clones were investigated by sequence analysis.

Figure 9 is a graphical presentation of the data derived from our cloning and sequencing work. The 370 bp satellite unit (equivalent to a dinucleosome) was divided into two equal halves, more or less arbitrarily. The left half (bp 213-27) is nearly identical to the satellite I' from the Oceanian black rat (see Fig. 3); the right half is unique to R. norvegicus, from which common laboratory strains are derived. Clones that start within the left part of the satellite unit are shown in the left column and clones starting with the second half of the satellite unit are shown in the right one. We want to emphasize that this kind of presentation does not necessarily imply a natural relationship between adjacent nucleosomes.

Clearly, the location of nucleosomes along the satellite sequence is nonrandom. The nucleosomes of the left part of the satellite unit are positioned in one preferred (c) and seven less preferred (a, b, d-h)

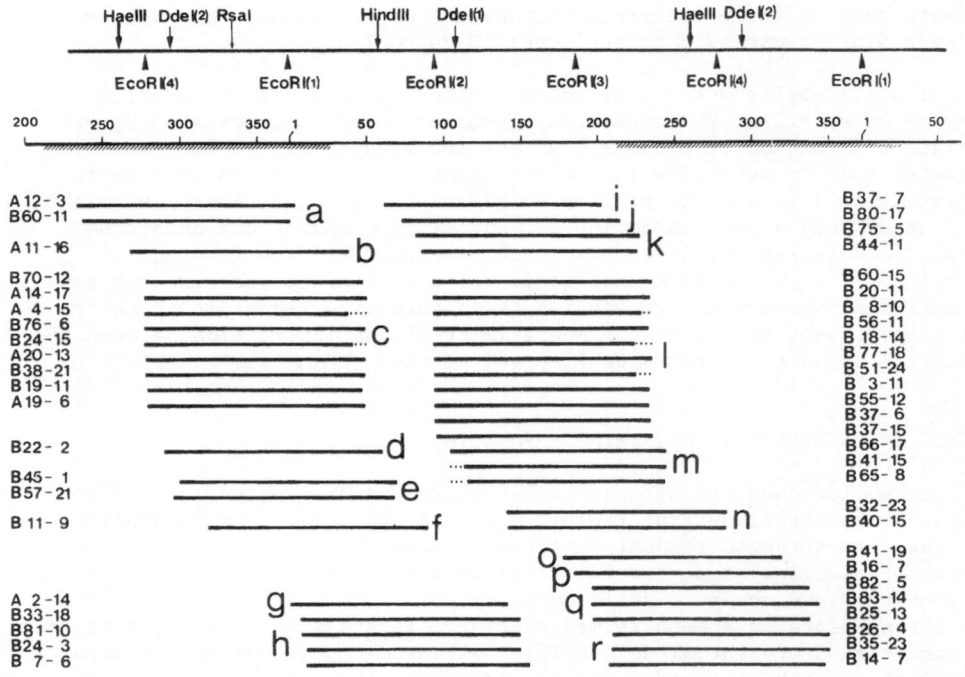

Fig. 9: Positioning of nucleosome cores on satellite I DNA. The first row represents a restriction nuclease map of satellite I. Only restriction sites relevant for this study are indicated. There are unique sites for Hae III (Bsp RI), Hind III and Rsa I within the 370 bp repeating satellite I unit. Restriction sites that occur twice (Dde I) or four times (Eco RI) within the satellite unit are appropriately labeled, labels given in parentheses. The numbering of the satellite I sequence (middle row) is according to Pech et al.[21] The satellite unit which can harbor two nucleosomes was divided in two equal halves (see text); the left half is underlined (hatched line). All clones which started within the underlined region are listed in the left column, the rest in the right one. The bars indicate the regions covered by each clone. In the two extreme columns the designation of the clones is given. Some bars are extended by dots. Although these clones are only approximately 133 bp long, they have been included in this figure since it seems clear from which side the bases were removed by exonuclease III overdigestion. Nucleosomes were found in eight defined sites (a-h) on the left part of the satellite and in 10 defined sites (i-r) on the right half. This figure is from reference 48.

positions. The same applies to the right part of the satellite unit where again one location is preferred (1) although other less preferred positions (i-k, m-r) exist.

## Nucleosome Positions are Strictly Defined

One of the most striking results of these investigations is the lack of microheterogeneity within the strongly preferred sites. Apparently, nucleosomes are located in strictly defined positions. On the left half of the 370 bp satellite unit the most preferred site (site c) spans the sequence between bp 276-50 (Fig. 10). No indication was obtained for positions shifted either to the right or to the left by one or only a few basepairs. We arrived at this conclusion since no clone was found that

```
          276       285        295              31        41        50
          *         *          *       105 bp   *         *         *
A14-17    CACGAATTCA CGAAGTTACT ..........      TTGAAACGTT GCTCTATCTT
B70-12    -CCGAATTCA CCATGTTACT ..........      TTAAAACGTT GCTCTACT--
A 4-15    ACCGAATTCA CCATGTCACT ..........      TTRRRRCT-- ----------
B76-06    ACCAAATTCA CCATGTTACT ..........      TTAAAACGCT GCTCTATCT-
B24-15    ACCGAATTCA CCATGTTACT ..........      ATAAAACGTT G---------
A20-13    -CCGAATTCA CCATGTTACT ..........      TTAAAACGTT GCTCTATCT-
B38-21    -CCGAATTCA CCATGTTACT ..........      TTAAAATGTT GCTCTATCT-
B19-11    --CGAATTCA CCATGTTATT ..........      TTAAAACGTT GCTCTAT---
A19-06    --TGAATTCA CCAAGGTACT ..........      TTAAAACGTT GCTCTATCT-
```

Fig. 10: Lack of a michroheterogeneity in nucleosome position of the prominent site c. The terminal nucleotide sequences of the clones corresponding to site c are listed. In the left column the designation of the clones is given. The numbering of the bases is according to reference 21. One sequencing gel (A4-15) could not be read unambiguously at every position: R was used for purine residues at such positions. This figure is from reference 48.

spanned the sequence, for example, from bp 274-48 or bp 272-46 (Fig. 10). Of course, our clones displayed another kind of heterogeneity: they showed some variation in length. This kind of heterogeneity, however, was attributed to overdigestion with exonuclease III, rather than to variation in nucleosome position. The lack of a microheterogeneity applies also for the right hand preferred site (site 1). The relatively low number of clones analyzed preclude similar conclusions concerning the less preferred sites, although we believe that these sites are also strictly defined.

## Mapping of Core-ends Relative to Restriction Nuclease Cleavage Sites

Our cloning approach for the mapping of nucleosome core positions on the satellite I DNA sequence is new, and we therefore wished to complement those experiments by other methods. Core DNA isolated by preparative gel electrophoresis was 5'-labeled with polynucleotide kinase, digested with restriction nucleases and enriched for satellite DNA sequences by exploiting the rapid rate of reassociation of highly repetitive DNA. This procedure has been successfully used for mapping the nucleosome positions of African Green Monkey α-satellite DNA[44] and mouse satellite DNA[45]. Separation of the renatured fraction from the bulk of single stranded DNA was achieved by hydroxyapatite chromatography.

Endlabeled core DNA digested either with Rsa I or Bsp RI (an isoschizomer of Hae III) was analyzed in 8% polyacrylamide high resolution sequencing type gels (Fig. 11). A pattern of discrete bands (due to satellite DNA) superimposed on a background was generated by both nucleases. Undigested DNA is composed of 141-145 nucleotide long fragments and some contaminating fragments 10 and 20 nucleotides shorter, resulting from overdigestion with exonuclease III. Digestion with Mnl I, for which no major site is present in the satellite, did not result in a striking pattern, although we detected some minor bands of unclear origin. The sizes of the fragments derived from Rsa I and Bsp RI digestion were determined by comparing their mobilities with known markers. The sizes add up pairwise to approximately 142 nucleotides. Each fragment-pair corresponds to one of the nucleosome positions detected by our cloning approach. The most prominent fragment-pair in the Rsa I digest (59/85 bases) corresponds to site c in perfect agreement with the cloning results. The less pronounced

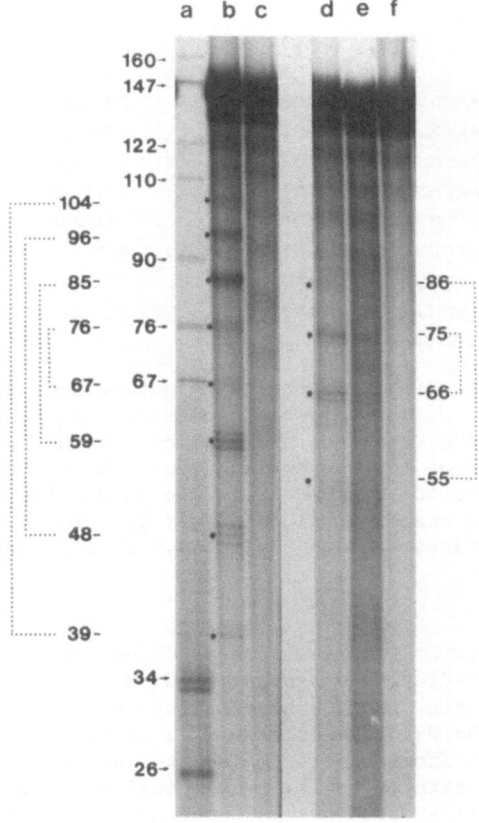

Fig. 11: Nucleosome cores occupy defined positions on the satellite I
repeat unit. 5'-endlabeled core DNA was digested with RSA I (b),
Mnl I (c) or Bsp RI (d,e), enriched for satellite I DNA by means
of rapid reassociation kinetics and hydroxyapatite chromatography
and analyzed in an 8% polyacrylamide sequencing-type gel. For
the Bsp RI digest both the enriched (d) and nonenriched (e)
fractions are shown. In (f) the 5'-endlabeled core DNA preparation without restriction nuclease digestion is shown. A 5'-
endlabeled Hpa II digest of pBR 322 DNA was used as a size marker
(a) with fragment lengths given in nucleotides. Clusters of
satellite bands are marked by a dot and coupled pairwise. The
sizes of the pairs add up to 143 bases. The pair 39 + 104 of
the RsaI digest corresponds to sites a and e, the pairs 48 + 96,
59 + 85, and 67 + 76 to the sites d, c and b, respectively. The
pair 55 + 86 of the Bsp RI digest corresponds to sites o and r,
and the pair 66 + 75 to sites p and q, as found with the cloning
and sequencing approach (Fig. 9). This figure is from reference
48.

fragment-pairs correspond to sites a, b, d and e. Fragments which would
result from an f-type nucleosome cannot be resolved on the gel. The bands
resulting from Bsp RI (Hae III) digestion correspond to sites o-r. Again,
the bands from a- and n-type nucleosomes cannot be resolved on the gel.

By this kind of analysis, the location of nucleosomes can be mapped
only on certain regions and not on the whole satellite unit. This is due
to the lack of additional restriction nucleases that cut only once within
the 370 bp satellite unit. The use of restriction nucleases that cut twice

70

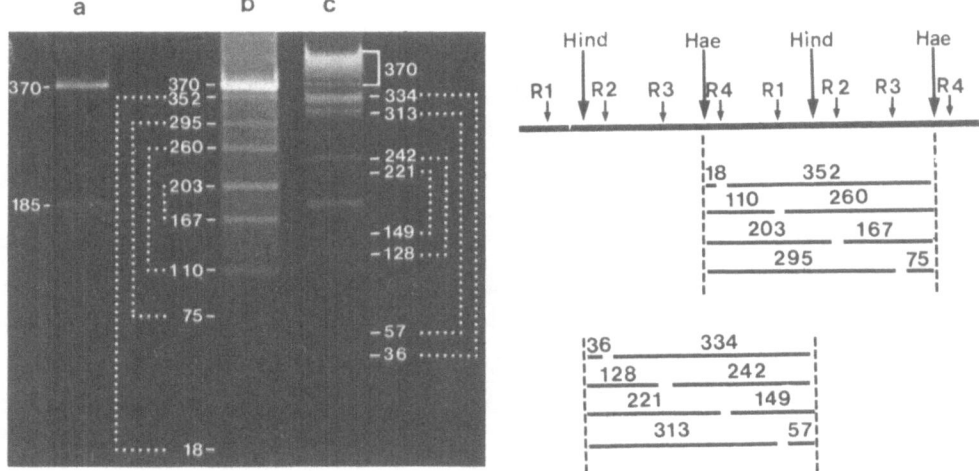

Fig. 12: The accessibility of the four Eco RI sites (R1-R4) of the 370 bp
repeating satellite I unit has been determined to be about 20%
on average. (A), rat liver nuclei were digested with Eco RI under
limit digestion conditions. After purification, the DNA was
digested to completion with either Hae III (b) or Hind III (c)
and subjected to gel electrophoresis on a 1.5% agarose slab gel;
(a), satellite I marker fragments. The lower part of the gel is
shown. (B), restriction nuclease map that shows the expected
fragment pairs. This figure is from reference 48.

or more within the unit leads to ambiguous results.

## Restriction Nuclease Digestion of Intact Nuclei

In order to confirm the reliability of the analyses presented so far,
we felt that the location of nucleosomes had to be investigated by other
independent experimental approaches as well. Restriction nucleases can be
used for this purpose. The accessibility of given restriction sites in
chromatin can be studied under the assumption that a site is protected when
located within the nucleosome core, but accessible if located in the linker
region. This has actually been shown to be the case for some enzymes[46,47].

The nucleosome positions deduced from our cloning experiments (Fig. 9)
lead to clear predictions concerning the accessibility of different restriction sites. Since 46 of the 49 analyzed clones contained a Dde I site, the
distribution of these sites between core and linker should be 46:3. Thus
we can predict that 6% of the Dde I sites are accessible and 94% protected
against cleavage. A similar estimation can be made for the accessibility
of the Eco RI sites. Since 17 clones contained only one site and 32 clones
contained two Eco RI sites, it follows that 17% should lie in linkers and be
accessible for cleavage with the rest of 83% occurring within cores and
inaccessible. The accessibilities of the Hae III and Hind III sites follow
directly from Figure 9. About 50% of these sites are found in linkers and
are accessible. We note, however, that some restriction sites are abolished
by sequence divergence leading to somewhat lower numbers.

The accessibility of the Eco RI sites in satellite I-containing chromatin could be measured directly. DNA was isolated from an Eco RI limit
digest of rat liver nuclei and cleaved to completion with either Hind III
or Hae III (Fig. 12). About 80% of the satellite is displayed as a 370 bp

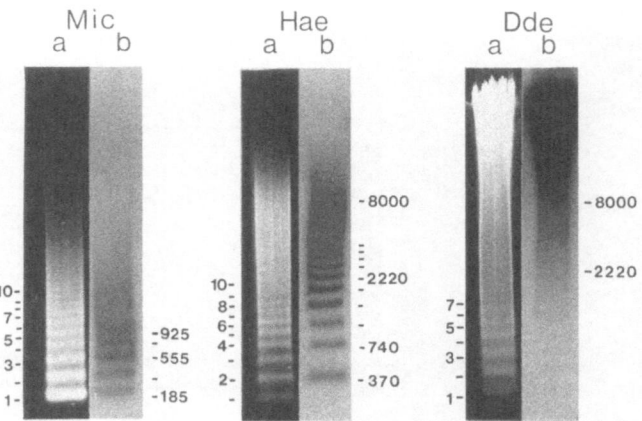

Fig. 13: Differential accessibility of restriction nuclease cleavage sites
in satellite I-containing chromatin. Rat liver nuclei were
digested with Hae III or Dde I, the DNA purified and 2-4 μg
subjected to 1% agarose gel electrophoresis. For comparison a
micrococcal nuclease digest is also included. (a) ethidium
bromide staining; (b) Southern transfer and hybridization with
[32]P-labeled nick-translated satellite I DNA. Numbers on the left:
mono- and oligonucleosomes; on the right: DNA sizes in base pairs.

Hae III or Hind III band indicating that about 80% of the Eco RI sites
remained uncleaved. About 20% of the satellite DNA appear as shorter bands
indicating a 20% accessibility of Eco RI sites in satellite I chromatin, in
fairly good agreement with our expectations. A similar double-digestion
experiment for estimating the accessibility of the Hae III sites in satellite chromatin (not shown) was in keeping with the expected value of 50%.

In Figure 13 the accessibility of Dde I and Hae III sites was compared.
To rigorously quantitate the accessibility of restriction sites in chromatin,
highly concentrated restriction nuclease preparations are necessary in order
to obtain limit digests within a reasonable short incubation time, under
which endogenous nuclease activities play only a minor role[46],[47]. Unfortunately, our Dde I preparations do not meet this criterion at present. In
this experiment a true limit digest could only be obtained with Hae III and
only a partial digest was obtained with Dde I. This became apparent upon
staining the gel with ethidium bromide. The amount of DNA in the low molecular weight region of the gel is a qualitative indication for the degree of
digestion. The DNA in the Hae III and Dde I digests showed a nucleosomal
ladder. It has been demonstrated previously[46],[47] that this banding pattern
is due to the restriction nuclease rather than to endogenous nuclease
activity(ies). The relative intensities of the nucleosomes derived from
the Hae III and Dde I digests are again indicative of the extent of
digestion.

The satellite digestion patterns were revealed upon transferring the
DNA to nitrocellulose and hybridization with a labeled satellite I probe.
The expected 370 bp ladder became apparent, characteristic for satellite I
digests with Hae III. With Dde I, however, only a very weak pattern was
obtained, indicative of a strongly limited accessibility of these sites in
satellite I-containing chromatin. The vast majority of the satellite DNA
was displayed in the high molecular weight region of the gel and was longer
than 8 kb. The limited accessibility of Dde I sites in satellite I-containing chromatin may become even clearer if one takes into account that in
order to compensate for the partial character of the Dde I digest, twice

the amount of DNA was loaded. Thus the amount of low molecular weight material, displayed as oligonucleosomal bands in the ethidium bromide stained gel, was comparable to the one in the Hae III-track.

We are fully aware of the problems which arise when an incomplete digest (Dde I) is compared with a complete one (Hae III) and conclusions are made about the accessibility of restriction sites from such comparisons. Semiquantitative estimations are still possible. It is fair to say that Dde I sites are much less accessible than Hae III sites and even less than Eco RI sites. The actual value may very likely be close to 6% as predicted on the basis of our cloning experiments. In conclusion we can say that the predicted susceptibilities of restriction nuclease cleavage sites in satellite I-containing chromatin could be experimentally verified.

## LONG-RANGE ARRANGEMENT OF NUCLEOSOMES ALONG THE CHROMATIN FIBER

The experiments presented so far give little information about the long-range organization of nucleosomes within the chromatin fiber. There are two basically different possibilities. First, any nucleosome, for example from the left column of Figure 9, might be flanked by any of the nucleosomes from the right column, with the only limitation being that overlapping nucleosomes be excluded. If all possible combinations existed, a rather complex picture of the satellite I-containing chromatin fiber has to be envisaged, despite the marked preference of nucleosomes for certain sites on the DNA.

Second, pairs of nucleosomes or more complex but specific oligo-nucleosome configurations, would give rise to "islands" or distinct nucleosome arrays. One array can be characterized easily in which all (or nearly all) Hae III sites are located in linkers and therefore are accessible to cleavage (Hae III susceptible arrays). Other arrays can be characterized in which Hae III sites are located in nucleosome cores (Hae III resistant arrays). Changes or switches from one kind of oligonucleosome array to another one may be due to occasional deletions or insertions of 92/93 bp satellite subunits that interrupt the monotonous regularity of tandem repetitions of the 370 bp satellite units. We now present data that favor this second view of alternating arrays with fixed mutual relationships between nucleosomes.

### Oligonucleosomal Arrangement in the Hae III Susceptible Array

Digestion of rat liver nuclei with Bsp (Hae III) gave rise to a bimodal distribution of satellite I DNA fragments (Fig. 14). The location of the nucleosomes on the shortest, 370 bp fragment as well as on the rather long fragments containing 10-14 nucleosomes has been analyzed separately. The location of nucleosomes on the 370 bp chromatin fragment has been determined by experiments in which the protruding DNA ends were trimmed by exonuclease III and S1 nuclease digestion. If the nucleosome cores were located on the DNA fragment in a random fashion, a broad band of shortened fragments would be expected. In case of specific location(s) one or several sharp bands should be observed. The exonuclease/S1 experiment is shown in Figure 15. The strategy of the experiments and the results are summarized in the graph of Figure 15.

The trimmed DNA fragments were subjected to gel electrophoresis (not shown) and the distribution of satellite fragments within the bulk of the digested material was revealed by blotting and hybridization. What was found were fairly narrow bands centered around 335 bp, 705 bp, etc. In some gels the shortened band of ca. 335 bp was resolved as a double band centered around 332 and 342 bp.

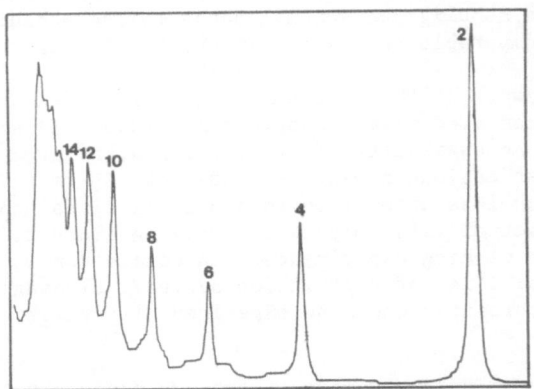

Fig. 14: Cleavage of satellite I-containing chromatin with Hae III leads
to a bimodal fragment distribution. This kind of distribution is
due to Hae III susceptible and Hae III resistant oligonucleosomal
arrays. DNA from a limit digest of rat liver nuclei with Hae III
was subjected to electrophoresis on a 1.2% agarose gel. The DNA
was then transferred to nitrocellulose and hybridized with labeled
satellite I DNA probe. Autoradiograms were scanned and a densito-
gram is shown. Numbers are multiples of 185 bp (the nucleosome
repeat in satellite I-containing chromatin). This figure is from
reference 48.

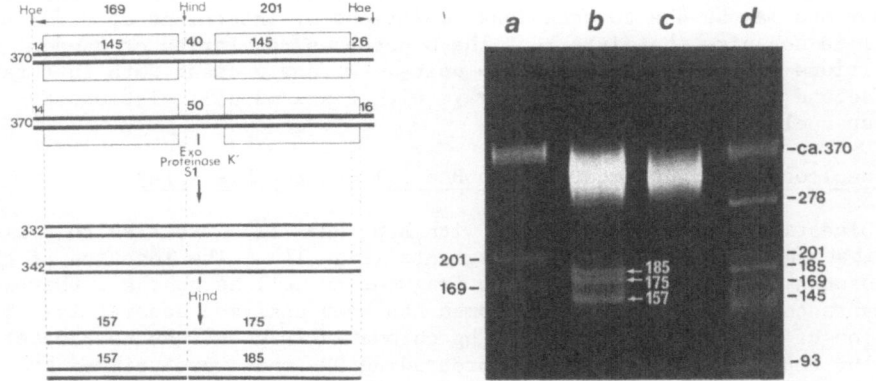

Fig. 15: Nucleosomes on the 370 bp satellite I fragment are located predominantly in three preferred positions. (A) The strategy of
the experiments and the interpretation of the results are shown
schematically. 14 bases were removed from the left and either
26 of 16 bases from the right of the 370 bp fragment by exonuclease III treatments. DNA is depicted as double bar and
nucleosome cores as boxes. After removal of the histones with
proteinase K the protruding single-stranded ends were removed
with nuclease S1. (B) Untrimmed dinucleosomal DNA (a) and
trimmed DNA (b) were digested with Hind III and loaded onto a
2% agarose slab gel. (c) Trimmed DNA without Hind III treatment.
(d) Marker fragments, lengths given in bp.

In order to determine the extent of trimming on either side of the dinucleosome fragment, we eluted to exonuclease III and S1 nuclease digested DNA from the 290-370 bp region of a preparative agarose gel and further digested with Hind III (Fig. 15 track b). Since the Hind III site is located asymmetrically on the 370 bp fragment, one can thus determine which of the two termini was trimmed and to what extent. The satellite I DNA was converted predominantly into three sharp bands with chain lengths of 157, 175 and 185 bp, in relative amounts of 1 : 0.7 : 0.3, respectively (track b of Fig. 15). Some additional faint bands were neglected in this quantitation. Most of the DNA, which was not satellite DNA, was cleaved by Hind III only to a small extent and remained at its original position on the gel.

Nucleosomes on the Hae III generated 370 bp fragment were found to be located in two alternative positions on the 201 bp Hind-Hae arm and in only one position on the 169 bp Hae-Hind arm of the fragment. The dinucleosomes with the 26 and 14 bp protruding ends comprise 67% of the population while the ones with the 16 and 14 bp termini are present in 33%. The respective linker lengths are inferred to be 40 and 50 bp in two types of dinucleosomes. The sites correspond to the prominent nucleosome sites (c) and (1), and the less prominent site (m) of Figure 9. This experiment also established relationships between nucleosomes of the c- and 1-type and c- and m-type, respectively. Such relationships could not be established by our cloning approach with core DNA.

Specific Nucleosome Positioning in the Multiple Hae III Resistant Arrays

How are nucleosomes located on the longer fragments? We digested nuclei with Bsp under limit digestion conditions and extracted soluble chromatin from the digested nuclei. The fragments were separated according to length by sucrose gradient centrifugation. Fractions corresponding to dodecameric nucleosomes were pooled and digested with Eco RI followed by agarose gel electrophoresis of the purified DNA. The satellite I bands were visualized by blot hybridization. The pattern obtained (Fig. 16 track b) is puzzling and different from that obtained by Eco RI digestion of unfractionated chromatin (d). Most remarkable is the high intensity of four bands which have mobilities corresponding to 3.5, 4.5, 5.5 and 6.5 nucleosomal lengths. Those bands are also prominent in the total chromatin digest; the interesting feature of the experiment is that other prominent bands in the total digest, namely those corresponding to the nucleosomal lengths (4.0, 5.0, 6.0, 7.0, etc.) became much less prominent in the pattern obtained from the high molecular weight sucrose gradient fraction. This means that the various bands of the rather complex Eco RI digestion pattern can be ascribed to arrays of the satellite-containing chromatin fiber that can be separated by Bsp RI digestion and sucrose gradient centrifugation. These arrays must have highly specific oligonucleosomal configurations since a very specific Eco RI digestion pattern was obtained.

Transition Sites Between Different Arrays

Transition from a certain array to another one may arise fortuitously. However, we isolated one clone that indicated a correlation between irregularities in the satellite DNA sequence and changes in the nucleosome arrangement. The sequence of the clone B67/10 is presented in Figure 17. The left boundary of the clone corresponds to the nucleosome site m, but the right border is different. This is due to a deletion of 93 bp of the DNA sequence; the right border of the nucleosome became shifted by 93 bp (Fig. 17) as compared to a normal m-type nucleosome site. This situation necessarily leads either to a new nucleosome arrangement or upon maintenance of the original nucleosome frame, to a rather long nucleosome-free gap. Such irregularities in the DNA subunit structure, which can also be seen

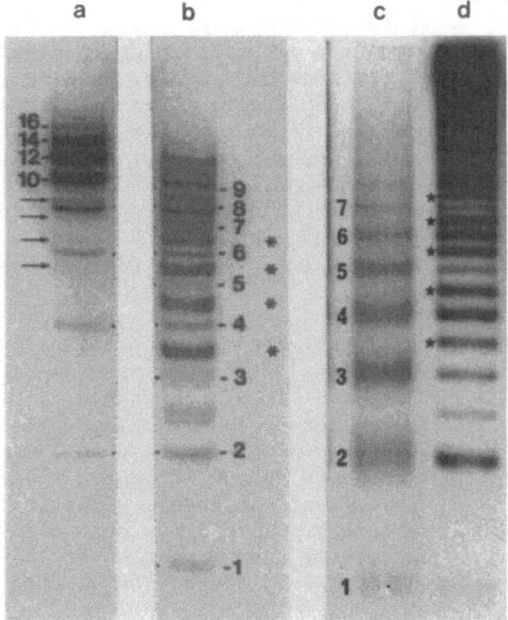

Fig. 16: Sucrose gradient separation of arrays of satellite I-containing
oligonucleosomes having specific nucleosome arrangements. Soluble
chromatin was prepared by Hae III digestion of rat liver nuclei
under limit digestion conditions and extraction with 10 mM Tris-
HCl pH 7.9, 0.2 mM EDTA. Hae III prepared chromatin was fractionated on a sucrose gradient (not shown). Oligonucleosome
fractions from the sucrose gradient corresponding to 10-14
nucleosomes were pooled (a) and digested to a limit with Eco RI
(b). For comparison, a micrococcal nuclease (c) and an Eco RI
digest of nuclei is included (d). Electrophoresis was done after
deproteinization. The autoradiogram of a Southern blot is shown.
The fragment lengths are given in nucleosomal lengths (n x 185
bp). Some bands in (b) are split into doublets or triplets;
this is due to either Eco RI ends alone or Eco RI and Hae III ends
of the fragments. Bands corresponding to (n + 0.5) x nucleosomal
lengths enriched in the sucrose gradient fraction are labeled with
asterisks. The arrows in (a) show Hae III bands which do not fit
properly into the n x 370 bp ladder. Such bands may arise by
deletions or insertions of 92/93 bp satellite subunits (see also
Fig. 17).

in restriction digestion patterns of satellite I DNA (arrows in Fig. 16
track a), provide a plausible explanation for changes in the chromatin
fiber structure and transitions from one kind of array to another. Needless
to say, much more work has to be done to rigorously solve the specific
nature of the long-range arrangement in satellite I-containing chromatin.


CONCLUDING REMARKS

The aim of this work was to give a review on experimental data concerning the organization, evolution, chromosome location and chromatin structure
of satellite I of the rat. Investigations at the DNA level have given clear
answers to the question of the internal architecture of this DNA and some
insight into the mechanisms by which satellite I DNA sequences changed

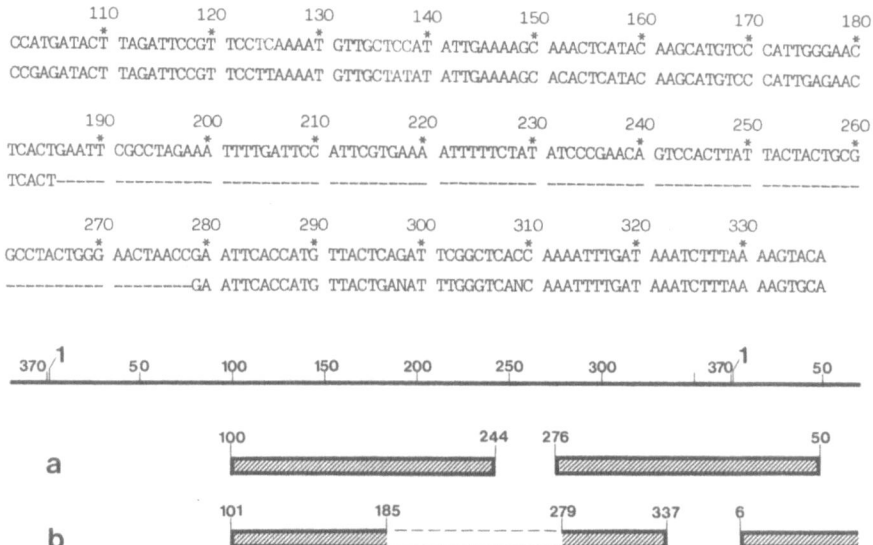

```
          110        120        130        140        150        160        170        180
          *          *          *               *          *          *          *          *
CCATGATACT TAGATTCCGT TCCTCAAAAT GTTGCTCCAT ATTGAAAAGC AAACTCATAC AAGCATGTCC CATTGGGAAC
CCGAGATACT TAGATTCCGT TCCTTAAAAT GTTGCTATAT ATTGAAAAGC ACACTCATAC AAGCATGTCC CATTGAGAAC

          190        200        210        220        230        240        250        260
          *          *          *          *                *          *          *          *
TCACTGAATT CGCCTAGAAA TTTTGATTCC ATTCGTGAAA ATTTTTCTAT ATCCCGAACA GTCCACTTAT TACTACTGCG
TCACT----- ---------- ---------- ---------- ---------- ---------- ---------- ----------

          270        280        290        300        310        320        330
          *          *          *          *          *          *          *
GCCTACTGGG AACTAACCGA ATTCACCATG TTACTCAGAT TCGGCTCACC AAAATTTGAT AAATCTTTAA AAGTACA
---------- --------GA ATTCACCATG TTACTGANAT TTGGGTCANC AAATTTTGAT AAATCTTTAA AAGTGCA
```

Fig. 17: Characterization of a mutant clone that may be involved in nucleosome phase transitions. The nucleotide sequence of clone B67-10 is presented in the lower line. In the upper line the average satellite sequence according to Pech et al.[21] is shown for comparison. This 144 bp long cloned DNA contains satellite I nucleotide sequences from bp 101-185 and 279-337; a complete 93 bp satellite subunit ranging from bp 186-278 was found to be deleted. The left end of the clone corresponds to an m-type nucleosome site (100-244) and the right end to a q-type site (195-337). The graph suggests how a nucleosome frame composed of m-type and c-type nucleosomes (a) may suffer a transition that leads to a new frame (b) due to a sequence deletion.

during evolution[21]. In situ hybridization has revealed the chromosomal location of these sequences[23]. Utilization of restriction nucleases for digestion of nuclei provided the basis for the isolation of satellite I-containing chromatin in pure form[32] and for the analysis of its protein composition[33,41]. We were unable to relate the condensed heterochromatic nature of satellite I-containing chromatin nor the difference in repeat lengths between satellite and bulk chromatin to differences in histone or nonhistone protein composition. Therefore, other features of satellite I-containing chromatin, possibly positioned nucleosomes, are responsible for these specific properties.

Our investigations clearly showed that histone octamers are located along the satellite I DNA in a nonrandom (phased or positioned) manner[37,48]. Nucleosomes occupy a number of preferred sites. The most preferred sites, but probably also other sites, are strictly defined with the precision of a single base pair. Good indications have also been obtained for a defined long-range organization of the satellite chromatin fiber in specific (Hae III susceptible and resistant) oligonucleosomal arrays.

We were surprised to find a specific chromatin structure of a DNA segment of the genome that has no coding function. These findings raise once again the question of the functional significance of satellites. Although the answer certainly will remain speculative, one new aspect has emerged. One of the consequences of folding a DNA chain around histone octamers is that DNA sequences that are distant in the unfolded DNA come into close proximity. The same applies for the formation of higher order chromatin structures. The spatial arrangement and the exposure of DNA sequences on the outside or inside of the solenoid would be different in a population of cells of the same cell type if the location of nucleosomes along the DNA chain were essentially random. On the other hand, specific spatial arrangements that are identical in all cells of a population may only be obtained with positioned nucleosomes. While specific spatial arrangements of DNA sequences may not be a necessary feature for some of the genomic DNA, they could be an important feature for others. Homologous pairing of chromosomes in meiosis may be one of the cases where such a specific exposure of particular DNA sequences to the surface of chromosomes is an essential property. It is hard to imagine how homologous chromosomes can be specifically aligned if the DNA sequences to be recognized are exposed on the surface of one chromosome but buried inside the fiber in the other chromosome.

Whether or not satellites participate in meiotic events or other chromosome functions remains to be seen. In favor of such a function is the observation that in some parasitic nematodes like Ascaris, satellites are largely eliminated in somatic cells, where they apparently have no function, but retained in germ line cells[49]. The specific location of satellites in pericentric and telomeric regions of chromosomes also point to a possible function in chromosome behavior. The rapid progress in gene technology and cell biology may help to solve the still open questions concerning heterochromatin and satellite-containing chromatin.

ACKNOWLEDGMENTS

The author would like to thank his coworkers and colleagues for their cooperation in the studies reported here. He is particularly thankful to H. G. Zachau, W. Hörz, and J. Robertson for reading the manuscript and for valuable discussions. The work was supported by Deutsche Forschungsgemeinschaft, "Forschergruppe Genomorganisation" and Fonds der Chemischen Industrie.

REFERENCES

1.  D. R. Hewish and L. A. Burgoyne, The digestion of chromatin DNA at regularly spaced sites by a nuclear deoxyribonuclease, Biochem. Biophys. Res. Commun. 52:504-510 (1973).

2.  M. Noll, Subunit structure of chromatin, Nature 251:249-251 (1974).

3.  R. D. Kornberg, Chromatin structure: A repeating unit of histones and DNA. Chromatin structure is based on a repeating unit of eight histone molecules and about 200 DNA base pairs, Science 184:868-871 (1974).

4.  A. L. Olins and D. E. Olins, Spheroid chromatin units (ν-bodies), Science 183:330-332 (1974).

5.  F. Thoma, T. Koller, and A. Klug, Involvement of histone H1 in the organization of the nucleosome and of the salt-dependent superstructures of chromatin, J. Cell Biol. 83: 403-427 (1979).

6. M. Renz, P. Nehls, and J. Hozier, Involvement of histone H1 in the organization of the chromatin fiber, Proc. Natl. Acad. Sci. USA 74: 1879-1883 (1977).

7. W. H. Straetling, U. Mueller, and H. Zentgraf, The higher order repeat structure of chromatin is built up of globular particles containing eight nucleosomes, Exp. Cell Res. 117:301-311 (1978).

8. C. Nicolini, Chromatin structure: from nuclei to genes, Anticancer Research 3:63-86 (1983).

9. C. Benyajati and A. Worcel, Isolation, characterization, and structure of the folded interphase genome of Drosophila melanogaster, Cell 9:393-407 (1976).

10. K. W. Adolph, S. M. Cheng, J. R. Paulson, and U. K. Laemmli, Isolation of a protein scaffold from mitotic HeLa cell chromosomes, Proc. Natl. Acad. Sci. USA 74:4937-4941 (1977).

11. T. Igo-Kemenes and H. G. Zachau, Domains in chromatin structure, Cold Spring Harbor Symp. Quant Biol. 42:109-118 (1978).

12. M. P. F. Marsden and U. K. Laemmli, Metaphase chromosome structure: evidence for a radial loop model, Cell 17:849-858 (1980).

13. A. L. Bak, J. Zeuthen, and G. H. C. Crick, Higher-order structure of human mitotic chromosomes, Proc. Natl. Acad. Sci. USA 74:1595-1599 (1977).

14. T. Igo-Kemenes, W. Hörz, and H. G.Zachau, Chromatin, Ann. Rev. Biochem. 51:89-121 (1982).

15. I. L. Cartwright, M. A. Keene, G. C. Howard, S. M. Abmayr, G. Fleischmann, K. Lowenhaupt, and S. C. R. Elgin, Chromatin structure and gene activity: the role of nonhistone chromosomal proteins, CRC Critical Reviews in Biochemistry 13:1-86 (1983).

16. J. J. Yunis, and W. G. Yasmineh, Satellite DNA in constitutive hetero-chromatin of the guinea pig, Science 168:263-265 (1970).

17. J. H. Frenster, V. G. Allfrey, and A. E. Mirsky, Repressed and active chromatin isolated from interphase lymphocyte, Proc. Natl. Acad. Sci. USA 50:1026-1032 (1963).

18. T. Igo-Kemenes, W. Greil, and H. G. Zachau, Preparation of soluble chromatin and specific chromatin fractions with restriction nucleases. Nucl. Acid Res. 4:3387-3400 (1977).

19. P. R. Musich, F. L. Brown, and J. J. Maio, Subunit structure of chro-matin and the organization of eukaryotic highly repetitive DNA: nucleosomal proteins associated with a highly repetitive mammalian DNA, Proc. Natl. Acad, Sci, USA 74:3297-3301 (1977).

20. X. Y. Zhang and W. Hörz, Analysis of highly purified satellite DNA contain-ing chromatin from the mouse, Nucl. Acids Res. 10:1481-1494 (1982).

21. M. Pech, T. Igo-Kemenes, and H. G. Zachau, Nucleotide sequence of a highly repetitive component of rat DNA, Nucl. Acids Res. 7:417-432 (1979).

22.  M. Fuke and H. Busch, Hind III-sensitive sites present once in every four repeats of EcoRI-sensitive sites in Novikoff rat hepatoma DNA, FEBS-Letters 99:136-140 (1979).

23.  L. Sealy, J. Hartley, J. Donelson, and R. Chalkley, Characterization of a highly repetitive sequence DNA family in rat, J. Mol. Biol. 145: 291-318 (1981).

24.  M. Singer, Highly repeated sequences in mammalian genomes, Int. Rev. Cytol. 76:67-112 (1982).

25.  J. -N. Lapeyre, W. G. Beattie, A. Dugaiczyk, D. Vizard, and F. F. Becker, Eco RI-generated reiterated components of the rat genome I. Sequence of two (92 and 93 bp) related DNA fragments, Gene 10:339-346 (1980).

26.  W. Hörz and W. Altenburger, Nucleotide sequence of mouse satellite DNA, Nucl. Acids Res. 9:683-696 (1981).

27.  F. R. Whitney and A. V. Furano, The independent evolution of two closely related satellite DNA elements in rats (Rattus), Nucl. Acids Res. 11: 291-304 (1983).

28.  E. M. Southern, Base sequence and evolution of guinea pig α-satellite DNA, Nature 227:794-798 (1970).

29.  T. H. Yosida, Chromosome differentiation and species evolution in rodents, in: "Chromosomes in Evolution of Eukaryotic Groups," A. K. Sharma and A. Sharma, eds. CRC Press, Boca Raton, FL (1983).

30.  T. H. Yosida, H. Kato, K. Tsuchiya, T. Sagai, and K. Moriwaki, Cytological survey of black rats, Rattus rattus, in southwest and central Asia, with specific regard to the evolutional relationship between three geographical types, Chromosoma (Berl.) 45:99-109 (1974).

31.  D. L. Brutlag, Molecular arrangement and evolution of heterochromatic DNA, Ann. Rev. Gent. 14:121-144 (1980).

32.  A. Omori, T. Igo-Kemenes, and H. G. Zachau, Different repeat lengths in rat satellite I DNA containing chromatin and bulk chromatin, Nucl. Acids Res. 8:5363-5375 (1980).

33.  T. Igo-Kemenes, W. Greil, and H. G. Zachau, Preparation of soluble chromatin and specific chromatin fractions with restriction nucleases, Nucl. Acids Res. 4:3387-3400 (1977).

34.  T. Igo-Kemenes, F. Miller, and H. G. Zachau, Use of restriction nucleases in the analysis of chromatin structure, in: "Gene Functions," 12th FEBS Meeting Dresden 51, S. Rosenthal et al., eds. Pergamon Press, 219-299 (1978).

35.  R. D. Kornberg, Structure of chromatin, Ann. Rev. Biochem. 46:931-1154 (1977).

36.  A. Prunell and R. D. Kornberg, Relation of nucleosomes to DNA sequences, Cold Spring Harbor Symp. Quant. Biol. 42;103-108 (1978).

37.  T. Igo-Kemenes, A. Omori, and H. G. Zachau, Nonrandom arrangement of
     nucleosomes in satellite I-containing chromatin of rat liver,
     Nucl. Acids Res. 8:5377-5390 (1980).

38.  T.-S. Hsieh and D. Brutlag, A protein that preferentially binds
     Drosophila satellite DNA, Proc. Natl. Acad. Sci USA 76:726-730
     (1979).

39.  L. Levinger and A. Varshavsky, Protein D1 preferentially binds A + T-
     rich DNA in vitro and is a component of Drosophila melanogaster
     nucleosomes containing A + T-rich satellite DNA, Proc. Natl. Acad.
     Sci. USA 79:7152-7156 (1982).

40.  L. Levinger and A. Varshavsky, Selective arrangement of ubiquitinated
     and D1 protein-containing nucleosomes within the Drosophila genome,
     Cell 28:375-385 (1982).

41.  C. G. P. Mathew, G. H. Goodwin, T. Igo-Kemenes, and E. W. Johns, The
     protein composition of rat satellite chromatin, FEBS-Letters 125:
     25-29 (1981).

42.  H. G. Zachau and T. Igo-Kemenes, Face to phase with nucleosomes, Cell
     24:597-598 (1981).

43.  R. Kornberg, The location of nucleosomes in chromatin:  specific or
     statistical?  Nature 292:579-581 (1981).

44.  X. -Y. Zhang, F. Fittler, and W. Hörz, Eight different highly specific
     nucleosome phases on α-satellite DNA in the African Green Monkey,
     Nucl. Acids Res. 11:4287-4306 (1983).

45.  X. -Y. Zhang and W. Hörz, Nucleosomes are positioned on mouse satellite
     DNA in multiple highly specific frames that are correlated with a
     diverged subrepeat of 9 bp. J. Mol. Biol.76:105-129 (1984).

46.  W. Pfeiffer, W. Hörz, T. Igo-Kemenes, and H. G. Zachau, Restriction
     nucleases as probes for chromatin structure, Nature 258:450-452
     (1975).

47.  W. Hörz, T. Igo-Kemenes, W. Pfeiffer, and H. G. Zachau, Specific
     cleavage of chromatin by restriction nucleases, Nucl. Acids Res.
     3:3213-3226 (1976).

48.  H. Boeck, S. Abler, X.-Y. Zhang, H. Fritton, and T. Igo-Kemenes,
     positioning of nucleosomes in satellite I-containing chromatin of
     rat liver, J. Mol. Biol. 76:131-154 (1984).

49.  K. Moritz and G.E. Roth, Complexity of germ line and somatic DNA in
     Ascaris, Nature 259:55-57 (1976).

THE NUCLEAR MATRIX:  AN ORGANIZING STRUCTURE FOR THE INTERPHASE NUCLEUS

AND CHROMOSOME

Kenneth J. Pienta and Donald S. Coffey

Departments of Urology, Oncology and Pharmacology
Johns Hopkins University School of Medicine
Baltimore, Maryland, USA  21205

ABSTRACT

The interphase nucleus is characterized by a nuclear matrix structure
that forms a residual scaffolding network composed of only 10% of the total
nuclear proteins.  The nuclear matrix contains residual elements of the
pore-complex lamina, the nucleolus, and an intranuclear fibrous network.
The matrix provides the basic shape and structure of the nucleus.  In the
interphase nucleus this nuclear matrix has been reported to be a central
element in the organization of DNA loop domains and contains fixed sites
for DNA replication and transcription.  In this study, we have analyzed
the role of the nuclear matrix and the DNA loop domains in the organization
and structure of the number four human chromosome.  A scale model is
proposed and constructed that closely approximates the observed structural
dimensions of this chromosome.  The model is composed of equivalent 30 nm
diameter filaments formed from solenoid with 6 nucleosomes per turn.  This
30 nm solenoid filament is organized into loops of DNA each containing
approximately 60,000 base pairs; each loop is anchored at its base to the
nuclear matrix structure.  A radial loop chromosome model containing 18 of
these loops per turn forms a new unit of chromosome structure termed the
miniband.  Each miniband contains approximately one million base pairs of
DNA and this is equivalent to a centimorgan in DNA content.  Approximately
106 of these minibands are stacked longitudinally along a central axis to
form the final chromatid.  The role of the nuclear matrix in this organization is presented.  The accuracy of the proposed model is tested by
comparing its features with the known properties of the number four human
chromosome.

INTRODUCTION

The nuclear matrix is an insoluble, structural framework that is
composed of residual elements of the pore complex-lamina, residual nucleolus
and internal network composed of RNP particles attached to a fibrous protein
mesh[1-10].  The nuclear matrix is obtained by extracting nuclei with Triton
X-100 which is a nonionic detergent, and then washing the nuclei in hypotonic
and hypertonic salt solutions (Fig. 1).  This yielded what is commonly
termed "chromatin", the soluble fraction of such a preparation containing
the bulk of the DNA and histones.  Very little attention has been given to
the insoluble residue from these preparations that contains the nuclear

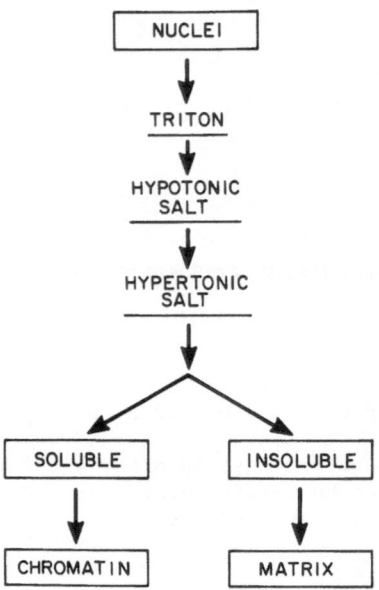

Fig. 1:  A schematic of the general steps in the isolation of the nuclear
         matrix [see reviews for specific details (8,9)].

matrix structures.  The upper portion of Figure 2 is an electron micrograph
of an isolated rat liver nucleus and the lower frame indicates the morphology of a single nuclear matrix sphere.  This matrix structure, that is
devoid of lipids, DNA, histones and has over 90% of the nuclear proteins
removed, still contains a residual scaffolding system composed of residual
elements of the nucleus.  The structure of the nuclear matrix may be
depicted in the schematic in Figure 3 that represents the various components
and lists some of the specific properties reported to be associated with
this nuclear structure.  The biological importance of the nuclear matrix is
emphasized by its reported role in DNA replication (3b, 11-16).  It appears
that the nuclear matrix contains fixed sites for DNA replication[13] and $\alpha$-DNA
polymerase[17].  In addition to its role in DNA replication, the nuclear matrix
also has a central function in transcription in that actively transcribed
genes are enriched on the nuclear matrix[17-19].  Other studies have indicated
that over 95% of the heterogeneous nuclear RNA is associated with the nuclear
matrix[20-25].  Similar to the DNA replication, it has also been reported that
RNA is synthesized at fixed transcriptional complexes on the nuclear
matrix[24].  It is still unknown how the functions associated in the nuclear
matrix are regulated, but insight has been provided by the reports that the
nuclear matrix contains specific receptors for steroid hormones 26a, 26b,
9, 10), as well as the acceptor sites for these steroid receptors[27].

    The higher order organization of DNA within the nucleus and within the
metaphase chromosome remains one of the major unsolved problems in molecular
biology.  At least three higher order levels of DNA organization have been
reported in the past decade, including the nucleosome, the 30 nm solenoid
and DNA loops.  Cook, Brazell and Jost in 1976[28] proposed that loop structures were involved in the superhelical organization of DNA.  In 1980,
Vogelstein, Pardoll and Coffey reported that the DNA loop.domains were
attached at their base to a nuclear skeleton structure termed the nuclear
matrix[14].

    It is the purpose of this report to analyze the concept of the DNA loop
attachment to the nuclear matrix and to determine how these loops can be

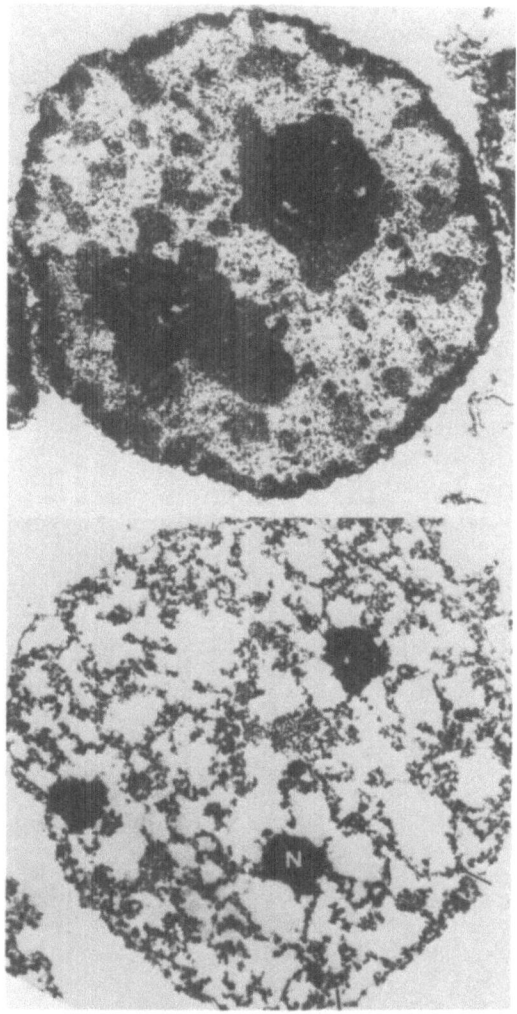

Fig. 2:  Electron micrographs of an isolated rat liver and nucleus (upper)
and the nuclear matrix (lower).  N is the residual nucleolus.


accommodated into chromosomal structure to meet the known spatial and
structural requirements of a given human chromosome.


RESULTS AND DISCUSSION

Vogelstein et al.[14] visualized DNA loop structures attached to the
nuclear matrix by releasing the supercoiled loops in the presence of a low
concentration of ethidium bromide (5 μg/ml).  These loops of DNA extended
out beyond the surface of the nuclear matrix structure forming a large DNA
halo region that surrounded the periphery of the nuclear matrix.  The
radius of this halo was approximately 15 microns.  This loop length was
calculated to contain 90,000 base pairs for each loop.  If the loop of DNA
was constrained at its base by attachment to the nuclear matrix, it should
be possible to rewind this loop by placing it in high concentrations (100
μg/ml) of ethidium bromide[29].  This was accomplished by Vogelstein et al.[14],
as depicted in Figure 4.  When the loops of DNA had been nicked, high

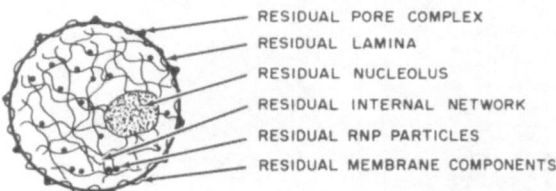

NUCLEAR MATRIX
(RESIDUAL NUCLEAR SKELETON)

RESIDUAL PORE COMPLEX
RESIDUAL LAMINA
RESIDUAL NUCLEOLUS
RESIDUAL INTERNAL NETWORK
RESIDUAL RNP PARTICLES
RESIDUAL MEMBRANE COMPONENTS

- LIPID FREE
- REPRESENTS ONLY 10% OF TOTAL NUCLEAR PROTEINS. CONTAINS RELATED PROTEINS
- SITE OF ATTACHMENTS OF DNA LOOPS
- CONTAINS FIXED SITES FOR DNA SYNTHESIS
- ASSOCIATED WITH HnRNA
- SPECIFIC BINDING OF HORMONES
- PROTEINS PHOSPHORYLATED
- MAY HAVE DYNAMIC PROPERTIES

Fig. 3:  A schematic of the structure and properties of the nuclear matrix.

ethidium bromide (100 μg/ml) did not rewind the halo, providing convincing evidence that the loop domains of DNA were anchored at their base to the nuclear matrix, thus forming a constrained DNA loop that is equivalent to circular DNA.  Therefore, an important role of the nuclear matrix is to constrain the loops of DNA for organization into the superhelical structure. This superhelical loop structure must be maintained even in the chromosome, since Paulson and Laemmli[30] have observed similar DNA loop domains attached to a residual chromosome core scaffold.

In interphase, another important role of the nuclear matrix is that it contains the fixed sites for DNA replication[13].  The loops of DNA observed by Pardoll et al.[13] were demonstrated to be equivalent in size to the

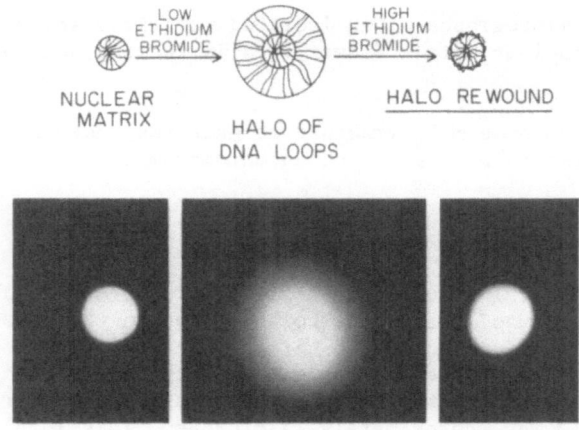

Fig. 4:  The release of DNA loops in low ethidium bromide (5 ug/ml) to form a DNA halo around the periphery of the nuclear matrix.  At high ethidium bromide concentration (100 ug/ml) the halo rewinds if the DNA loops are not nicked (adapted from Vogelstein et al.[14]).

86

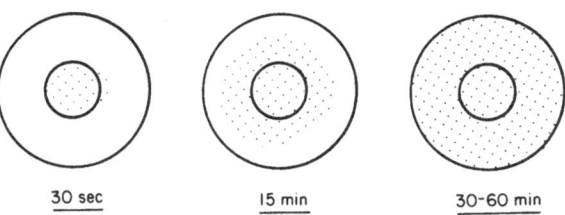

30 sec         15 min         30-60 min

Fig. 5:  A schematic of the autoradiography of grains from labeled
DNA ($^3$H-thymidine incorporation) moving into the DNA halo region
surrounding the nuclear matrix.  Each cell was labeled for 30
seconds to one hour (adapted from original data of Vogelstein
et al.[14]).

replicon units which are the basic lengths of DNA synthesized as continuous
units[31].  During DNA replication, the loops are reeled down through these
fixed sites of synthesis located on the matrix; during this process they
form two new loops of DNA.  It was possible to visualize the rate of movement of this newly synthesized DNA by direct autoradiography and to determine the distance that the grains ($^3$H-thymidine) had moved into the DNA
halo region with increasing periods of labeling.  This concept is depicted
in the schematic in Figure 5, where the label of the newly synthesized DNA
molecules can be monitored with time as it moves out into the DNA halo
region surrounding the nuclear matrix[14].

It is apparent that the DNA loop domain is a basic unit of higher
order structure of DNA in eukaryotic cells.  As can be observed in Table 1,
measurements of these loops by various authors have placed their DNA
content in a range from 10-180 kilobase pairs with an average of 63 kilobase
pairs for all studies combined.  Table 2 lists the properties of these DNA
loop domains.  There are approximately 63,000 base pairs of DNA per loop
contained in 21 microns of DNA double helix.  Each loop is large enough to
contain approximately 315 nucleosomes that are wound with 6 nucleosomes
per turn into a solenoid as proposed by Finch and Klug[32].  This solenoid is
30 nm in diameter and forms the filament of the loop.  Based on a total DNA
content of 6 x 10$^9$ base pairs per diploid nucleus, there are approximately
95,000 of these loops within a cell, and each of these loops of DNA is
synthesized in approximately 30-60 minutes and represents the length of DNA
in a replicon.

It is unknown how these loop domains are organized within the interphase nucleus.  The two theories that have been suggested are represented
in Figure 6.  Some studies suggest that the DNA loops hang like draperies

Table 1:  Average Number of Base Pairs Per Loops of DNA.

| AVERAGE LOOPS (Kilobase Pairs) | RANGE OF LOOPS (Kilobase Pairs) | REFERENCE |
|---|---|---|
| 62 | 30–70 | Georgiev et al.[38] |
| 53 | 10–180 | Hancock and Boulikas[46] |
| 54 | 35–85 | Igo-Kemenes et al.[47] |
| 83 ± 29 | – | Earnshaw & Laemmli[40] |
| 63 ± 14 Average | | |

Table 2:  Properties of an Average DNA Loop Domain.

| PROPERTIES | AVERAGE VALUE | RANGE |
|---|---|---|
| Base pairs/loop | 63,000 | 30,000–100,000 |
| Total length of DNA in loop | 21.4 μm | 10–34 μm |
| Total nucleosomes/loop | 315 | 150–500 |
| Diameter of loop filament | 30 nm | 30 nm |
| Turns of solenoid/loop | 52 | 25–83 |
| Total length of loop | 0.52 μm | 0.25–0.83 |
| Height of loop | 0.26 μm | 0.12–0.41 |
| DNA packing ratio | 40 | 40 |
| Total number of loops per human diploid cells | 95,000 | 60,000–200,000 |

from the nuclear lamina[33-35].  Kendall et al.[36] have demonstrated a densely populated nuclear region 0.5 microns thick around the nuclear periphery. However, we believe that this explanation is inadequate to fully explain the chromatin pattern of interphase nuclei.  Figure 7 compares the length of a DNA loop to the dimensions of a typical nucleus of 7 microns in diameter.  In its fully extended double helix form, a 60,000 b.p. loop is 10.2 microns long.  Winding the DNA into its 10 nm beads-on-a-string form would yield loops 1.5 microns in length, leaving a DNA-free central sphere area equivalent to 33% of the nucleus.  Further compaction of the DNA into the 30 nm solenoid form would leave the nucleus 86% devoid of DNA and would

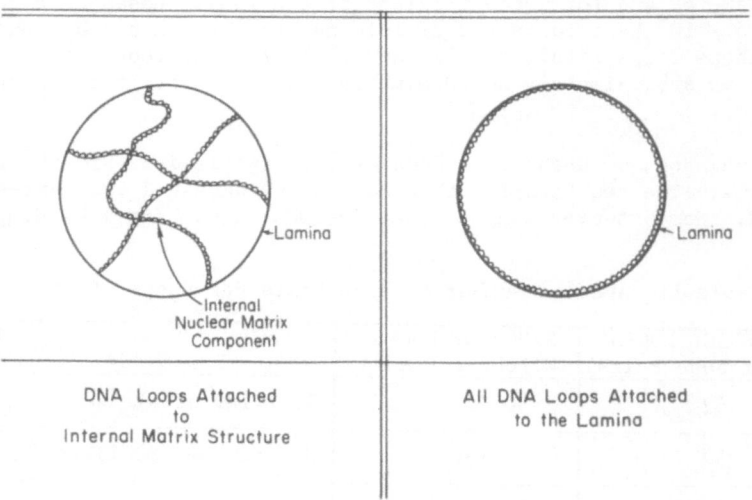

DNA Loops Attached
to
Internal Matrix Structure

All DNA Loops Attached
to the Lamina

Fig. 6:  A comparison of two concepts for the attachment of DNA loops in the nucleus.  Left concept shows attachment of the DNA loops at their base to the nuclear matrix component.  The concept on the right limits the attachment of the DNA to the peripheral lamina components.

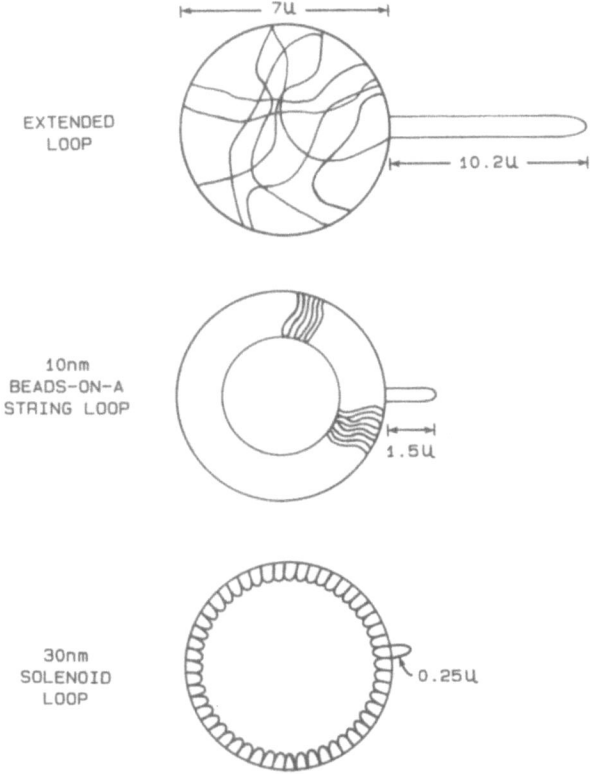

Fig. 7:  A scale comparison of DNA structure dimensions in relation to a
typical nucleus of 7 microns in diameter.


line the nuclear sphere with a chromatin band only 0.25 microns in diameter.
Since both of these higher order DNA structures can be isolated from interphase nuclei[37], another explanation may be required other than restriction
of DNA loop binding only to the nuclear lamina.  Pardoll, Vogelstein and
Coffey[13] demonstrated that newly synthesized DNA was attached to an internal
network of the nuclear matrix.  This makes more feasible a model based upon
DNA loops attached at their bases to the internal nuclear matrix that courses
throughout the interior of the interphase nucleus.  Since the DNA loops
domains are still preserved in metaphase chromosomes and the metaphase
chromosomes are devoid of nuclear envelope lamina proteins, it would appear
that the loops of the chromosome are anchored to other structural elements
of the nucleus besides the lamina[38].  Earnshaw and Laemmli[40] have isolated
the scaffold proteins of the metaphase chromosome and have shown that they
are non-lamina proteins of 135K and 170K molecular weight and are similar
to those present in the interphase nucleus as components of the nuclear
matrix.

     It is unknown how DNA loops are organized to form chromosomes.  Knowing
the amount of DNA in a chromatid of the #4 human chromosome, we attempted to
construct scale models of this chromatid equivalent to a 30 nm filament
organized into loop domains.  Of four previously proposed models of chromosome structure[41-44], [39], [45], we could accommodate these loops into the
actual chromatid dimensions only by utilizing the radial loop model suggested by Marsden and Laemmli[44] and Adolph and Kreisman[43].  The radial loop
model proposes that loops are organized into radial structures wrapped
around the central axis of the chromatid as they are wound and stacked to

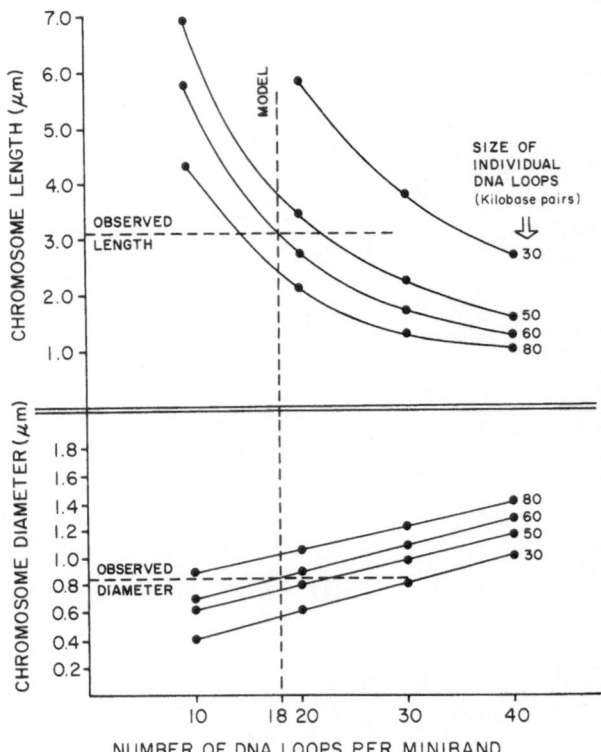

Fig. 8:  Human chromosome #4 dimensions as determined by DNA loop size and
         number of radial loops per miniband (see text).  The y-axis is the
         calculated chromosome length and chromatid diameter in microns that
         would be required to accommodate the $1.15 \times 10^8$ base pairs in a
         chromatid of the #4 chromosome at various loop sizes and number of
         loops per turn.  The horizontal broken lines are the actual
         observed dimensions of the chromatid.  The x-axis is the number
         of DNA loops per chromosome turn (miniband).  The optimal fit to
         the observed length and diameter was found to be 18 loops of
         60,000 bases pairs per loop (see text).  We have termed this unit
         of 18 radial loops per turn on the chromosome a 'miniband'.

achieve the overall chromosome length.  We then determined how many of these
DNA loops would be required for each full turn of the chromatid (defined as
a miniband) to fit the total amount of DNA into the known dimensions of the
#4 chromatid.  To fit the known chromatid dimensions, we varied the amount
of DNA per loop from 30,000 to 80,000 base pairs per individual loop as
shown in Figure 8.  The observed length and diameter dimensions of the
chromatid were realized when 18 loops per turn were utilized, with each loop
containing 60 kilobase pairs of DNA.  Therefore, this model of chromatid of
the #4 human chromosome predicts that each level of the chromatid contains
18 loops of 60,000 base pairs per loop.  This 18 loop unit forms another
higher order structure of DNA organization that we termed the miniband.
Therefore, the miniband is equivalent to one full turn of loops around the
chromatid and contains approximately one million base pairs.  In Table 3 we
compare the properties of the #4 human chromosome predicted from our model
with those that have actually been experimentally observed.  The 60 kilobase
pairs in this loop model can be compared to the 62 kilobase loop reported by
Georgiev et al.[38]; the 53 kilobase pairs loop by Hancock and Boulikas[46]; 54
kilobase loop by Igo-Kemenes et al.[47]; and 83 $\pm$ 29 kilobase loop by Earnshaw

Table 3:  Comparison of Experimentally Observed Values of Chromosome Properties with those Predicted form Proposed Model.

| | LOOP DIMENSIONS | | CHROMATID DIMENSIONS | #4 Human Chromosome | | |
| --- | --- | --- | --- | --- | --- | --- |
| | Base pairs/ loop | Length of DNA (µm)/loop | DNA loops/ miniband | DNA packing ratio | Length (µm) | Chromatid Diameter (µm) |
| Observed | $63 \pm 14$ K[a] | $21.4$[b] | $16.9 \pm 1.9$[c] | $12,400$[d] | $3.15$[e] | $0.85$[e] |
| Model (predicted) | 60 K | 20.4 | 18 | 12,260 | 3.19 | 0.84 |

[a] Average value $\pm$ S.E.M. from following studies: Georgiev et al., (38); Hancock and Boulikas, (46); Igo-Kemenes, et al., (47); Earnshaw and Laemmli, (40).

[b] 63,000 base pairs x 3.4 angstroms per base pair = 21.4 microns.

[c] Average number of loops per turn on chromatids counted from micrographs published in the following studies: Utsumi, (48); Adolph, (49); Laemmli, (50); Dupraw, (45).

[d] Length of DNA double strand divided by chromatid length ($3.91 \times 10^4$ microns divided by 3.15 microns).

[e] Measured by Dr. G. F. Bahr of Armed Forces Institute of Pathology, Washington, D. C.

Table 4:  The Number of DNA Loops per Chromosome Level (Miniband) Observed
by Direct Counting from Scanning Electron Micrographs.

| AVERAGE NUMBER OF DNA LOOPS/LEVEL (± S.D.) | REFERENCE |
|---|---|
| 17 ± 1.4 | Utsumi[48] |
| 17.8 ± 2.1 | Adolph[49] |
| 16.8 ± 3.4 | Laemmli[50] |
| 16 ± 1.3 | Depraw[45] |
| AVERAGE:  16.9 ± 1.9 DNA LOOPS PER MIMIBAND | |

and Laemmli[40].  The average value for all of the above studies is 63 ± 14
kilobase pairs per DNA loop, a length of DNA that would be equal to 21.4
microns assuming 3.4 angstroms per base pair.  The 18 loops per miniband
in the model was tested by actually counting the number of loops per turn
on the chromatids from scanning electron micrographs published in 4 previous studies.  The following values were determined:  17 ± 1.4 from the
studies of Utsumi[48]; 17.8 ± 2.1, Adolph[49]; 16.8 ± 3.4, Laemmli[50]; 16 ± 1.3,
Dupraw[45].  The average value for the number of loops per turn of the
chromatid in the above studies is 16.9 ± 1.9 (see Table 4).  The actual
dimensions of the fully condensed chromatid of the #4 human chromosome have
been provided to us by Dr. G. F. Bahr of the Armed Forces Institute of
Pathology in Washington, D.C., who has determined that the total length of
the chromatid is 3.15 microns and the diameter is 0.85 microns.  This
chromatid contains $1.15 \times 10^8$ base pairs equivalent to a total length of
DNA of $3.91 \times 10^4$ microns.  The observed packing ratio for the #4 chromatid
is 12,400 as determined by dividing the length of the free DNA ($3.91 \times 10^4$
μm) by the length of the chromatid (3.15 μm).  It is apparent from Table 2
that the proposed model agrees closely with all of the actual measured
values.

The various levels of organization of a chromatid of a chromosome and
the dimensions of each of the subunits are summarized in Figure 9.  First,
the 20 angstrom DNA helix is wound twice around the histone octamers that
form the well known 10 nm nucleosomes that each contain 160 base pairs.
These nucleosomes form the beads-on-a-string fiber.  These nucleosomes are
then wound in a solenoid fashion with 6 nucleosomes per turn to form the
30 nm filament.  The 30 nm solenoid filament forms the 60 kilobase pair DNA
loops that are attached at their base to the nuclear matrix structure.  The
loops attached to the nuclear matrix are then wound into the 18 radial loops
that form the miniband unit.  Approximately 106 of these minibands are
arranged along a central axis to form each chromatid of the final #4 human
chromosome.

We then constructed a scale model of a chromatid of the #4 human chromosome, minus the centromere region, based on the structural units outlined
above.  This scale model is shown in Figure 10.

Therefore, we propose that the miniband is a newly defined subunit of
chromosome structure.  Its width, 0.3 microns, is approximately equivalent
to the smallest bands seen in cytological Giemsa banding of metaphase chromosomes.  The number of base pairs, $1.08 \times 10^6$, is approximately equivalent to
the genetic unit, the centimorgan.  Therefore, the miniband not only explains
how DNA is packaged within the metaphase chromosomes, but also provides a

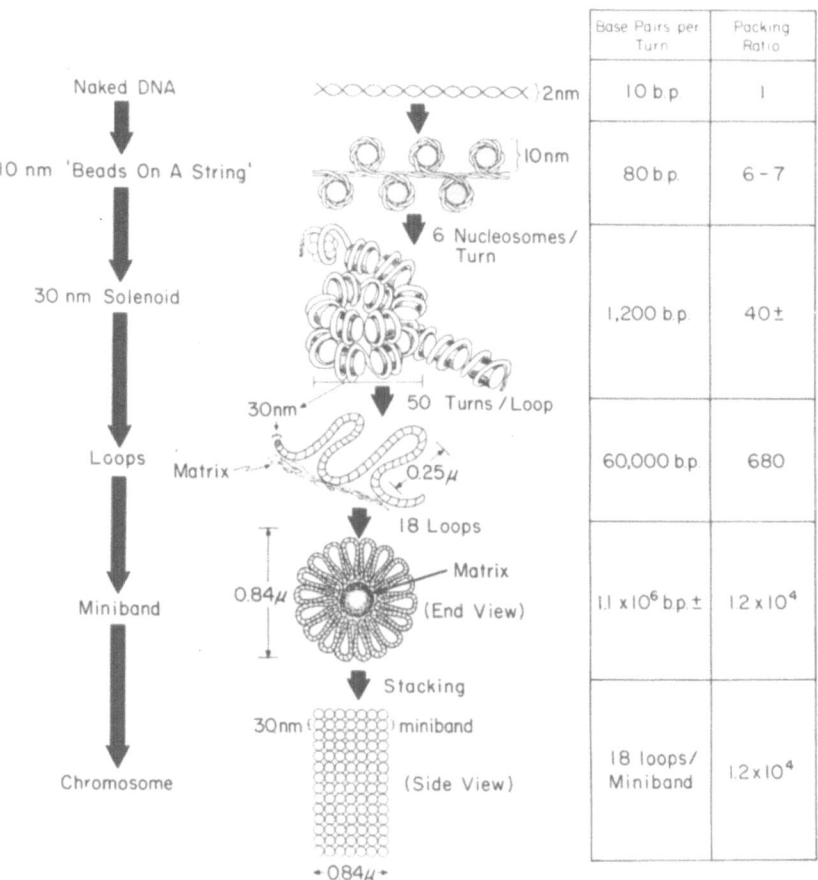

| Base Pairs per Turn | Packing Ratio |
|---|---|
| 10 b.p. | 1 |
| 80 b.p. | 6 - 7 |
| 1,200 b.p. | 40± |
| 60,000 b.p. | 680 |
| $1.1 \times 10^6$ b.p. ± | $1.2 \times 10^4$ |
| 18 loops/ Miniband | $1.2 \times 10^4$ |

Naked DNA — )2nm

10 nm 'Beads On A String' — )10nm

6 Nucleosomes/ Turn

30 nm Solenoid

30nm — 50 Turns/Loop

Loops  Matrix — 0.25μ

18 Loops

0.84μ — Matrix (End View)

Miniband

Stacking

30nm ( )miniband

(Side View)

Chromosome

← 0.84μ →

Fig. 9:  A schematic of the higher order organization of a chromatid of a
chromosome.

structural unit for the centimorgan, since the number of minibands is
equivalent to the number of centimorgans in the human genome.

Cook et al.[28] and Vogelstein et al.[14] have demonstrated that even
though chromosome structure is not visible during interphase, the loop
domains of DNA are preserved.  The integrity of these DNA loops is maintained in the interphase nucleus as well as in the chromosomes by attachment
to the nuclear matrix.  Figure 11 depicts our concept of the organization of
the DNA loops through the cell cycle.  During DNA synthesis the loops are
reeled down through their fixed sites of DNA synthesis that are located on
the nuclear matrix, and this process forms a new paired loop.  During
prophase, the paired loops with their associated matrix separate and
condense to form the metaphase chromosome with elements of the nuclear
matrix forming the core portion of the chromosome scaffold.  Recently,
Laemmli has reported that the interphase nuclear matrix and the core proteins
of the chromosome  scaffold contain a similar protein of 170 K molecular
weight[50].  Since the DNA loop organization is maintained throughout chromosome expansion and condensation, it would appear that chemomechanical interactions will be required to bring about these events.

In summary, this study has analyzed chromosome structure in relation to
the DNA loop model and its attachment to the nuclear matrix.  A new unit of
hierarchical chromosome structure has been defined, the miniband, that

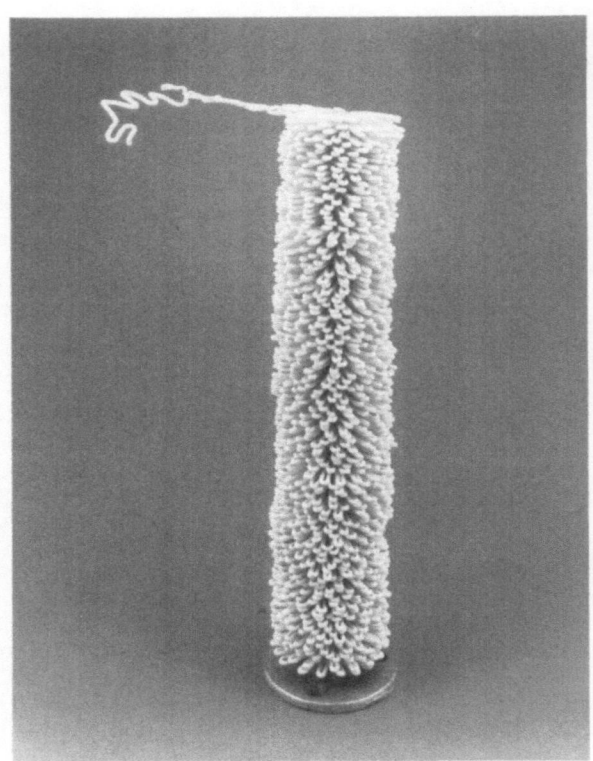

Fig. 10: A scale model of the #4 human metaphase chromatid, without cento-
mere, that contains 106 minibands stacked vertically along a
central axis in a radial loop model with 18 loops per miniband.
The white fiber in the model is equivalent in scale to the 30 nm
filament. This fiber forms individual loops each equivalent to
60,000 base pairs. The model contains a total of 1908 of these
loops. The scale model is 26.5 cm in length and is equivalent to
an actual chromatid of 3.19 microns.

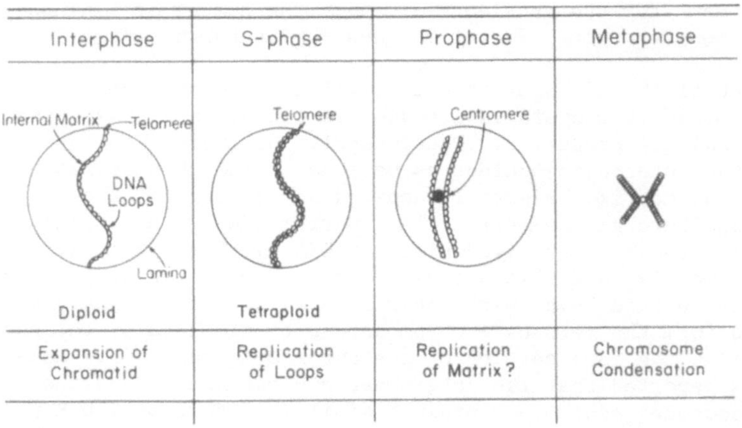

| Interphase | S-phase | Prophase | Metaphase |
|---|---|---|---|
| Internal Matrix —Telomere / DNA Loops / Lamina | Telomere | Centromere | X |
| Diploid | Tetraploid | | |
| Expansion of Chromatid | Replication of Loops | Replication of Matrix? | Chromosome Condensation |

Fig. 11: A schematic of the concept of the role of the nuclear matrix in
organizing a single chromatid in the interphase nucleus. During
S phase the DNA loops replicate. During prophase the matrix
separates and disengages the telomere from the lamina. The matrix
attached to the DNA loops condenses during metaphase to organize
the chromosome.

94

contains approximately 18 radial loops, each composed of approximately 60 kilobase pairs of DNA. This miniband may be equivalent to the centimorgan. Insight into the next order of higher structure will require a more complex understanding of how these minibands are clustered into groups to form the well known chromosomal bands that are visualized at the light microscopic level.

REFERENCES

1.  R. Berezney and D. S. Coffey, Identification of a nuclear protein matrix, Biochem. Biophys. Res. Commun. 60:1410-1417 (1974).

2.  R. Berezney and D. S. Coffey, The nuclear protein matrix, isolation, structure and function, Advances in Enzyme Regulation 14:63-100 (1976).

3a. R. Berezney and D. S. Coffey, Nuclear matrix: isolation and characterization of a framework structure from rat liver nuclei, J. Cell Biol. 73:616-637 (1977).

3b. R. Berezney and D. S. Coffey, Nuclear protein matrix: association with newly synthesized DNA, Science 189:291-293 (1975).

4.  D. E. Comings and T. A. Okada, Nuclear proteins. III. The fibrillar nature of the nuclear matrix, Exp. Cell Res. 103:341-360 (1976).

5.  F. Wunderlich and G. Herlan, A reversible contractile nuclear matrix, its isolation, structure and composition, J. Cell Biol. 73:271-278 (1977).

6.  L. D. Hodge, P. Mancini, F. M. Davis, and P. Heywood, Nuclear matrix of HeLa $S_3$ cells, J. Cell Biol. 72:192-208 (1977).

7.  P. A. Fisher, M. Berrios, and G. Blobel. Isolation and characterization of a proteinaceous subnuclear fraction composed of nuclear matrix, peripheral lamina, and nuclear pore complexes from embryos of Drosophila melanogaster, J. Cell Biol. 92:674-686 (1982).

8.  J. H. Shaper, D. M. Pardoll, S. H. Kaufmann, E. R. Barrack, B. Vogelstein, and D. S. Coffey, The relationship of the nuclear matrix to cellular structure and function, Adv. Enz. Reg. 17:213-248 (1979).

9.  E. R. Barrack, and D. S. Coffey, Biological properties of the nuclear matrix: steriod hormone binding, Recent Prog. Horm. Res. 38:133-195 (1982).

10. E. R. Barrack and D. S. Coffey, Hormone receptors and the nuclear matrix, in: "Gene Regulation by Steroid Hormones II," A. K. Roy and J. H. Clark, eds., Springer-Verlag, New York (1983).

11. V. M. Dvorkin and B. D. Vanyushin, Replication and kinetics of the reassociation of DNA of the nuclear matrix of the regenerating rat liver, Biochem. (USSR) 43:1297-1301 (1978).

12. P. Dijkwel, L. Mullenders, and F. Wanka, Eucaryotic chromosome replication, in: "Annual Review of Genetics," 9, E. Roman, ed., Annual Reviews, Inc., Palo Alto (1979).

13. D. M. Pardoll, B. Vogelstein, and D. S. Coffey, A fixed site of DNA replication in eucaryotic cells, Cell 19:527-536 (1980).

14. B. Vogelstein, D. M. Pardoll, and D. S. Coffey, Supercoiled loops and eucaryotic DNA replication, Cell 22:79-85 (1980).

15. S. J. McCready, J. Godwin, D. W. Mason, I. A. Brazell, and P. R. Cook, DNA is replicated at the nuclear cage, J. Cell Sci. 46: 365-386 (1980).

16. R. Berezney and L. A. Buchholtz, Dynamic association of replicating DNA fragments with the nuclear matrix of regenerating liver, Exp. Cell Res. 132:1-13 (1981).

17. H. C. Smith and R. Berezney, DNA polymerase is tightly bound to the nuclear matrix of actively replicating liver, Biochem. Biophys. Res. Commun. 97:1541-1547 (1980).

18. B. D. Nelkin, D. M. Pardoll, and B. Vogelstein, Localization of SV40 genes within supercoiled loop domains, Nucleic Acids Res. 8:5623-5633 (1980).

19. S. I. Robinson, B. D. Nelkin, and B. Vogelstein, The ovalbumin gene is associated with the nuclear matrix of chicken oviduct cells, Cell 28:99-106 (1982).

20. T. E. Miller, C. Huang, and A. O. Pogo, Rat liver nuclear skeleton and ribonucleoprotein complexes containing hnRNA, J. Cell Biol. 76: 675-691 (1978).

21. R. Herman, L. Weymouth, and S. Penman, Heterogeneous nuclear RNA-protein fibers in chromatin-depleted nuclei, J. Cell Biol. 78:663 674 (1978).

22. B. H. Long, C.-Y. Huang, and A. O. Pogo, Isolation and characterization of the nuclear matrix in Friend erythroleukemia cells: chromatin and hnRNA interactions with the nuclear matrix, Cell 18:1079-1090 (1979).

23. C. A. G. van Eekelen and W. J. van Venrooij, hnRNA and its attachment to a nuclear protein matrix, J. Cell Biol. 88:554-563 (1981).

24. D. A. Jackson, S. J. McCready, and P. R. Cook, RNA is synthesized at the nuclear cage, Nature 292:552-555 (1981).

25. E. C. M. Mariman, C. A. G. van Eekelen, R. J. Reinders, A. J. M. Berns, and W. J. van Venrooij, Adenoviral heterogeneous nuclear RNA is associated with the host nuclear matrix during splicing, J. Mol. Biol. 154:102-119 (1982).

26a. E. R. Barrack, E. F. Hawkins, S. L. Allen, L. L. Hicks, and D. S. Coffey, Concepts related to salt resistant estradiol receptors in rat uterine nuclei: nuclear matrix, Biochem. Biophys. Res. Commun. 79:829-836 (1977).

26b. E. R. Barrack and D. S. Coffey, The specific binding of estrogens and androgens to the nuclear matrix of sex hormone responsive tissues, J. Biol. Chem. 255:7265-7275 (1980).

27. E. R. Barrack, The nuclear matrix of the prostate contains acceptor sites for androgen receptors, Endocrinology 113:430-432 (1983).

28. P. R. Cook, I. A. Brazell, and E. Jost, Characterization of nuclear structures containing superhelical DNA, J. Cell Sci. 22:303-324 (1976).

29. C. Benyajati and A. Worcel, Isolation, characterization and structure of the folded interphase genome of Drosophila melanogaster, Cell 9:393-407 (1976).

30. J. R. Paulson and U. K. Laemmli, The structure of histone-depleted metaphase chromosomes, Cell 12:817-828 (1977).

31. J. A. Huberman and A. D. Riggs, On the mechanism of DNA replication in mammalian chromosomes, J. Mol. Biol. 32:327-341 (1968).

32. J. T. Finch and A. Klug, Solenoid model for superstructure in chromatin, Proc. Natl. Acad, Sci. USA 73:1897-1901 (1976).

33. C. Nicolini, Chromatin structure: From nuclei to genes (Review), Anticancer Research 3:63-86 (1983).

34. B. Cavazza, V. Trefiletti, F. Piolo, E. Ricci, and E. Patrone, Higher-order structure of chromatin from calf thymus, J. Cell Sci. 62:81-102 (1983).

35. A. L. Olins and D. E. Olins, Stereo electron microscopy of the 23 nm chromatin fibers in isolated nuclei, J. Cell Biol. 81:260-265 (1979).

36. F. Kendall, F. Beltsame, S. Zictz, A. Belmont, and C. Nicolini, The quinternary chromatin-DNA structure. Three-dimensional reconstruction and functional significance, Cell Biophys. 2:373-404 (1980).

37. F. Thoma, I. M. Koller, and A. Klug, Involvement of histone H1 in the organization of the nucleosome and of the salt-dependent super-structures of chromatin, J. Cell Biol. 83:403-427 (1979).

38. G. P. Georgiev, S. A. Nedspasov, and V. U. Bakayev, Supranucleosomal levels of chromatin organization, in: "The Cell Nucleus," 6, H. Busch, ed., Academic Press, New York (1978).

39. U. K. Laemmli, Levels of organization of the DNA in eukaryotic chromosomes, Pharmacol. Revs. 30:469-476 (1979).

40. W. C. Earnshaw and U. K. Laemmli, Architecture of metaphase chromosomes and chromosome scaffolds, J. Cell Biol. 96:84-93 (1983).

41. A. Leth Bak, J. Zeuthen, and F. H. C. Crick, Higher-order structure of human mitotic chromosomes, Proc. Natl. Acad. Sci. USA 74:1595-1599 (1977).

42. J. Sedat and L. Manuelidis, A direct approach to the structure of eukaryotic chromosomes, CSHSQB XII:331-350 (1977).

43. K. W. Adolph and L. R. Kreisman, Surface structure and isolated meta-phase chromosomes, Exp. Cell Res. 147:155-166 (1983).

44. M. P. F. Marsden and U. K. Laemmli, Metaphase chromosome structure: evidence for a radial loop model, Cell 17:849-858 (1979).

45. E. J. Dupraw, "DNA and Chromosomes," Holt, Rinehart, Winston, New York (1970).

46. R. Hancock and T. Boulikas, Functional organization in the nucleus, Int. Rev. Cytol. 79:165-214 (1982).

47.  T. Igo-Kemenes, W. Horz, and M. G. Zachau, Chromatin, <u>Ann. Rev. Biochem.</u> 51:89-121 (1982).

48.  K. R. Utsumi, Studies on the structure of chromosomes. II. Chromosome fibers as revealed by scanning electron microscopy, <u>Cell Structure and Function</u> 6:395-401 (1981).

49.  K. W. Adolph, Isolation and structural organization of human mitotic chromosomes, <u>Chromosoma</u> 76:23-33 (1980).

50.  U. K. Laemmli, <u>J. Cell Sci.</u>, Suppl. 1 (1984).

# NUCLEAR STRUCTURE MODIFICATIONS IN THE CONTROL OF GENE EXPRESSION AND CELL FUNCTION

Claudio Nicolini

Chair of Biophysics
University of Genova

In a recent review[1] we have presented evidence for the organization of DNA from its lowest (bp sequence) to its highest structure, as emerging from a wide variety of biophysical and biochemical measurements conducted on cells of diversified functional states. The changes occurring at the level of the nuclear structure were determinant in building a firm basis for the high order chromatin structure, from the nucleus to the genes, namely the "fibrosome" model which identified within the 300 Å chromosome-sized fiber a fundamental repeating unit about 17 Kbp long, arranged drapery-like near the nuclear envelope or the nucleoli and capable of undergoing transitions between three discrete states of DNA superpacking[1]. Without such a working model to be constantly challenged and updated, any exploration of the numerous modifications occurring during cell proliferation and transformation could be nothing more than a fishing expedition. Some of the changes induced are indeed horrifying in their complexity (cycles within cycles) and heterogeneity (membrane versus cytoskeleton, cytoplasmic proteins versus nuclear chromatin, acetylation versus phosphorylation of histones, HMG versus H1). An excellent account of most recent findings is given in multi-authored books[2-4]. Despite the jungle of "descriptive" cellular events (with recurrent logic where viral oncogenes are now substituting for serum stimulation) and the "zoo" of specific molecules (such as cyclic nucleotides, HMG, "growth factors", H1, viral proteins, microtubules, glycoproteins), critical steps can be identified, and where feasible, will be summarized here within a coherent framework for gene expression compatible with the above model for chromatin and gene structure.

## CELL PROLIFERATION

### Continuously Dividing Cells

The life of a cell cycle includes a series of metabolic events which may be temporarily and sequentially related, including protein, RNA and DNA synthesis, and which are important in the overall process of cell division and growth. Namely, while total RNA synthesis and total protein synthesis increase at a constant rate during the cell cycle until they double their original content, DNA replication appears to occur - in mammalian cells at least - only during a finite time interval of 7-10 hours (called S-phase). Cell division into two identical daughter cells occurs instead during a short time frame of 0.5-1 hour, called mitosis, which is well understood in terms of a sequential progression of morphological events through four distinct subphases, i.e. prophase, anaphase, metaphase (during which individual chromosomes become visible) and telophase. Two less understood periods of quite variable duration, from a few hours to several hours are G1 (postmitotic and prereplicative) and G2 (postreplicative and premitotic), names which well characterize our present "knowledge gap" of the molecular events unique to them, and possibly critically related to the control of DNA replication and cell division.

By now it is apparent that genetic sequences are differentially expressed during cell cycle progression[5] and that regulation of a specific set of genetic sequences, as those coding for human histones, resides at least in part at the transcriptional level.

The availability of human histone genes, or any other gene, is determined by changes in chromatin structure, a subject which has indeed received considerable attention from the beginning, though in varying degrees of sophistication.

In parallel and independent studies[6,7] using synchronized cells at frequent time intervals after mitosis, it has been established recently that the time-sequence and the nature of chromatin pattern alterations (namely nuclear shape in addition to chromatin condensation and supercoil) in the course of the cell cycle are much more complicated than revealed by earlier reports.

Despite the wide range of values for all parameters at every time interval, multiparameter analysis reveals clear clusters around homogeneous labeling patterns and morphometric data, unique for each time interval, as cells progress through two cycles of nuclear DNA condensation-decondensation and roundness/elongation, as revealed by a compartmental (FPI) analysis.

When this compartmental analysis is applied to synchronized HeLa cells, we can see that a double cycle of chromatin condensation and decondensation occurs in the 2C compartment, as nuclei move from a very condensed state, followed by an abrupt relaxation (in early G1), through a progressive condensation until mid-late G1, where an abrupt relaxation again takes place just prior to DNA synthesis. The flow of cells through S phase with progressive condensation up to G2-M is also obvious[7].

As previously shown, these data reflect abrupt and continuous changes in intranuclear-DNA distribution, not just nuclear volume. Moreover, time-lapse photography of phase-contrast on single viable cells and scanning cytometry on single cells[8], A.O.-stained to differential monitor changes in chromatin-DNA primary binding sites, suggest that two cycles per cell cycle are indeed present in all mammalian cells so far analyzed (HeLa, CHO, fibrosarcoma, WI-38) and that they refer to changes in chromatin structure at a tertiary-quaternary level. Actually, the temporal sequence of events is such that within 0.5 and 1 hours after mitosis (as can be seen in fibroscarcoma cells released from a colchicine block) nuclei change their size twice in a dramatic and previously unsuspected fashion. Such biphasic behavior (see also Fig. 1) was implicit in the original structural characterization[9] of chromatin biochemically isolated from the same synchronized HeLa cells and probed by circular dichroism at 272 nm and by EB spectropolarimetric titration: it could not be made explicit then, due to the wide heterogeneity in G1 residence times and to the continuous abrupt changes in the chromatin which "a posteriori" explain the limited resolving power of such characterization on "bulk" preparation. Average variation on both nuclear morphometry and chromatin conformation from "bulk" synchronized populations at various times after mitosis are in the same direction and on the order of 40-60%, while the same variations at the single nuclei level are on the order of 400-600%.

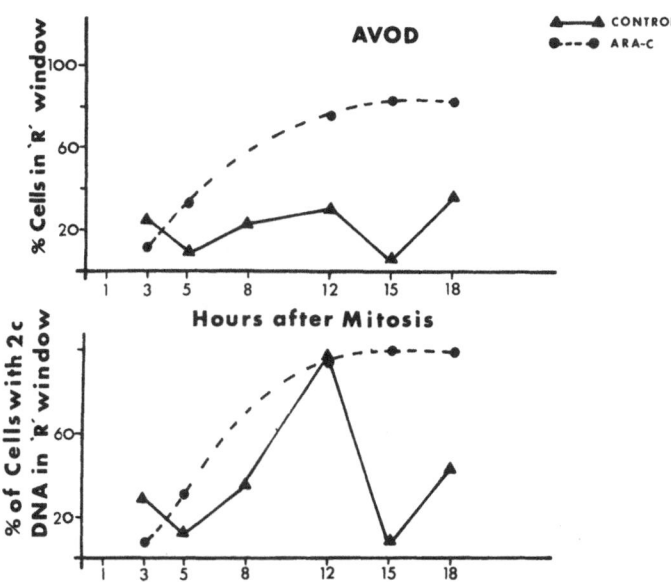

Fig. 1:  Cell-cycle variation in the percentage of HeLa cells displaying
high chromatin decondensation, i.e. characterized by Feulgen-
stained nuclei with very low average optical density ("R" window
in the AVOD distribution).  The progressive accumulation of cells
in such a state of diffuse chromatin, following ARA-C administra-
tion to a synchronized culture of HeLa cells, appears evident by
comparing the untreated (△—△) with the ARA-C treated (o—o) cells,
both for the overall population (above) and for the 2C subpopulation (below) at various time intervals after selective mitotic
detachment.


Parallel experiments with synchronized HeLa[9a] showed that the addition
of theophylline at 1-2 hours post-detachment progressively blocked all cells
in a highly packed chromatin state, yielding a homogeneous population of
nuclei at 5 hours, which began to enter S phase much later at 12-15 hours
after spontaneous release of the block and subsequent chromatin decondensation.  On the other hand (Fig. 1), ARA-C treated HeLa accumulated at the
G1-S interface with highly dispersed 2C DNA content and they did not progress into the S phase, compatible with the ARA-C inhibition of the enzymes
(DNA polymerase and ligase) required for DNA synthesis.  The prevention of
the normal relaxation in chromatin structure, as induced by theophylline
through inhibition of H1 phosphorylation (with c-AMP levels, NHCP phosphorylation and total histone synthesis proceeding uncorrelated), is then
not a direct result of inhibition of DNA synthesis, but is rather temporally
and causally related to the onset of DNA synthesis.  If inhibition of H1-
phosphorylation occurs behind the point of normal chromatin relaxation, no
inhibition of DNA synthesis takes place, compatible with the idea that this
represents a restriction point within the G1 period.

It is interesting that the high level of nuclear condensation is
achieved both in very early G1 (120-71 IOD per unit area) and late G1 (63
IOD per unit area), just prior to a dramatic increase in nuclear DNA dis-
persion (24-25 IOD per unit area) which in turn precedes initiation of RNA
synthesis (early G1) and DNA synthesis (early S).  The high level of condensation (and perfectly round shape) immediately prior to the first and

second transitions is identical to the one displayed in other human nuclei such as WI-38 fibroblasts[10] and lymphocytes[11] in the "non-cycling" phases, respectively in Q (non-readily reversible into cycle) and G0 (readily reversible). All of the above findings point to a role of "higher order" chromatin-DNA organization in the control of DNA replication and transcription. These two abrupt nuclear-DNA decondensations could correspond to the two random transitions postulated to account for the responses of quiescent cells to stimulation by growth factors. More strikingly, these two abrupt changes in nuclear chromatin condensation and volume correspond exactly to the two cycles of transient deciliation of the centriole during G1[12] and to the biphasic changes in the nuclear pore frequency for the same synchronized HeLa, previously shown to form pores at the highest rate in the first hour after mitosis and shortly before S phase[13].

Experiments are presently in progress to verify if whenever a cell line, as Chinese hamster V79-8, does not exhibit G1 period, entry into S is preceded only by one abrupt chromatin relaxation from an extremely condensed 2C state and lacks the second cycle of condensation and decondensation. In such cells the presence of proper enzymatic substrates (possibly provided in most other cells by one or more cycles of condensation-decondensation) and chemical environment could warrant a direct entry into S from mitosis: fusion of V79-8 cells with fibroblasts G+ produces hybrids that are all G-, indicating the presence of some condition in G- cells that is deficient in G+ cells.

Initiation of DNA Synthesis

The cell fusion experiments provide a compatible perspective on the initiation of DNA synthesis. When HeLa cell in the S period was fused with a cell in G1 to make a binucleated cell, the G1 nucleus was induced to begin DNA synthesis precociously. Fusion of a S with a G2 cell did not instead induce DNA synthesis in the G2 nucleus. The cytoplasmic origin of the inducer was suggested by fusing S cytoplasts (enucleated S cells) with intact G1 cells, which resulted in DNA synthesis initiation in the G1 nuclei. Apparently, initiation of S phase requires a cytoplasmic inducer and a responsive state of the DNA, uniquely present in G1 but lacking in G2 and mitosis.

The highly condensed mitotic and G2 chromosomes fail indeed to respond to the inducing S signal, a factor which appears intermittently present in cells with a G1 period as opposed to constitutively present in cells without G1. The critical role of higher order DNA structure thus appears confirmed by these observations.

On reviewing the autoradiography slides (defining as labeled only those nuclei with grain numbers well above the background), labeling indexes of approximately 5%, 17%, and 66% where determined at 5, 8, and 10 hours after mitosis (Fig. 2). What was also determined was the presence of several different labeling patterns which were present in different fractions at the three time points examined. In order to maximally reduce any subjectivity involved in the classification of nuclei, these patterns can be grouped independently of grain density into only two categories: Those in which the grains were distributed circularly and sparing a central region (Pattern I), and those in which the grains were variously distributed throughout the nucleus (Patterns II-IV). In this case, very few labeled nuclei could be considered to have questionable classifications.

At 5 hours after selective detachment, of the labeled nuclei 66% had Pattern I, and 25% Patterns II-IV; at 8 hours, these proportions had changed to 29% for Pattern I and 68% for Pattern II, while at 10 hours 21% were now in Pattern I, with 74% in Patterns II-IV. By analyzing the area distri-

3H-THYMIDINE GRAIN DISTRIBUTION
HeLa Synchronized

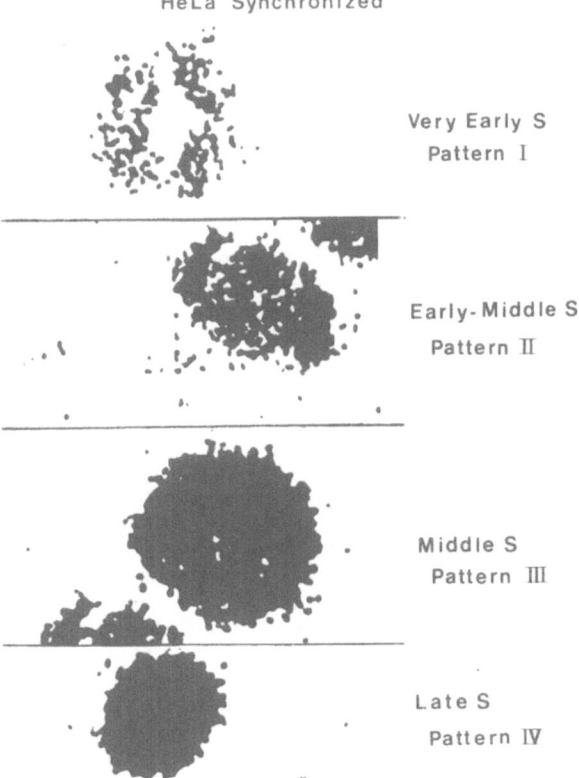

Very Early S
Pattern I

Early-Middle S
Pattern II

Middle S
Pattern III

Late S
Pattern IV

Fig. 2: Typical autoradiographic labeling patterns of [3]H-thymidine pulsed
cells as they enter and then progress along S-phase. Both in
vitro (i.e., synchronized HeLa) and in vivo (i.e., rat hepatocytes
after partial hepatectomy). A critical nuclear size and an anular
ring pattern are always associated with the initiation of DNA
replication.

butions at each time point of labeling Patterns I and II-IV, it appears that
the distribution of Pattern I is remarkably invariant for each of the time
points. This, in combination with the large differences between the area
distributions of the entire Feulgen stained populations at the different
time points, would argue that nuclei undergoing a pattern of DNA synthesis
to produce this pattern are not distributed randomly in regard to nuclear
area among the general population. Rather, it means that only nuclei of a
characteristic size (or intranuclear distribution of the replicating DNA)
will undergo the pattern of DNA synthesis to produce Pattern I, and that
this would determine S-phase initiation. Furthermore, the sites of DNA
initiation, contrary to previous suggestions, must be mostly near the
nuclear envelope to induce a circular ring of [3]H-thymidine incorporation
around the nuclear border. As shown from rigorous modeling[14], a homogeneous
distribution within the nucleus would yield patterns similar to types II-IV,
which are found only at later times.

Fixed sites of DNA replication have been observed by other investigators (see chapter by Coffey, et al. in this volume), who associated them
to the nuclear matrix, and mainly to the internal fibrogranular network

rather than to the peripheral lamina. A possible source of this disagreement could be not the different cell system utilized (rat liver after partial hepatectomy), but the failure to correctly identify the pattern truly representative of DNA synthesis initiation: pattern II which would be compatible with fixed sites associated to the nuclear matrix, is indeed also occurring in the early part of S phase, but immediately following the anular ring pattern. This conclusion also appears confirmed by experiments on rat-liver, closely monitoring the thickness of the emulsion, the time of exposure and the amount of [3]H-thymidine (all factors which critically determine the observed pattern) and focusing our attention on the early times after partial hepatectomy.

I must emphasize that the abrupt changes in nuclear-DNA morphometry at the beginning of G1 and at the end, prior to S phase, and so pronounced at the single cell level (3-6 fold increase in area and dye uptake), reduce to only 40-70% the alterations in average value of "synchronized" populations. Similarly, the structural alterations between late G1 and middle S-phase cause significant but finite differences in differential light scattering in isolated bulk chromatin[15] which then becomes a "yes versus no" phenomenon on individual nuclei. The sign and magnitude of the differential scattering of left versus right circularly polarized light (CDLS), outside the DNA absorptive band, is indeed explainable only with a "left-handed" helical folding of one or more nucleofilaments (with the multifibrilar "rope" giving a higher CDLS signal than the unifibrilar "solenoid"); transition to a linear "unfolded" nucleofilament would be accompanied by a null differential light scattering[16], as indeed found for S phase nuclei. Thermal denaturation and circular dichroism studies in "bulk" preparation of a S versus G1 phase chromatin from rat liver after partial hepatectomy or from synchronized HeLa (Fig. 3) are indeed suggestive of a much more stable G1 chromatin in both the main helix-coil (characterized by a decrease in molar ellipticity) and in the superhelix-helix (characterized by an increase in molar ellipticity) transitions. Upon cooling down to room temperature, chromatin ellipticites (contrary to B-form DNA) do not return to their starting values, which are representative of differentially packed supercoiled DNA maintained by the chromosomal proteins and irreversibly denatured during the heating process.

Interestingly, the structural differences between two given chromatins (G1 versus S, or from G0 versus G1) remain quantitatively unaltered after the disruption induced by shearing, which causes a generalized increase in molar ellipticity (after correction for differential light scattering) and dye intercalation. Since, after shearing, we are left only with nucleofilaments, the persistent difference can only be attributed to changes occurring also at the level of each nucleosomal DNA, i.e. state I versus state II of the fibrosome model (Fig. 7). The modulation of these two-order superhelical foldings of DNA around the nucleosomal axis and around a quaternary "rope-like" axis can be detected in the bimodal derivative plot of positive molar ellipticity changes with temperature and more clearly in the multimodal microcalorimetric enthalphy changes in the same chromatin isolated from cells in different functional states[17].

This is apparent also at the electron microscope level, where in 500 Å sections from liver nuclei the degree of chromatin supercoil can be monitored for individual fibers[17].

Finally, a higher number of negative superhelical turns per 10 base pairs is observed in middle G1 with respect to middle-S phase unsheared chromatin, or in G0 versus early G1, as monitored by the intercalation kinetics of low concentrations of ethidium bromide (Fig. 4). Their functional significance, in terms of additional free energy, will be addressed later; at present it is worthwhile to notice that higher numbers of negative

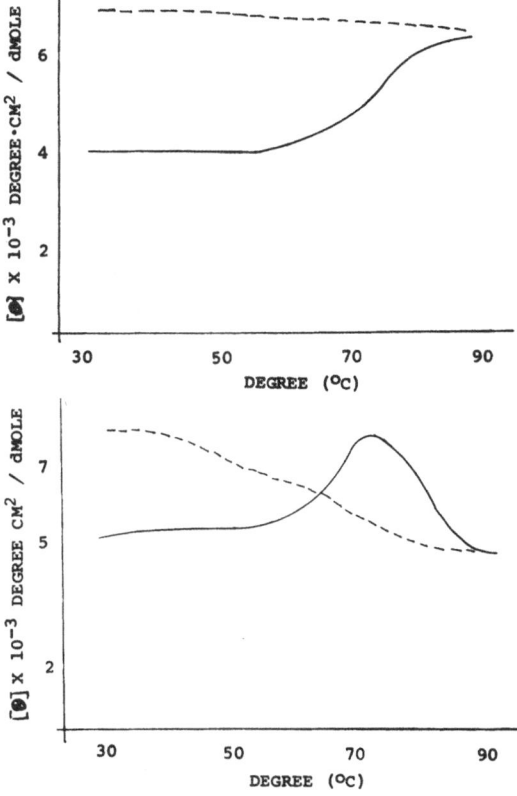

Fig. 3:  Thermal denaturation profiles by molar ellipticity at 276 nm for
G1 (above) and S-phase (below) chromatin.


superhelical turns are present also in "G0" resting cells; they decrease
substantially whenever the cell increases its metabolic activity during
the G0-G1 transition.

Few other events correlate as well with DNA synthesis and are worthy
of comment.  Hybridization of histone cDNA with cell-cycle specific mRNAs
points to a temporal correlation in HeLa between the expression of H4, H3,
H2A and H2B histone genes and DNA replication.  However, in addition to
being questioned by similar experimentation in other cell systems, a functional causal coupling could not be established.

Similarly, the cycle variations of a poorly understood structure, the
centriole[12], have been correlated to DNA replication and mitosis, postulating their critical role in modulating the contractile machinery of the cell
through cycles of ciliation and deciliation.  Quiescent cells serum-
stimulated to enter DNA synthesis lose their cilia in the centrioles 1-2
hours later, regain them by 5-8 hours and lose them again for the second
and final time in association with DNA synthesis initiation.  The timing
of these two cycles of deciliation, present also in continuously dividing
cells, exactly parallels the two cycles of chromatin conformation and
points to their close association with DNA synthesis initiation and subsequent mitosis.

It is worthy of note that, among numerous other factors, short RNA
fragments have been suggested as possible primers of DNA replication,

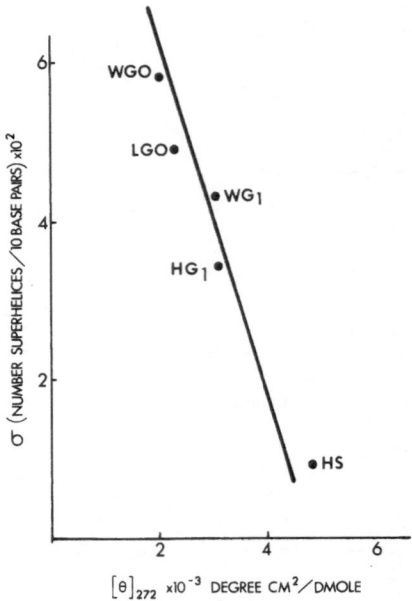

Fig. 4: Number of DNA superhelices per 10 base pairs versus molar ellipticity at 272 nm for native chromatin isolation from confluent
(WGO) and 3 hours after stimulation (WG1) human fibroblasts.
HeLa cells synchronized at 3 (HG1), 11 (HS) and 0 (HM) hours
after selective mitotic detachment, and from rat liver (LGO).

confirming early studies of Okasaki on E. coli. Short DNA chains in Erlich
ascites tumor cells in vivo appear to be formed by extension of even shorter
covalently linked RNA chains, which seem synthesized on the parental DNA
strand and removed before the DNA fragments are joined by ligases[18]. Following initiation, replication of eukaryotic DNA proceeds by means of a
continuous sequence of disassembly, reproduction and reassembly, which
passes through each DNA sequence and originates simultaneously in many sites
near the envelope, propagating in both directions as a replication fork[19].
The "fibrosome" with its drapery-like structure, may provide an excellent
topological constraint for this process, warranting that prior to replication, chromatin locally relaxes to condense again after replication, but
in such a way to yield daughter chromosomes quite disentangled to allow
their segregation into the daughter cells of mitosis (Fig. 5).

Chromosomal Protein Modifications

Several biochemical mechanisms have been associated with the cell
progressing through the cycle, at the level of histone and nonhistone
chromosomal proteins, both quantitatively (synthesis of new non-histone
proteins or a different amount of the existing proteins) and qualitatively,
in terms of specific chemical modifications such as acetylation, methylation and phosphorylation. Recent data indicate that histones are phosphorylated through the cell cycle, but apparently only histone H1 and H3
can be phosphorylated at multiple sites. In the case of histone H1, the
mono- and unphosphorylated forms increase through the cell cycle and
reach a maximum at M phase. Gel electrophoresis profiles show furthermore that a new class of non-histone chromosomal protein is synthesized
during S phase, while phosphorylation of H1 histone increases and shows a
biphasic behavior which parallels the two cycles of chromatin condensation
per cell cycle. In a crucial experiment with theophylline, a selective

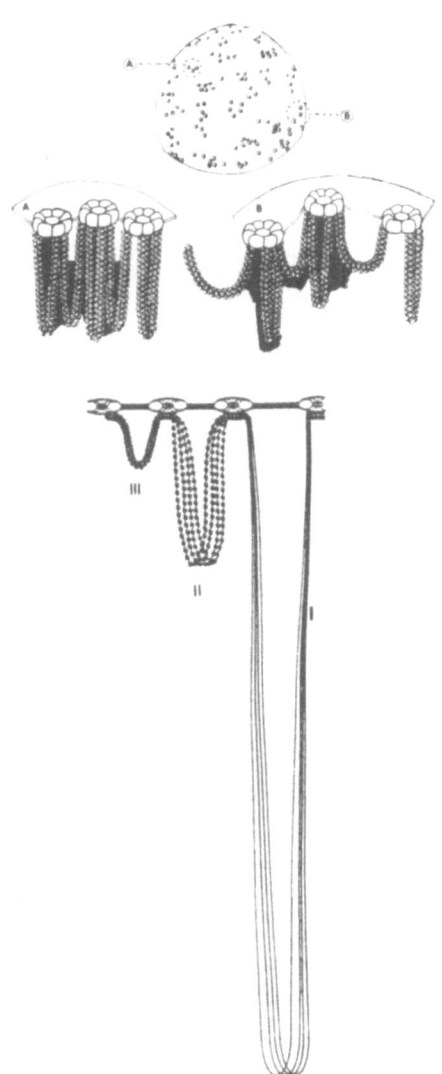

Fig. 5:  A model for the high order chromatin-DNA structure during the in-
         terphase, based on numerous recent experimental evidence (for a
         review see Ref. 1).  Multifilament fibers supercoiled rope-like,
         most with a similar size of about 17 Kbp, suggesting the existence
         of a fundamental repeating unit, appear to lay down from the
         envelope near the pores (and from the nucleoli) and to alternate
         with highly packed regions attached to the nuclear membrane.  Only
         up to three discrete states (I, II, III) of higher order chromatin
         structure, leading to three levels of DNA packing ratios (1, 7,
         19) appear present within mammalian nuclei[1].

inhibition of H1 phosphorylation (Fig. 6) was causally correlated with the
inhibition of both the natural chromatin structure (at the end of G1) and
the onset of DNA synthesis, while nonhistone chromosomal protein phosphorylation, c-AMP level and overall histone synthesis (H-lysine incorporation) proceeded uncorrelated.  The latter effect would confine the
reported correlation between total histone gene expression and S-phase to
a consequence of a prior chromatin relaxation, rather than to a cause-

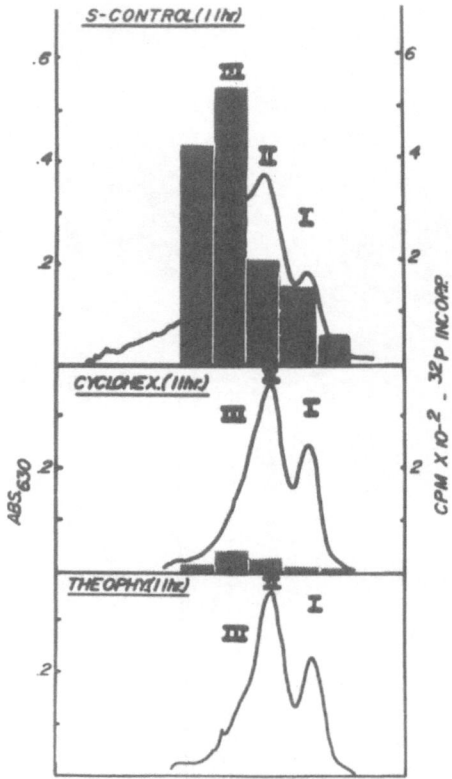

Fig. 6: Effect of theophylline (below) and cyclohexamide (center) treatment beginning in G1 on subsequent histone H1 phosphorylation
during the G1-S transition. As a reference the corresponding gel
electrophoresis of H1 histones obtained from the untreated cell
population, at the same time interval (11 hours or middle S) after
mitosis, is shown in the upper panel.

effect relationship. This histone synthesis was related to initiation of
DNA synthesis, which is instead apparently causally correlated with enzymatic modification of preexisting H1 histone. Other specific enzymatic
modifications such as acetylation of H4 and undermethylation of DNA have
been linked to DNA synthesis initiation and gene transcription. Among the
non-histone chromosomal proteins a small group (HMG) bound to chromatin by
weak ionic linkages and dissociated by 0.25 - 0.35 M NaCl have been extensively characterized: their recent association[20] with the expression of
DNase I sensitivity by active genes, for which their presence is needed, is
consistent with the old observation[21] on their selective removal being
capable of abolishing the structural and functional differences between GO
(inactive) and G1 (metabolicly active) chromatin. Recently, HMG proteins
have been also shown to affect DNA supercoil, by lowering the topological
linking number of circular DNA molecules when incubated with topoisomerase.
Comfortingly, all the above protein modifications do alter the electrostatic interaction with DNA in the same direction of an increased H1 phosphorylation, which has so far been the one change more clearly and causally
correlated to a relaxation of chromatin structure and to an increased metabolic activity. Disturbingly, however, in separate experiments with synchronized Physarum and CHO cells, an increase in H1 phosphorylation,
causally preceded by an increased activity in histone kinase, has conclusively shown to be correlated with the onset of mitotic condensation.
These contradicting and apparently irreconciable phenomena have been

108

either ignored, or have been empirically explained by involving an hydrophobic component in the H1 binding which is not supported experimentally. Recent developments[22] in the Manning formulation of polyelectrolyte theory may furnish the explanation; where the two opposite effects, condensation versus relaxation of chromatin, DNA, induced by a similar increase in H1 phosphorylation, can be reconciled by the presence of two different sites being phosphorylation, can be reconciled by the presence of two different sites being phosphorylated at the end of G1 and G2 within the H1 molecule, the first one directly interacting with the DNA backbone and the other not.

According to polyelectrolyte theory, the first phosphorylation would indeed yield a decrease in the neutralization of negative DNA phosphates and consequently a decrease in the spontaneous bending angle (or nucleofilament supercoiling), while the second phosphorylation would cause a conformational change in H1 leading to an opposite effect, namely an increased DNA neutralization and higher order supercoil. Strikingly, this prediction has been upheld by recent examination of the intramolecular sites of phosphorylation of H1A and H1B labeled with $^{32}P$ during the S phase and mitosis of synchronized HeLa-S3. In S-phase cells, most of the $^{32}P$ incorporated was at two places in the C-terminal cationic tail of each subtype, an H1 region directly binding to DNA, while in mitotic cells major phosphorylation occurs in the opposite N terminal regions of both H1B and H1A.

At this point, I wish to insert a personal reflection: when the correlations between various chromosomal protein modifications and gene expression were first discovered ten years ago, I was fortunate to work with two of the leading pioneering groups, active in two opposite camps. One group was committed to the cause of H1 phosphorylation and the other to that of weakly bound nonhistones then nick named "Snoopy", and now "rebaptized" HMG. Since then I have witnessed a progressive acquisition of data in a wide number of cell type and functional alterations, alternatively fitting either one of the two molecular schemes, but none justifying an absolute faith, at the exclusion of other molecular events independently reported which lead to a similar alteration in the electrostatic interaction with the DNA phosphates. Unfortunately, the tendency still remains to ignore what cannot be explained or properly addressed by available "in house" technology.

The only common denominator was the sign and magnitude of the structural alterations in chromatin-DNA, causally linked to cell cycle progression. Similar structural differences between cells in any two different functional states (G0 versus G1 or G1 versus S phase) can be observed: 1) in native chromatin probed by spectropolarimetry, thermal denaturation, or intercalating dyes; 2) in isolated nuclei probed by microcalorimetry in a physiological buffer; 3) in nuclear lysates in the presence of detergent and high ionic strength as probed by viscoelastometry and 4) even in situ following crude fixation and Feulgen staining or after removal of all histones. The basic intranuclear DNA distribution in three orders of superpacking and the existence of discrete transitions among them thus appear similar in all of the above conditions being preserved, even after complete removal of both H1 and HMG.

The first level of control appears exercised by other factors, namely: 1) by the strongly bound nonhistones still present at 2 M NaCl, which maintain the DNA supercoil; 2) by nicking-closing enzymes such as topoisomerase which is known to vary its activity during the cell cycle and critically determines negative DNA superhelix and therefore transcription; 3) by local changes in ions (those interacting with DNA phosphates and thereby affecting DNA bending and cell function; and 4) by the level of DNA methylation or hydration (critically determining secondary structure and gene activation).  It would then seem that H1 histone phosphorylation, H4 acetylation and HMG nonhistones represent only the second level of control of gene experssion, being a sufficient but not necessary co-factor for the lower order transitions, possibly between state II (nucleofilament) and state I (free-DNA or modified nucleofilament) leading to local gene activation.


## CELL TRANSFORMATION

Immunological, biophysical, and biochemical differences have been described between neoplastic cells and their counterparts.  Differences extend to the whole chromatin and to nonhistones, but not to histones, which (at least quantitatively) seem indistinguishable in normal and transformed cells.  Several criticisms can be raised when a tumor is compared to its tissue of origin, since a difference may reflect cell type rather than manifestation of cell transformation.  Similarly, studies in culture (with transformed cells grossly aneuploid) may reflect changes subsequent to, rather than concomitant, with transformation.

### Cancer Genes

In all cases the metabolic events accompanying tumor cell cycle progression are similar to or identical with those occurring in normal cell replication, implying that normal cells bear genetic information that is similar in quality (if not quantity) to the transformed one, as that contained in a transforming virus gene, for instance.  Indeed, the normal chicken possesses a gene, called sarc, that is biochemically and functionally similar to the Rous Sarcoma Virus (RSV) sarc-gene[23]; an increased cell proliferation as during embryogenesis may then be related to an increased expression of the proto sarc-gene during that period, as confirmed in normal chicken by the increased amount of a phosphoprotein (60,000 Daltons) with properties similar to the viral pp60.  More than a dozen transforming viral genes have been identified in the past which all are homologous in normal cells.  For some authors, actually, the degree of homology is such that only less than 1-3% of mRNA in transformed cells had sequences which were not present in the normal parental line, with the increase in abundance at certain sequences accompanied by a decrease in the abundance of other RNA sequences.

Among the rapidly transforming RNA retroviruses, RSV is unique in its ability to replicate independently of a helper virus, since it contains all the genes necessary for virus replication; after cell infection, the RNA is transcribed by the viral reverse transcriptase into a double-stranded DNA which is then integrated in the cellular DNA.

An important question is, how do the cancer-causing and normal oncogenes differ?  By genetic engineering exchanges of definite segments of the normal and "cancer" gene (from malignant bladder tumor) were made to isolate the small region capable to confer on a normal gene the ability to trigger malignancy.  Sequencing the nucleotides present in this region, among the 4,600 nucleotide pairs present, no differences could be detected, with the exception of a single change of one nucleotide (CGC in normal versus GTC in malignant).  Related genes in three animal cancer viruses also differ from the normal cellular gene at the same location.  In each virus the glycine of the protein encoded is replaced with a different amino acid. The quality (change in a protein coding sequence, rather than in the sequence regulating the amount of a protein being produced) and extent of this change makes it doubtful that the lengthy development of most human cancer is controlled by a single genetic alteration.

It would appear that despite recent excitement for the biochemical identification of proteins which are coded for by the oncogenes of the various tumor viruses (such as Rous Sarcoma Virus), the oncogenes and their products are multifunctional and the emerging picture is much more complex than most may have previously hoped. In the next few lines, rather than address the cyclic and frustrating empirical search for chimeric specific molecules or enzymes "unique" for cancer cells, I will summarize the common alterations reported for chromatin and nuclear constituents upon neoplastic transformation induced by virus and chemicals or spontaneously occurring in animals.

## Viral and Spontaneous Neoplastic Transformation

When comparing quiescent WI-38 fibroblasts to their stationary SV-40 virus transformed counterparts (2RA), the findings are apparently contrary to the common expectation that 2RA cells are in a more active state. Nuclear morphometry did show, in fact, that the chromatin of the stationary 2RA cells is more condensed than that of confluent WI-38 cells, which is quite compatible with the surprising fact that the template activity of chromatin from stationary 2RA cells is less than that of quiescent WI-38 cells. Also, the reported immunological differences between chromatin of normal cells and their transformed counterparts was proved to be due to changes in chromatin structure as well as to differences in chromosomal proteins, whose immunological activity is a critical function of DNA structure. Reduced template activity has also been observed in walker tumor chromatin when compared to rat liver and mammalian chromatin.

More recently, (Fig. 7), the same increase in average chromatin condensation has been reported when comparing (I) "fibroblast-like" cAMP reverse-transformed to transformed CHO-K1 cells; (II) low metastatic cell variants (F1) to high metastatic variants (F10) from the same B16 tumor in mice; (III) human fibroblasts versus their cytomegalovirus-infected counterparts. It must be stressed that the differences are only among mean values of kinetically matched cell populations, since normal and transformed cells display identical cycles of chromatin condensation and decondensation per cell cycle. It then appears that regardless of the mode of cell transformation (either spontaneous, viral or chemical) and regardless of an occasional increase in DNA content (as in 2RA cells, where the number of chromosomes is highly heterogeneous) a dramatic increase in chromatin condensation (for the average population or a given cell cycle phase) characterized the expression or enhancement of any "abnormal growth" behavior, and was consistent with the idea that a limited transcription of the genome is necessary to maintain the transformed phenotypes. This is compatible with a recent observation that, upon cell transformation, the observed increase in the abundance of certain messenger RNA sequences is accompanied by a substantial reduction in the abundance of other sequences. This finding did not emerge earlier by traditional biochemical or biophysical studies, perhaps because any technique which measures a chemical or physical parameter of bulk preparation necessarily combines the tunnel vision of single parameter observation with a loss of that distributional information that would exist if each contributor could be observed independently (as with multiparameter image analysis).

## Chemically Induced Neoplastic Transformation

Cancer production by treatment with chemicals is discussed in a vast amount of literature[24]. The processes of somatic mutation (point mutation of a single gene) and neoplastic transformation in vitro (measured by colony formation in agar or tumorigeneity), while spontaneously occurring at a $10^{-7}$ and $10^{-8}$ frequency respectively, can both be initiated and enhanced to $10^{-5}$ by specific chemically induced damage to various

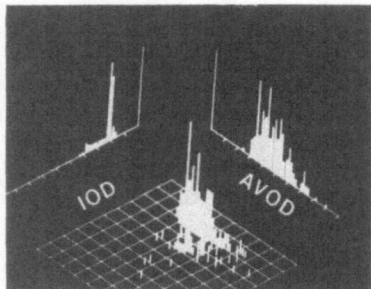
Low Metastatic  F1

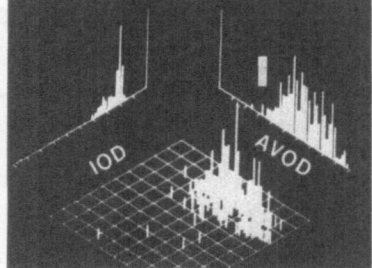
High Metastatic  F10

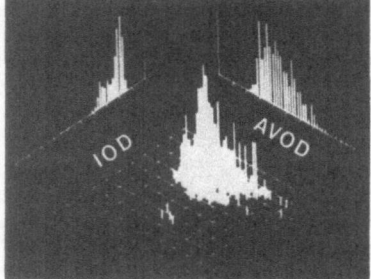
Reversed Transformed  CHO

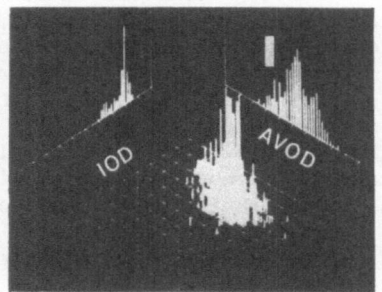
Transformed  CHO

Fig. 7:   DNA amount (integrated optical density, IOD) versus chromatin-DNA
condensation (average optical density, AVOD, of Feulgen-stained
nuclei) of low versus high metastatic clone variants from B16
melanoma cells (upper panels) and of transformed versus fibroblast-like CHO-K1 cells (lower panels).


macromolecules (mainly DNA, but also protein and RNA).  The time required
for the expression goes from 5-10 population doublings for somatic mutation
to 35-150 population doublings for neoplastic transformation, pointing to
a lengthy cascading effect of successive highly coupled processes (see
also Chapter by Ts'o, et al. in this book).  This long period for cancer
progression mimics the human situation and may be explained in terms of a
single gene mutation, which is an adequate model for the complexity of the
neoplastic transformation only if such mutation is recessive and triggers
the chromosomal variability needed to alter gene balances and the overall
structure of the genetic apparatus.  Keeping in mind that chemically-in-
duced transformation is a progressive multistep process, and early changes
after treatment (i.e., morphology and DNA strand breaks) are not sufficient
to indicate tumorogenicity, it is useful to summarize at this stage the
present knowledge on the early nuclear alterations induced by the chemical
carcinogens.

DNA adducts appear to be the common result of cell interaction with
most chemical carcinogens, leading possibly through other cell cofactors to
initiation and promotion of the neoplastic process.  Generally, the biochemical lesion in DNA most relevant to cancer initiation is a miscoding
one; experimental evidence to justify such a presumption are, however,
circumstantial and inconclusive.  Conceivably, other types of alterations
in DNA, such as genetic combination, gaps, translation, and transposition,
are also important.  Among them, the structural alterations occurring in
chromatin, either isolated or in situ are apparent even after short exposure
to a relatively small dose of a carcinogenic agent such as DMNA, and are
paralleled by a reduction in DNA length and flexibility through the creation
of single-strand breaks.  When we induce the formation of preneoplastic

nodules in rat liver by the Solt-Farber method, namely a 0.02% 2-acetylamino-fluorene (2-AAF) diet coupled with partial epatectomy, the selected carcinogen-initiated hepatocytes from the focal islands appear to have completely different properties with respect to cycling and early carcinogen-altered hepatocytes, i.e., a decreased diffusion and increased microviscosity of the nuclear environment combined with a decreased bound water per unit DNA, which is compatible with the apparent increase in chromatin condensation.

## Negative Superhelical Turns and Z-DNA

Interestingly, this apparent increase in chromatin condensation for preneoplastic hepatocytes, usually associated with a change in chromatin tertiary-quaternary structure toward a higher DNA packing ratio, is a common denominator in all transformed cells (either genetically, spontaneously, chemically or virally induced) when compared to their normal counterparts. This suggests that in neoplastic transformation, a decrease in DNA template activity and site availability is an early prerequisite for the expression of the transformed phenotype. A few characteristics of transformed cells, which unequivocally discriminate them from the normal counterparts at the single cell level rather than as "average" property (such as chromatin structure which indeed modulates significantly during the cycle of both normal and abnormal cells) can be identified, namely: 1) the uncoupling between changes in nuclear morphometry and changes in cell morphometry[25]; 2) the disruption and/or disorganization of microtubles/microfilaments[26]; and 3) the anchorage-independent growth and the uncoupling between cell geometry and cell growth[27].

The higher chromatin superpacking can be shown to be accompanied by a higher number of negative superhelical turns in the DNA of unsheared chromatin isolated from the same SV-40 transformed WI-38 cells, when compared to the normal counterparts as monitored by spectropolarimetric titration of low concentration of ethidium bromide.

Strikingly similar results were obtained by independent determination of the density of DNA topological linking turns per unit length of DNA by means of sedimentation of "nucleoid structures" containing loops of superhelical DNA held by nonhistones[28], in gradients of 15-30% sucrose containing 12.95M NaCl and various similarly low concentrations of ethidium bromide. In four malignantly transformed Syrian hamster cell lines (three SV-40-transformed and one spontaneous) the density of DNA topological turns was higher than the equivalent density in the normal counterparts. Furthermore, contrary to normal cells, malignant cells display a persistently higher density of turns even upon subcultivation. The author proposed that it is the persistence in such higher numbers of "titrable negative superhelical turns" that is responsible for the activation of a large number of given genes during malignant transformation. How this may reconcile with the repression of other genes also apparent during transformation, will be discussed later. Considering that alternating regions of the native chromatin fiber are fixed at both ends, any protein enzyme, or protein modifications capable of inducing a twist in the DNA molecule may lead to an enhancement in the preexisting negative superhelical turns, and then trigger gene expression. Interestingly, a similar event could be primed also by a single local change in DNA secondary structure.

Even if most DNA is in the B-form, locally induced transitions to Z-DNA have been observed recently for up to 5-10% of the genome, by means of specific immunoflourescence. A mechanism for the observed enhancement in superhelical DNA density could then be the transition from the preexisting Z-form to a B-form, possibly controlled by DNA undermethylation. Active genes are indeed frequently undermethylated, with a significant DNA methylation being present in inactive genes. The more stable Z-form DNA is characterized by a zig-zag arrangement of the phosphate backbone, due to the different torsion angles of phosphodiester G-C and C-G linkages, and is localized to short G-C rich DNA sequences. Local Z-DNA, within the fibrosome unit, could be induced by binding to specific DNA sites of multi-valent cations, for instance.

A causative relationship between DNA methylation and increased gene expression was actually proven for transferred thymidine kinase genes[29].

## Water

Specific enzymatic modifications in H1 histone and nonhistone proteins have been correlated with chromatin alterations and gene expression, but a search for possible modifications in ions and mainly in water (which makes up to 90% of each nucleus and could also explain the involvement of overall genome and pores) was hampered by the lack of available and appropriate probes.

The intracellular water has long been known to play an important role in cellular organization and function, and the data recently reported on the electric properties of intact nuclei show for the first time that macro-molecular hydration is an early event during cell proliferation. Previously, a decrease in water content and relaxation time (assessed by NMR) have been reported during the transition from the G1 to S phase of synchronized HeLa S3 cells, in conjunction with a parallel increase in chromatin-DNA primary binding sites. At 18 hours after partial hepatectomy, when the liver cells also enter S phase, an increase in tightly bound water per unit DNA (Table I) occurs on a scale similar to what is found for the number of chromatin primary binding sites per unit DNA. For a G0 resting cell the electricity derived volumetric fraction of tightly bound water per unit DNA is 0.22, identical to the molar ratio of bound ethidium bromide (E.B.) per unit DNA. A shown in Table I, both parameters then increase dramatically when the

Table 1:  Electrical properties of nuclei from rat liver preneoplastic nodules, being developed using the Solt-Farber method. Data have been acquired between 50 and 100 MHz, with 50 MHz interval (o), or between 100 and 2000 MHz with 100 MHz interval (+).

| SAMPLE | N | T/V | F |
|---|---|---|---|
| Control | 98±2 | 0.24$^{+}$ -0.22° | 71 |
| Preneoplastic lesions | 91±1 | 0.12$^{+}$ | 69 |
| Partial Hepatectomy | 90±5 | 0.38° -0.49$^{+}$ | 81 |
| DMNA (5.6 mg/kg) | 107±2 | 0.27° | – |

-F = relaxation frequency in MHz

-T/V is the volumetric ratio of tightly bound water to DNA per unit DNA.

-N = equivalent normality in mM NaCl

*The values are extimated normalizing to a constant control value (Nicolini, C., et al., in ref. 24).

cells enter G1 and early S phase upon stimulation by partial hepatectomy. This increase parallels a substantial decrease in free (NF) and total (WT) water content and relaxation frequency (F), as also shown by NMR in a similar G1-S transition of synchronized HeLa, where a decrease in the proton spin-lattice relaxation time (increased bound water) was reported.

It has been shown recently that certain physical properties (NMR relaxation times of hydrogen protons) of water are altered in tumor cells, even independently of water contentration, which since early in this century was known to be elevated in tumors (apparently in the cytoplasm) above that of normal tissue of origin. It has been also suggested that a change in the physical state of water (decrease in bound water or increase in the relaxation times of water protons), reflecting a change in chromatin condensation, precedes the increase in water concentaation and a change in cell function. Conversely, as shown earlier, DNA hydration related to an increased water concentration could be one of the initial critical factors determining changes in the local secondary DNA structure, namely a transition from B- to Z- and A-DNA, which in turn causes changes in chromatin supercoil (and bound water) with profound implications on cell function.

## MOLECULAR MECHANISMS AND MODELS FOR GENE EXPRESSION

What are the molecular modifications that may eventually lead to cell proliferation and to cell transformation? In this chapter, a wide number of candidates have been proposed, but only a few appear linked with cell function in general and particularly with gene expression, the onset of DNA replication and/or mitotic condensation. They are: change in the physical state of water; centriole deciliation; level of H4 acetylation; level of H1 phosphorylation; nuclear matrix; ions, such as $Mg^{++}$, $Ca^{++}$, $Na^+$ and $K^+$ both in absolute concentration and in their redistribution among free and bound compartments; HMG nonhistone chromosomal proteins; cell geometry in normal cells, but not in transformed cells, which is apparently related to the presence of a direct coupling between nuclear and cellular geometry and possibly of oriented-organized microtubules-microfilaments; localized regions of right-handed A-DNA; DNA undermethylation; localized regions of left-handed Z-DNA; negative DNA superhelical turns; and strongly bound nonhistones. All the above changes have as a common denominator a dramatic effect on chromatin structure which abruptly relaxes/uncoils immediately before a cell increases its metabolic activity, both in terms of RNA and DNA synthesis or when a cell is "initiated" by a chemical carcinogen. Actually, the existence of a cause-effect relationship between abrupt changes in chromatin structure and cell function (as DNA replication or mitotic condensation) has been shown rather conclusively. It is now also clear and predictable quantitatively from polyelectrolyte theory, as to how changes in neutralization of phosphate negative charges, induced either by modification in bound positive ions or by enzymatic protein modifications, can cause abrupt changes in the spontaneous bending of supercoiled DNA at the quaternary level (being a rope-like or solenoid-like structure).

A packing of DNA into superstructures mimicking the in vivo behavior, where it is complexed with histones or nonhistones, can be induced in free DNA by the use of salt and alcohol alone, which determines changes in the electrostatic charge density and water activity of the immediate microenvironment of the helix[30]. Naked DNA can indeed be compacted into a beaded structure virtually indistinguishable from that of a nucleofilament in the presence of a dehydrating agent such as 95% ethanol, and at low ionic strength.

Chromatin appears closely interlinked to nuclear volume and permeability and any alteration of the genome organization caused by "localized" nick-closing enzymes, A-DNA sequences, proteins or Z-DNA enzymatic modifications, or by "generalized" redistribution of free versus bound water and ions, could then sequentially trigger, through the creation of thermodynamic favorable highly negative superhelical turns, the random expression of specific genes (yielding the transformed phenotypes) and, through induced changes in $Ca^{++}$ cytoplasmic concentration or tyrosine phosphorylation, the disruption of microtubules-microfilaments (leading to the uncoupling between cells and nuclear geometry and eventually to the uncontrolled abnormal cells growth).

Positive control of normal cell growth by the physical constraint imposed by a round cell shape (eventually acquired upon cell crowding or upon growth on a given substrate) on nuclei and on chromatin structure and function can indeed be warranted by the integrity and orientation of the cytoskeleton, which is lost only upon cell transformation. In the absence of such positive constraint (as during normal embryogenesis and during neoplastic transformation) and in the presence of the needed uninhibited enzymatic substrates, the abrupt complete relaxation of a few "fibrosomes" from a highly coiled rope (State III) to an extended DNA (State I) is taking place at the two restriction points, cyclically leading to gene activation and DNA replication.

The second level of positive control of cell function is given by the degree of chromatin supercoil and negative DNA superhelix, which per se is known to yield changes in some protein-enzyme affinities and to cause gene activation through the creation of particularly favorable thermodynamic conditions. This control could be originally exercised by the strongly bound nonhistones and lipids, which through the formation of a highly resistant chromosome skeleton present in both metaphase and interphase, create fixed sites of attachment for the "tetrafilament" loops[1]. The resulting highly twisted DNA with negative superhelical turns can then be maintained and modulated by topoisomerase or gyrase, by ions, by the hydration and by the enzymatic modifications on the DNA itself, and (only as a final, sufficient but unnecessary, step) by modifications in HMG nonhistones and in the H4-H1 histones.

It appears, paradoxically, that it is through highly coiled DNA superstructures (being larger even in normal cells immediately prior to the initiation of RNA and DNA synthesis) that gene expression, i.e. the local "complete" unfolding of the "fibrosome" unit, is normally taking place and enhanced. A further increase in negative superhelical turns and DNA supercoil, as that occurring during neoplastic transformation for all phases of the cell cycle, would then yield a further increase in the number of the same genes being expressed, including the few specific ones characteristic of the transformed phenotype.

Through the mechanism of induced high twisting of the DNA molecule, the cell apparently develops a type of energy storage which is then transferred during transcription. Astonishingly, cells possess enzymes such as topoisomerase or gyrase, which decrease or further increase the linking number of each "fibrosome", depending on the state of chromatin DNA structure prior to its interaction with an enzyme. In certain conditions, as those determined by an increase in chromatin condensation followed by a strand nicking and closing with topoisomerase, super-superhelical twists are created in individual fibrosomes with stored energy quite above the normal "threshold" level, which could then trigger the transcription (or replication) of the corresponding DNA sequences, also through an enhanced binding of RNA (or DNA) polymerases (Fig. 8). Alternatively, similar conditions, depending on the critical interplay among enzymes, pre-existing chromatin structure and other co-factors, may induce a repression of genes which otherwise are normally transcribed (Fig. 8).

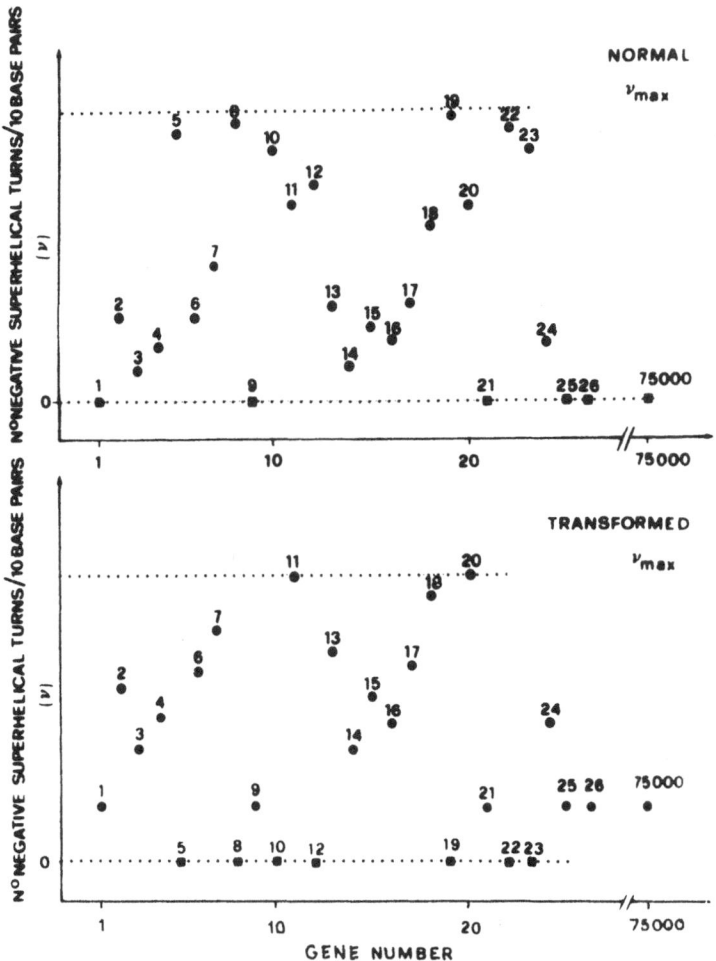

Fig. 8: Model for differential gene expression associated with the global
increase in nuclear DNA condensation apparent during neoplastic
transformation and at the onset of DNA or RNA synthesis. Normal
cell (above) would display for each of its 75,000 fibrosomes
("genes") a varying number of DNA negative superhelical turns σ
from zero (unfolded and transcribing) to a maximum "threshold"
value (highly packed nucleofilament) behind which DNA would undergo
an abrupt transition to a relaxed form (zero σ) releasing all its
stored energy. This excess energy would in turn trigger the
transcription (or replication) of the corresponding DNA sequences,
now accessible in the state I, also through an enhanced binding
of RNA (or DNA) polymerases. The increased condensation in the
overall genoma (below) causes a similar increase in negative
superhelical turns for each of the 75,000 fibrosome units, which
in turn may lead either to gene repression (for those with σ near
the initial threshold value).


It does not escape our notice that the model for the control of gene
expression, proposed here to fit all available experimental data, is at
odds with the widely accepted operon model described by Jacob and Monot[31].
Indeed, regulation of gene activity depends upon the cytoskeleton and the
local conformational changes of the DNA molecule itself at the level of the
individual "fibrosome", rather than upon the structural alteration of the

protein which controls (lack-repressor) or performs (RNA polymerase) the transcription following the interaction with an effector molecule. Furthermore, it would appear that the nuclear scaffold or cage, still present after histone and lipid removal and possibly determined by the spherically distributed folded regions of the chromatin rope at the pores (maintained by nuclear lamina proteins and metal ions), may have a critical role in controlling gene expression, not only in creating local supercoil but also because of its unique and close association with transcribed segments. Indeed, while the view that transcription occurs as RNA polymerase moves along the DNA remains unchallenged, an alternative provocative view has been recently presented, whereby the DNA passes through a transcription complex fixed to nuclear cage[32].

ACKNOWLEDGEMENT

    This work was supported by a grant from the C.N.R. Finalized Project "Oncology" (Contract 84.00702.44).

REFERENCES

1.  C. Nicolini, Anticancer Research 3:63-86 (1983).

2.  C. Nicolini, ed., "Nobel Symposium on New Frontiers at the Crossing of Life and Physical Sciences,"Plenum Publishing Corp., New York (1984).

3.  C. Nicolini, ed., "Chromatin Structure and Function," NATO Life Sciences Series, Plenum Publishing Corp., New York (1979).

4.  C. Nicolini, ed., "Cell Growth," NATO Life Sciences Series, Plenum Publishing Corp., New York (1982).

5.  G. Stein and J. Stein, in: "Cell Growth", NATO Life Sciences Series, C. Nicolini, ed., Plenum Publishing Corp., New York (1982).

6.  C. Nicolini, F. Kendall, and W. Giarretti, Biophysical Journal 19:163-179 (1977).

7.  F. Kendall, F. Beltrame, A. Belmont, S. Zieta, and C. Nicolini, Cell Biophysics 4:19-38 (1980).

8.  C. Nicolini and A. Belmont, Cell Biophysics 5:79-94 (1983).

9.  C. Nicolini, A. Kozu, T. Borun, and R. Baserga, Journal of Biological Chemistry 250:3381-3385 (1975).

9a. T. Dolby, A. Belmont, T. Borun, and C. Nicolini, Journal of Cell Biology 89:78-85 (1981).

10. C. Nicolini, F. Kendall, C. Desaive, B. Clarkson, and J. Fried, Experimental Cell Research 106:111-117 (1977).

11. S. Abraham, S. Lessin, E. Vonderheid, and C. Nicolini, Cell Biophysics 4:51-67 (1980).

12. R. Tucker, A. Pardee, and K. Fujaware, Cell 18:527-538 (1979).

13. G. Maul, J. Scogma, M. Lieberman, G. Stein, and T. Borum, Journal of Cell Biology 55:433-447 (1972).

14.  A. Belmont, F. Kendall, and C. Nicolini, Journal of Cell Science 65: 123-138 (1984).

15.  T. Dolby, T. Borun, S. Zweidler, S. Cohen, P. Miller, and C. Nicolini, Biochemistry 18:1333-1345 (1979).

16.  A. Belmont, S. Zietz, and C. Nicolini, Cell Biophysics 5:163-189 (1983).

17.  C. Nicolini, P. Carlo, R. Finollo, M. Bignone, E. Patrone, and G. Brambilla, Journal of Molecular Biology 161:155-178 (1982).

18.  C. Nicolini and R. Baserga, Exper. Mol. Pathology 21:74-78 (1974).

19.  A. Howell and R. Sager, Proc. Natl. Acad. Sci. USA 75: 2358-2362 (1978).

20.  S. Weisbrod and H. Weintraub, Proc. Natl. Acad. Sci. USA 76:630-635 (1979).

21.  C. Nicolini, N. Sally and R. Baserga, Proc. Natl. Acad. Sci. USA 72: 2361-2365 (1975).

22.  A. Belmont and C. Nicolini, J. Theoret. Biol. 90:169-179 (1981).

23.  A. Wang, P. Snyder, and H. Hemafusa, Journal of Virology 35:52-65 (1980).

24.  C. Nicolini, ed., "Chemical Carcinogenesis," NATO Life Sciences Series, Plenum Publishing Co., New York (1982).

25.  C. Nicolini and F. Beltrame, Cell Biol. Int. Rep. 6:63-71 (1982).

26.  B. Brinkley, G. Fuller and D. Highfield, Proc. Natl. Acad. Sci. USA 72:4981-4985 (1975).

27.  J. Filkman and A. Moscona, Nature 273:345-348 (1978).

28.  A. Lucknick and W. Glaser, Molecular Gen. Genet. 183:553-556 (1981).

29.  R. Christy and G. Scangos, Proc. Natl. Acad. Sci. USA 79:6299-6303 (1982).

30.  T. Eickbush and E. Moudrianakis, Cell 13:295-306 (1978).

31.  F. Jacob and J. Monod, J. Molec. Biol. 3:318-356 (1961).

32.  D. Jackson, S. McCready and P. Cook, Nature 292:552-555 (1981).

# ORGANIZATION AND CELL CYCLE PERIODIC EXPRESSION OF HUMAN HISTONE GENES

G. S. Stein, J. L. Stein, and F. Marashi

Department of Biochemistry and Molecular Biology
and Department of Immunology and Medical Microbiology
University of Florida College of Medicine
Gainesville, Florida 32610

## INTRODUCTION

In this chapter we will summarize several of the experimental approaches we have been taking to examine human histone genes. The structure and organization of human histone genes will be discussed, particularly within the context of the putative relationships of specific regions of the genes to their expression. Approaches to assessing the levels at which control of histone gene expression resides will also be considered. Results will be presented which suggest that: a) Human histone genes are a family of moderately reiterated sequences with variations in the structure, organization, and possibly in the regulation of the various copies. b) At least 15 different, though not necessarily all, human histone genes are coordinately expressed during the S phase of the cell cycle and appear to be temporally and functionally coupled with DNA replication. c) There are both transcriptional and post-transcriptional components to the regulation of those histone genes expressed in conjunction with DNA replication.

## STRUCTURE AND ORGANIZATION OF HUMAN HISTONE GENES

### The General Organization of Human Histone Genes

Several years ago when we initially screened a λCh4A human gene library (constructed by Lawn et al.[1]) and isolated clones containing genomic human histone sequences, our expectation for the organization of the human histone genes was a simple tandem repeat such as had been observed for _Drosophila_[2] and "early" sea urchin histone genes[3,4], i.e., a repeated unit of approximately 7Kb in length containing one of each of the five histone genes (H2A, H2B, H3, H4 and H1) with a nontranscribed spacer sequence between each mRNA coding region. We anticipated this type of organization because it was known at the time that the human histone genes were moderately reiterated (approximately 40 copies per haploid genome for each of the five histone proteins[5]) and _in situ_ hybridization studies, in which human chromosomes were hybridized with radiolabeled human mRNA[6] or sea urchin histone cRNA[7], suggested clustering of the histone genes.

However, it soon became apparent that although the human histone genes were clustered, they were not organized in the form of a simple tandem

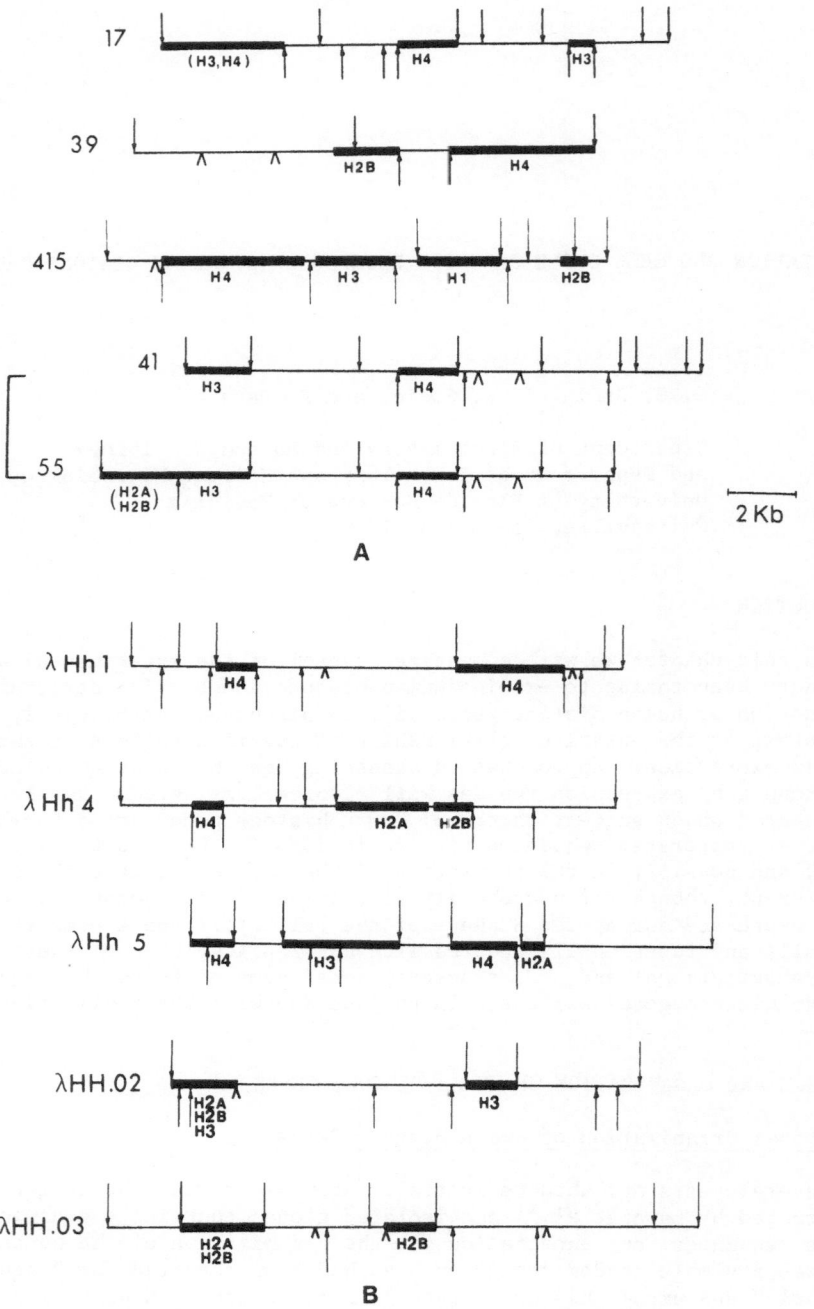

Fig. 1:  Restriction maps of cloned human histone genes.
A. λHHG clones isolated by Sierra et al.[8]  λHHG clones were mapped
with respect to Eco RI (↓) and Bam HI (↑) restriction endonucleases.
The bar at the bottom of the figure indicates the scale.  Boxes indicate restriction fragments that hybridize with heterologous
histone gene probes.  The locations of histone coding regions within
the λHHG phage have been confirmed by hybrid selection - in vitro
translation.  B. Clones isolated in other laboratories.  λHh clones
were isolated by Heintz et al.[10] λHH clones by Clark and Wells[11].

repeat[8]. Rather, as shown in the restriction maps in Figure 1A, the human histone gene clones we have isolated and characterized exhibit at least four types of arrangements with respect to restriction sites and the representation and order of coding sequences; each of these arrangements is totally distinguishable from the others. In all the clones we have studied, at least two different histone genes are found adjacent to each other (within a few kilobases). Clones λHHG 5, λHHG 55 and λHHG 415 (Fig. 1A) each contain one of each of the four core histone genes, H2A, H2B, H3 and H4. On the other hand, clones λHHG 6, λHHG 17, and λHHG 22 each contain two genes coding for each of the inner core histones, H3 and H4 (Fig. 1A). Clone λHHG 415, which was isolated by screening the human library with a chicken genomic H1 histone DNA probe, contains an H1 coding region, as well as at least one of each of the other histone genes[9]. This indicates that in human at least some some H1 histone genes are clustered together with the core histone gene sequences.

Two other laboratories have reported the isolation and characterization of human histone genes. Shown in Figure 1B are maps of those clones isolated by Heintz et al.[10] and by Clark[11] in which the organization of histone genes differs from those in our clones. Thus far, a total of nine different types of human histone gene clusters have been reported (Clones λHh2 and λHh7 isolated by Heintz et al. appear to be identical to clones λHHG 39 and λHHG 17, respectively). It is likely that the clones identified to date are not a representative sample of the entire spectrum of possible arrangements of the histone genes in the human genome, because the selection was strongly biased toward clones containing H4 histone genes. Heintz et al. used a cloned human H4 probe to select their clones, while most of our clones were isolated using a probe containing chicken H3 plus H4 coding sequences (provided by Dr. J. R. E. Wells). Clark used a probe containing sequences for all four core histone genes from chicken (H2A, H2B, H3 and H4) and selected two human histone gene clones, neither of which contains H4 coding sequences[11]. Interestingly, there is no obvious overlap between the various types of clusters that have been isolated.

Analysis of histone genes in several other organisms has shown that a polymorphic organization of these genes is prevalent in eucaryotes. In yeast, two copies of each histone gene have been found per haploid genome[12]. Cloning of these DNA fragments has shown that the H2A and H2B genes are adjacent to each other with divergent transcriptional polarity[12,13] and that the H3 and H4 genes are not adjacent to the H2A and H2B genes[12,14]. More recent work has shown that the organization of histone genes in vertebrates is far more complicated than shown for yeast. In Xenopus laevis, the genes appear to be clustered[15,16] and some clusters are tandemly repeated[17]; however, more than one gene order has been found, each one associated with a different H1 variant[15]. The newt Notophthalamus viridescens has homogeneous 9Kb clusters containing one each of the five histone genes; however, these clusters are not arranged in tandem repeats, but are separated by up to 50Kb of unrelated DNA sequences[18-20]. Chicken[21,22] and mouse[23,24] histone genes, like human, have a polymorphic organization with no obvious simple tandem repeats.

Of course, the possibility that tandem repeats exist in higher vertebrates cannot be formally excluded based on the available information. It is conceivable that some of the clones which have been studied represent fragments derived from a larger tandem repeat. Detailed studies of genomic histone gene organization (in progress) should resolve whether any of the histone gene clusters observed in higher vertebrates (chicken, mouse and human) are tandemly repeated.

It has been known for several years that the genomes of higher eucaryotes contain, in addition to single copy sequences, large amounts

of DNA of moderate to high repetition[25,26]. In most eucaryotes, repeated
sequences approximately 300 nucleotides long have been found interspersed
throughout the genome[27,28]. In humans, the Alu DNA family is predominant
among these reiterated sequences, with a repetition frequency of approximately $3 \times 10^5$ per haploid genome[29]. Experiments in which EcoRI-restricted
λHHG phage DNA was hybridized to an Alu I DNA sequence cloned into pBR322
(generously provided to us by Dr. S. Weissman) have shown that the histone
genes are interspersed with several members of the Alu family of repetitive
DNA sequences, as well as with other DNA sequences whose transcripts are
represented in the polysomes of HeLa S3 cells[30]. Of particular interest is
the location of Alu sequences in the regions flanking several H4 histone
genes (P. Kroeger, M. Plumb, J. Stein and G. Stein, unpublished observations).

The last point we will consider with regard to the general organization
of human histone genes is some of the experimental evidence for sequence
variations in the different copies of the H4 histone genes, despite the
stringent evolutionary conservation of the amino acid sequence of the H4
histone proteins. Histone protein amino acid sequences are well conserved
evolutionarily; however, variant proteins have been detected for all histones
except H4[31].

Our first indication of the polymorphic nature of human H4 histone
genes preceded the availability of cloned genomic human histone sequences
and was based on direct analysis of the H4 histone mRNAs[32]. By electrophoretically fractionating H4 histone mRNAs, initially on the basis of size
under nondenaturing conditions, Lichtler et al.[32] identified at least seven
different H4 histone mRNA species in S-phase HeLa S3 cells. Presumably,
these different species of H4 mRNA are all functional, as they were isolated
from polysomes. In vitro translation of the individual mRNA species in a
wheat germ system gave rise to acid-soluble proteins that comigrated with
HeLa cell H4 histone proteins in an acetic acid-urea polyacrylamide gel.
In addition, tryptic peptide mapping of in vitro translation products from
several of the H4 histone mRNAs gave patterns that were indistinguishable
from one another or from in vivo synthesized HeLa H4 histone mRNA species,
all of which code for identical or very similar polypeptides[32,33].

Two lines of experimental evidence indicate that the various H4 histone
mRNAs are encoded in individual genes. Initially we demonstrated differences
in the two-dimensional "fingerprints" of the T1 ribonuclease oligonucleotides
from the seven H4 histone mRNA species. The oligonucleotides obtained from
the smaller molecular weight H4 mRNAs were not subsets of those generated
from the larger H4 mRNAs, which rules out a simple product-precursor relationship. The results are similar to Grunstein's findings for H4 histone
mRNA fractions from sea urchin[34]. More direct evidence that the human H4
histone mRNAs are independently encoded comes from experiments in which
various H4 histone mRNA species were assigned to specific H4 histone genes.
By hybridizing a mixture of all the HeLa H4 histone mRNAs to various cloned
genomic human H4 histone DNA sequences, we were able to demonstrate that
each H4 histone gene formed an S1 nuclease-resistant hybrid with only one
H4 mRNA. Furthermore, where two H4 histone genes are present in the same
cluster, as in clones λHHG6 and λHHG17, different H4 histone mRNA sequences
are encoded in the adjacent genes (Fig. 1A). We have initiated studies
directed towards the identification, isolation and characterization of
multiple forms of the other core histone mRNAs. We have been able to
identify at least four distinct H2A, H2B or H3 histone mRNAs including
normal diploid, transformed and tumor cells.

The obvious question that arises is the biological significance of
multiple forms of H4 histone mRNAs which are genetically encoded and serve
as templates for the synthesis of apparently identical histone polypeptides.

Our current thinking encompasses a working model with the following components: All histone genes in a cluster are coordinately controlled, with their expression being modulated by common regulatory sequences and/or regulatory molecules. Only a subset of the reiterated histone genes are expressed in any given cell at any given time, with variations in those histone genes (gene clusters) expressed in different cells and/or in different biological circumstances. Selection of clusters to be transcribed would be based on a requirement for a histone H2A, H2B, H3 or H1 subspecies for which differences in the mRNAs and in the histone proteins have been observed. The H4 genes expressed would be predicated on location within a cluster containing coding sequences for a specific H2A, H2B, H3 or H1 histone subspecies - with the possibility that all genes in such a cluster contain similar regulatory sequences.

Alternatively, multiple forms of H4 histone mRNAs in HeLa cells and other human cell lines may have arisen by conservative nucleotide substitutions occurring in multiple genes. For example, two H4 histone genes expressed during the same early developmental stages of the sea urchin Psammechinus miliaris show as much as 10.3% divergence in the nucleotide sequences of the H4 coding region[35,36], yet both code for identical H4 proteins.

## Specific Human Histone Coding Sequences

To facilitate detailed analysis of specific human histone genes and their flanking regions, we have subcloned essentially all EcoRI fragments from our genomic histone clones (λHHG) into pBR322. Many of these subclones have been further characterized by restriction endonuclease mapping and DNA sequencing.

DNA sequences are available (Figure 2) for the H4 histone gene present in λHHG41 (pF0108A), the H3 gene in λHHG17 (pST519) and the H2B gene in λHHG39 (pTN521 + pTN402), and partial sequences have been determined for the H3 gene in λHHG41 (pF0535) the H2B and H2A pseudogenes in λHHG55 (pFF435D), and the H1 gene in λHHG415 (pFNC16A). Because the amino acid sequence is available for only one human histone protein[37], the nucleotide sequences of the human H1, H2A, H3 and H4 histone genes have provided the first direct information pertaining to the primary structures of these proteins.

Except for the H2B and H2A genes present in λHHG55 (described below), the human histone genes we have sequenced have the capacity to code for typical histone proteins that do not differ greatly from their counterparts in other species. As shown in Table I, the H4 gene in λHHG41 codes for an H4 histone protein that does not differ at all from that of calf[31]. Similarly the regions of the two human H3 genes we have sequenced code for the same amino acid sequence found in the calf H3 histone protein. In comparing the carboxy terminal 40 amino acids predicted from the nucleotide sequences of the two human H2B genes, we find only 7.5% divergence, consistent with the conservation of the carboxy termini of H2B proteins from other species[31].

Careful examination of the H2B sequences present in λHHG55 (pFF435D) (Fig. 2) indicates that, despite the extensive homology with other H2B coding sequences, this gene cannot express a functional H2B protein because it contains at least one frame-shift mutation located at the position coding for amino acid 92(Arg) and a nucleotide substitution (C to G transversion) resulting in replacement of serine 55 with tryptophan (an amino acid not present in histones). Furthermore, putative regulatory sequences are absent from the flanking regions of this gene[38]. 1) While TATA boxes are usually located 65-90 bases upstream from the ATG initiation codon of H2B genes[39], there is none within 130 nucleotides of the ATG of the λHHG55 H2B gene;

```
  -240        -230       -220       -210         -200       -190
  AATTC TCCCG GGGAC CGTTG CGTAG GCGTT AAAAA AAAAA AAGAG TGAGA GAGGG ACTGA

  -180       -170       -160        -150         -140       -130
  GCAGA GTGGA GGAGG AGGGA GAGGA AAACA GAAAA GAAAT GACGA AATGT CGAGA GGGCG

  -120        -110       -100        -90          -80        -70
  GGGAC AATTG AGAAC GCTTC CCGCC GGCGC GCTTT CGGTT TTCAA TCTGG TCCGA TATCt

  -60        -50        -40         -30          -20        -10
  CtGTA TATtA CGGGG AAGaC GGtGa CGCtC CGatC GaNcN Nctat CGGGC TCCtG CGGTC

  ATG TCC GGC tGt GGa aAG GGC GGA AAG GGC TTA GGC AAA GGT GGC GCT AAG CGC
  Met Ser Gly Arg Gly Lys Gly Gly Lys Gly Leu Gly Lys Gly Gly Ala Lys Arg
     0    1                5              10                 15

  CAC CGC AAG GTC TTG AGA GAC AAC ATT CaG GGC ATC ACC aAG CCT GCC aTT CGG
  His Arg Lys Val Leu Arg Asp Asn Ile Gln Gly Ile Thr Lys Pro Ala Ile Arg
          20              25              30              35

  CGT NTA GCT CGG CGT GGC GGC GTT AAG CGG ATC TCT GGC CTC ATT TAC GAG GAG
  Arg Leu Ala Arg Arg Gly Gly Val Lys Arg Ile Ser Gly Leu Ile Tyr Glu Glu
                      40              45              50

  ACC CGC GGT GTG CTG AAa GTG TTC TTG GAG AAT GTG ATT CGG GAC GCA GTC ACC
  Thr Arg Gly Val Leu Lys Val Phe Leu Glu Asn Val Ile Arg Asp Ala Val Thr
          55              60              65              70

  TAC ACC GAG CAC GCC AAG CGC AAG ACC GTC ACA GCC ATG GAT GTG GTG TAC GCG
  Tyr Thr Glu His Ala Lys Arg Lys Thr Val Thr Ala Met Asp Val Val Tyr Ala
                  75              80              85

  CTC AAG CGN CAG GGG AGN aCC CtC TAC GGC TTC GGA GGC TAG GCCGC CGCTC
  Leu Lys Arg Gln Gly Arg Thr Leu Tyr Gly Phe Gly Gly Stop
      90              95              100  102
                                     mRNA 3' end

  CAGCT TTGCA CGTTT CGATC CCAAA GGCCC TTTTT GGGCC GACCA CTTGC TCAtC CTGAG

  GAGTT GGACA CTTGA CTGCG TAAAG TGCAA CAGTA ACGAT GTTGG AAGGT AACTT TGGCA

  GTGGG GCGAC AATCG GATCT GAAGT TAACG GAAAG acata accgc
```

**A**

Figure 2: Nucleotide sequence of several human histone genes.
A. The H4 gene present in λHHG41 (pF0108A) and its flanking
regions. Lower case letters indicate residues that were not
definitively resolved. An "N" indicates an undetermined nucleotide. The boxes at 5' end of the gene indicate the location of
the tandem "CAAT" boxes, while the box just preceding the 3' end
of the mRNA coding region indicates the T hyphenated dyad symmetry. The box located just past these nucleotides indicates
the histone-related purine box. Wavy underlines in the 5' flanking region indicate, in order from 5' to 3': 1) twenty-one base
pairs of purines; 2) histone-related GGTCC motif; and 3) TATA box.
Horizontal arrows indicate short direct repeats. B. The H3 gene
present in λHHG17 (pST519) and the 5' end of the H3 genes in
λHHG41 (pF0535). C. The H2B gene present in λHHG39 (pTN521 +
pTN402) and a partial sequence of the H2B pseudogene in λHHG55
(pFF435D). D. The partial sequence of the H2A (pseudo)gene is
λHHG55. E. The nucleotide sequence of the N terminal region of
the H1 histone gene in λHHG415 (pFNC16).


2) No translation stop codon occurs at or near the end of the amino acid
coding region of the gene.

   We extended our nucleotide sequence analysis to the region of the H2A
gene present within pFF435D. Figure 2 shows the nucleotide sequence which
codes for the amino terminus of the H2A protein, and a comparison with the
nucleotide sequence of chicken (λCH-01)[40] and the protein sequences of
calf, trout and the sea urchin, P. miliaris[31]. In spite of the frequent
third base substitutions between the H2A gene in pFF435D and that in λCH-01,
the polypeptide sequence is completely conserved, in calf thymus, human
spleen, trout and P. miliaris except for amino acids 11-14 (Arg-Ala-Lys-Ala)
which are absent in pFF435D. It is tempting to speculate that the absence

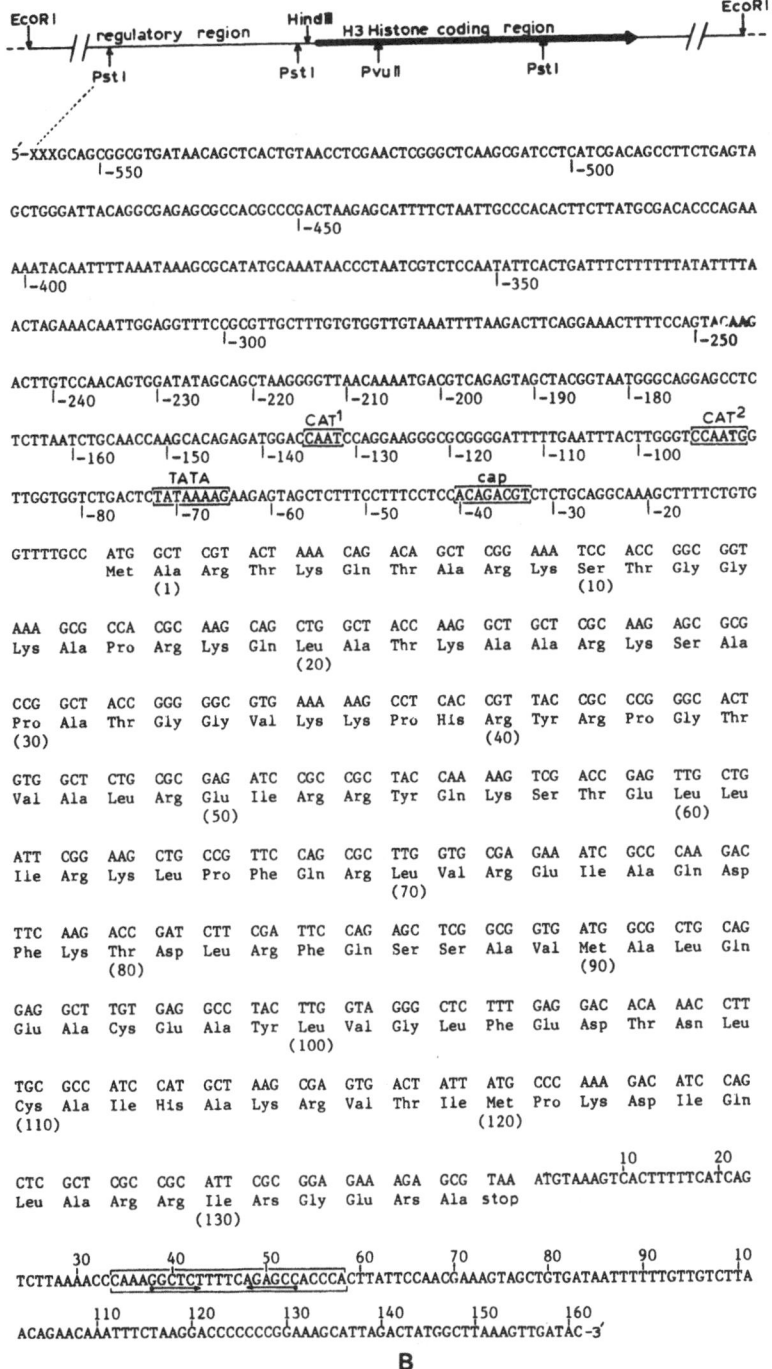

EcoRI ─ ─ ╫ / / ─ regulatory region ─ HindⅢ H3 Histone coding region ────▶ / / EcoRI ─ ─
PstI        PstI   PvuⅡ        PstI

5'–XXXGCAGCGGCGTGATAACAGCTCACTGTAACCTCGAACTCGGGCTCAAGCGATCCTCATCGACAGCCTTCTGAGTA
     |–550                                          |–500

GCTGGGATTACAGGCGCGAGAGCGCCACGCCCGACTAAGAGCATTTTCTAATTGCCCACACTTCTTATGCGACACCCAGAA
                  |–450

AAATACAATTTTAAATAAAGCGCATATGCAAATAACCCTAATCGTCTCCAATATTCACTGATTTCTTTTTTATATTTTA
|–400                                    |–350

ACTAGAAACAATTGGAGGTTTCCGCGTTGCTTTGTGTGGTTGTAAATTTTAAGACTTCAGGAAACTTTTCCAGTACAAG
           |–300                                          |–250

ACTTGTCCAACAGTGGATATAGCAGCTAAGGGGTTAACAAAATGACGTCAGAGTAGCTACGGTAATGGGCAGGAGCCTC
  |–240    |–230    |–220    |–210    |–200    |–190    |–180

                              CAT¹                                        CAT²
TCTTAATCTGCAACCAAGCACAGAGATGGAC̲C̲A̲A̲T̲CCAGGAAGGGCGCGGGGATTTTTGAATTTACTTGGGT̲C̲C̲A̲A̲T̲G̲G̲
  |–160    |–150    |–140    |–130    |–120    |–110    |–100

          TATA                              cap
TTGGTGGTCTGACTC̲T̲A̲T̲A̲A̲A̲A̲G̲AAGAGTAGCTCTTTCCTTTCCTCC̲A̲C̲A̲G̲A̲C̲G̲T̲CTCTGCAGGCAAAGCTTTTCTGTG
  |–80      |–70      |–60      |–50      |–40      |–30      |–20

GTTTTGCC ATG GCT CGT ACT AAA CAG ACA GCT CGG AAA TCC ACC GGC GGT
         Met Ala Arg Thr Lys Gln Thr Ala Arg Lys Ser Thr Gly Gly
         (1)                                 (10)

AAA GCG CCA CGC AAG CAG CTG GCT ACC AAG GCT GCT CGC AAG AGC GCG
Lys Ala Pro Arg Lys Gln Leu Ala Thr Lys Ala Ala Arg Lys Ser Ala
                    (20)

CCG GCT ACC GGG GGC GTG AAA AAG CCT CAC CGT TAC CGC CCG GGC ACT
Pro Ala Thr Gly Gly Val Lys Lys Pro His Arg Tyr Arg Pro Gly Thr
(30)                              (40)

GTG GCT CTG CGC GAG ATC CGC CGC TAC CAA AAG TCG ACC GAG TTG CTG
Val Ala Leu Arg Glu Ile Arg Arg Tyr Gln Lys Ser Thr Glu Leu Leu
                    (50)                              (60)

ATT CGG AAG CTG CCG TTC CAG CGC TTG GTG CGA GAA ATC GCC CAA GAC
Ile Arg Lys Leu Pro Phe Gln Arg Leu Val Arg Glu Ile Ala Gln Asp
                              (70)

TTC AAG ACC GAT CTT CGA TTC CAG AGC TCG GCG GTG ATG GCG CTG CAG
Phe Lys Thr Asp Leu Arg Phe Gln Ser Ser Ala Val Met Ala Leu Gln
        (80)                              (90)

GAG GCT TGT GAG GCC TAC TTG GTA GGG CTC TTT GAG GAC ACA AAC CTT
Glu Ala Cys Glu Ala Tyr Leu Val Gly Leu Phe Glu Asp Thr Asn Leu
                    (100)

TGC GCC ATC CAT GCT AAG CGA GTG ACT ATT ATG CCC AAA GAC ATC CAG
Cys Ala Ile His Ala Lys Arg Val Thr Ile Met Pro Lys Asp Ile Gln
(110)                              (120)

                                              10        20
CTC GCT CGC CGC ATT CGC GGA GAA AGA GCG TAA ATGTAAAGTCACTTTTTCATCAG
Leu Ala Arg Arg Ile Arg Gly Glu Arg Ala stop
                (130)

      30        40        50        60        70        80        90        10
TCTTAAAACC̲C̲A̲A̲A̲G̲G̲C̲T̲C̲T̲T̲T̲T̲C̲A̲G̲A̲G̲C̲C̲A̲C̲C̲C̲A̲CTTATTCCAACGAAAGTAGCTGTGATAATTTTTTGTTGTCTTA

     110      120      130      140      150      160
ACAGAACAAATTTCTAAGGACCCCCCCGGAAAGCATTAGACTATGGCTTAAAGTTGATAC–3'

B

(continued)

```
         130          120          110          100           90           80           70           60           50           40           30
          |            |            |            |            |            |            |            |            |            |            |
5' - GGAAAACTCGCGAACCATAACGCAGCGTCATGCGCACCAGCCTCTGTAAGTACACAGTCGTTTCCGGTAGACCCCGAGCCTACCGCTCTGCTTGCGTTCTCGGGGGT

             20         10
     CGGTCTCGGTCTTGGGTCTGGCC                        met  (1)
                              pFF435D        1     ATG  CCC(Pro)  GAG(Glu)    CCT(Pro)  GCA      AAG(Lys)  TTC(Phe)  GCG(Ala)
                              λHHG-39         2          T                    A         G        A         C (Ser)   T
                              λCH-02          3          T                    G         C        C         C (Ser)
                              λCH-05          4          G                    T                   C         C (Ser)
                   Yeast(S.cerviciae)         5          T T(Ser) GCT(Ala)    CA(Pro)   AAA(Lys)  C G A(Glu) AAG(Lys)  AAA(Lys)
                      P.miliaris h22          6          G T(Ala) CA(Pro)     A A(Thr)  T C A(Gln) ————————  TT(Val)

           Pro  Ala       (10)          Lys  Lys  Gly                                                                            (20)
     1     CCG  GCT  CCC(Pro)  AAG  AAG  GGC  TCC(Ser)  AAG(Lys)  AAA(Lys)  GCC(Ala)  GTC(Val)  ACC(Thr)  AAA(Lys)
     2          C        G                    T                   G                   G                   G (Ser)   G
     3          C    C                                            G                                                 G
     4          C    C                    T                       G         G                             G         G
     5          A    C    T (Ser)    A  ——  ——  G (Ala)  CCA(Pro)  GCT(Ala)  AA(Glu)  AAG(Lys)            AA(Lys)  CC (Pro)
     6     ——   T                         A                       G         A                            ————————  G

     1     GCC  CAG(Gln)  AAG(Lys)  AAG(Lys)  ————————  (25) GAC(Asp)  GGC(Gly)  AAG(Lys)  AAG(Lys)  CGC(Arg)  ————————
     2     A                                              G (Gly)   A (Asp)                            ————————
     3     A                                              G (Gly)   A (Asp)                            ————————
     4          GCT(Ala)      A                 ACT(Thr)  TCC(Ser)  ACT(Thr)  TC (Ser)  CT(Thr)  G T(Asp)  G T(Gly)  ————————
     5          CT(Pro)    CG(Arg)  CCC(Pro)               GC(Ser)  GT(Gly)                      A G(Arg)  CAT(His)
     6

                     (30)                                                                              (40)
           Lys  Arg  Ser                      Arg  Lys  Glu             (Tyr)                      Tyr
     1          AAG  CGC  AGC                  CGC  AAG  GAG  AGC(Ser)  TAC  TCC(Ser)  ATC(Ile)  TAC  GTG(Val)
     2                                                                                G A(Val)
     3     AAG(Lys)       ———                                                         G
     4     AAG(Lys)       ———                                                         G
     5     AAG(Lys)       A       AAG(Lys)  GCT(Ala)  A       A   CA(Thr)             T       CT(Ser)       A T(Ile)
     6     G (Arg)   A    ———                         A G                            GT(Gly)                C(Ile)

           Tyr  Lys  Val  Leu  Lys                (50) His  (Pro) Asp  Thr  Gly                  ┌─────────┐
     1     TAC  AAG  GTC  CTG  AAG  CGG(Arg)  GTC(Val)  CAC  CCC  GAC  ACC  GGC  ATC(Ile)  │TGG(Trp) │ TGC(Cys)  AAG(Lys)
     2          A    G         A    A (Gln)              CC(Pro)                            │CC (Ser) │ CT(Ser)   A
     3          G              A    A (Gln)   G                                             │C  (Ser) │ C (Ser)
     4          G                   A (Gln)                                                │C  (Ser) │ C (Ser)
     5          A    T    T    A    AA (Gln)  ACT(Thr)   T          T    T    T            │CC (Ser) │ CAA(Gln)
     6          A         C    A    A (Gln)   T          T          T    T  GTC(Val)       │CC (Ser) │ A (Ser)   CG (Arg)
                                                                                           └─────────┘

                Met  (60)            Ile            Asn  Ser  Phe                 Asn  Asp  Ile  Phe  Glu  Arg  Ile   (70)
     1     GCC(Ala)  ATG  GGC(Gly)  ATC  ATG(Met)  AAC  TCC  TTC  CTC(Leu)       AAC  GAC  ATC  TTC  ———  ———  ATC
     2                    G                         T         T   G (Val)                               GAG  CGC  ATC
     3                                                            G (Val)
     4                                              G             G (Val)
     5     T (Ser)        TCT(Ser)        T (Leu)   T             G T(Val)        T         T    A    A
     6                    A A(Thr)                  AG       T    G (Val)         T                   G    G

           Ala             Glu  Ala  Ser       (80) Leu                 Tyr  Asn  Lys            Ser  Thr  Ile
     1     ———  ————————   ———  ———  ———  ————————  CTG  ACA(Thr)  CAC(His)  TAC  AAC  AAG  CGC(Arg)  TCC  ACC  ATC
     2     GCC  GGC(Gly)   GAG  GCT  TCC  CGC(Arg)  T    G G(Ala)  T                                       G
     3                              G    G          T    G G(Ala)                                         G
     4                              G    G          T    G G(Ala)                                         G
     5          A T(Thr)   A        A    T          AAA(Lys)  T    G T(Ala)  GCG(Ala)  T         AAG(Lys)  G    T    T
     6          A          C             T          C        C    G(Gln)               A    AAG(Lys)      A

              (90)  ┌─────┐
           Thr  Ser │Arg  │ Glu       Gln  Thr  Ala            Arg  Leu  Leu  Leu  Pro  Gly  Glu  Leu  Ala  Lys  (100)
     1     ACG  TCC │CG(*)│ GAG  ATC(Ile)  CAG  ACG  GCC  GCG(Ala)  CGC  CTG  CTG  CTG  CCC  GGC  GAG  CTG  GCC  AAG
     2     C        │T│A  │ G    G (Val)                       T (Val)                      G
     3              │G│   │ G                                  T (Val)  G
     4              │G│   │ G             A                    T (Val)  G
     5     T T   G T│A│A  │ A    A       T         A   C   T   TT(Val)  A A   T   A C T A   A   T   A   T        T
     6     GC   AGT │C│   │ C             T                    TC(Val)       C   A T   C        A               A
                    └─────┘

              (110)                            Ser  Glu  Gly  Thr  Lys  Ala  Val  Thr  Lys  Tyr  Thr  Ser            Lys
           His  Ala  CTG(Leu)  TCC  GAG  GGC  ACC  AAG  GCG  GTC  ACC  AAG  TAC  GCC  AGC  TCC(Ser)  AAG  ————————
     1     CAC  GCC                                                                                            (120)
     2          T    G  (Val)  A                                C    T                   A         TT(Lys)  ————————
     3          G    G  (Val)                                                                      A         ————————
     4          G    G  (Val)            G                                                         A         ————————
     5     T    T    G C(Val)   T    A   T   T   GA(Arg)T   T                             T T  TC   T         CT  CAA(Gln)  GCA(Ala)
     6          T    G  (Val)  AG         T                      A    G    G    A         A T  C

        ┌─────┐                                        ~90
        │Stop │                                          |
     1  │ ————│CTGTTCCTGCCG————————————~75 bases————CTCCAAAGGCTCTTTTCAGGGCCACTTAACCCCGTTAGTGAAATAAGCT
     2    TAA │————————————————————————————————————ACCCAAAGGCTCTTTTCAGAGCCACTCA————————
     3    TAG │———————————————————— 24 bases————ACCCAAAGGCTCTTTTCAGAGCCACCATTTGTTCTAATAAAAGGGCTGT
     4    TAA │———————————————————— 32 bases————ACCCAAAGGCTCTTTTCAGAGCCACCCCCCACCTTGCCAGAGAAAGAGC
     5    TAA │TGAAATCACTTC————————————————————————————
     6  │ TAG │———————————————————— 29 bases————TGACAACGGCCCTTTTCAGGGGCCACCAAACATCCAAGAAAGAATTGTGT
        └─────┘                                                            |
                                                                   mRNA terminus

                                          C
```

128

```
            70          60          50          40          30          20          10
            |           |           |           |           |           |           |
          5'-GGTAGGCAGCGGCGTTTTCGGCGCCCTTTCCGATTGCCAAGCAGGAGTTTCTCTCGGTGACTACTATCGCTGTC
```

```
                   Met Ser Gly Arg Gly Lys Gln Gly Gly Lys Ala (10)
pFF435D      1     ATG TCT GGT CGT GGC AAG CAA GGA GGC AAG GCC  ---
λCH-01       2         G   G   C   A       G   C   G       G    CGC(Arg)
Calf         3                                                   Arg
Trout        4                                 Thr               Arg
P. Miliaris  5                                 ---         Ala  Gly  Lys
                                               (20)
```

```
                   --- --- --- Lys Ser Arg Ser Ser Arg Ala Gly Leu Gln Phe
           1                   AAG TCG CGC TCG TCC CGC GCT GGC CTT CAG TTC
                   Ala Lys Ala
           2       GCC AAG GCC              C           C   G   G
           3       Ala Lys Ala         Thr
           4       Ala Lys Ala         Thr
           5       Ala Lys Ala         Ser
```

```
                                       (30)
                   Pro Val Gly Arg Val His Arg Leu Leu Arg Lys Gly Asn Tyr
           1       CCG GTA GGG CGA GTG CAT CGC TTG CTG CGC AAA GGC AAC TAC
           2        C   G       C   C       C   G   C           G
           3
           4
           5                                       Phe
```

```
                   (40)
                   Ala Glu Arg Val Gly Ala Gly Ala Pro Val (50)
                                                            Tyr
           1       GCG GAG CGA GTG GGG GCC GGC GCG CCC GTC TAC
           2               G       C           C   G   G
           3
           4
           5           Asn
```

**D**

```
     -80      -70      -60      -50      -40      -30      -20      -10
      |        |        |        |        |        |        |        |
  CCCGGGCCCGAGCATAGCAGCAACGCAAAACCTGCTCTTTAGATTTCGAGCTTATTCTCTTCTAGCAGTTTCTTGCCACC ATG TCG GAA ACC
                                                                                     Met Ser Glu Thr
```

```
GCT CCT GCC GAG ACA GCC ACC CCA GCG CCG GTG GAG AAA TCC CCG GCT AAG AAG AAG GCA ACT AAG AAG GCT
Ala Pro Ala Glu Thr Ala Thr Pro Ala Pro Val Glu Lys Ser Pro Ala Lys Lys Lys Ala Thr Lys Lys Ala
                (10)                                           (20)
```

```
GCC GGC GCC GGC GCT GCT AAG CGC ATA GCG GCG GGG CCC CCA GTC TCA GAG CTG ATC ACC AAG GCT GTG CCT
Ala Gly Ala Gly Ala Ala Lys Arg Ile Ala Ala Gly Pro Pro Val Ser Glu Leu Ile Thr Lys Ala Val Pro
        (30)                                     (40)                                     (50)
```

```
GCT TCT AAG GAG CGC AAT GCC C
Ala Ser Lys Glu Arg Asn Ala
```

```
Human    Ser Glu Thr Ala Pro Ala Glu Thr --- --- Ala Thr Pro Ala Pro Val Glu Lys Ser Pro Ala Lys ---
Rabbit   Ser Glu --- Ala Pro Ala Glu Thr --- --- Ala Ala Pro Ala Pro Glu Lys Ser Pro Ala Lys ---
Xenopus  Ala Glu Thr Ala Ser Thr Glu Thr Thr Pro Ala Ala Pro --- Pro Ala Glu --- Pro Lys Gln Lys ---
Trout    Ala Glu --- Ala Pro Ala Glu Val --- --- Ala --- Pro Ala Pro Ala Ala Ala Pro Ala Ala Lys Ala
```

```
Human    --- --- Lys Lys Ala Thr --- Lys Lys --- Ala Ala Gly Ala Gly Ala Ala Lys Arg Ile --- Ala Ala
Rabbit   --- Lys Lys Lys Ala Ala --- Lys Lys Pro --- --- Gly Ala Gly Ala Ala Lys Arg Lys --- Ala Ala
Xenopus  --- Lys Lys Lys Gln Gln Pro Lys Lys --- Ala Ala Gly --- Gly Ala --- Lys Ala Lys Lys Pro Ser
Trout    Pro Lys Lys Lys Ala Ala --- Ala Lys Pro --- Lys Lys Ala Gly --- --- --- --- --- --- --- ---
```

```
Human    Gly Pro Pro Val Ser Glu Leu Ile Thr Lys Ala Val Pro Ala Ser Lys Glu Arg Asn Ala
Rabbit   Gly Pro Pro Val Ser Glu Leu Ile Thr Lys Ala Val Ala Ala Ser Lys Glu Arg Asn Gly
Xenopus  Gly Pro Ser Ala Ser Glu Leu Ile Val Lys Ser Val Ser Ala Ser Lys Glu Arg Gly Gly
Trout    Gly Pro Ala Val Gly Glu Leu Ile Gly Lys Ala Val Ala Ala Ser Lys Glu Arg Ser Gly
```

**E**

129

Table I:  Nucleotide Sequence Comparison for Different Organisms

| Histone | Clone Designation | Literature Reference | # of nucleotides compared | % nucleotide divergence | | % amino acid divergence | |
|---|---|---|---|---|---|---|---|
| | | | | pFF435D | pTN521 | pFF435D | pTN521 |
| H2B | pFF435D (human pseudogene) | 38 | 117 | - | 13.8 | - | 7.5 |
| | pTN521 (human) | 38 | 117 | 13.8 | - | 9.5 | - |
| | λCH-02 (chicken) | 40 | 116 | 11.0 | 12.4 | 9 | 0 |
| | λCH-03 (chicken) | 40 | 117 | 10.8 | 15.0 | 10 | 2.5 |
| | λCH-05 (chicken) | 40 | 117 | 11.0 | 11.9 | 9 | 7.5 |
| | (yeast) | 13 | 117 | 43.0 | 42.9 | 29 | 2.5 |
| | (sea urchin) (P. miliaris) | 121 | 117 | 26.0 | 24.1 | 18 | 2.5 |
| | | | | pF0535 | pF0535 | | |
| H3 | pST519 (human) | 122 | 111 | 18.0 | 0 | | |
| | pHU 2.6 (chicken) | 11 | 78 | 19.2 | 0 | | |
| | pCH 3dR (chicken) | 53 | 156 | 14.7 | 0 | | |
| | h 22 (early sea urchin) | 35, 36 | 156 | 23.0 | 0 | | |
| | λLph (late sea urchin) | 123 | 156 | 19.9 | 0 | | |
| | | | | pF0108A | pF0108A | | |
| H4 | pHU4A (human) | 10 | 193 | 14.1 | 3 | | |
| | mus-hi-1 (mouse) | 23 | 303 | 13.2 | 0 | | |
| | pxl ch4 (Xenopus) | 124, 125 | 186 | 19.3 | 0 | | |
| | xl-hi-1 (Xenopus) | 124, 125 | 303 | 18.1 | 0 | | |
| | pcxlH4W2 (Xenopus) | 124, 125 | 303 | 17.5 | 0 | | |
| | pcxlH4W1 (Xenopus) | 124, 125 | 303 | 18.1 | 0 | | |
| | Nv 51 (Notophtha-lamus) | 126 | 138 | 19.2 | 0 | | |
| | h 22 (sea urchin) | 35, 36 | 181 | 20.0 | 0 | | |
| | h 19 (sea urchin) | 35, 36 | 303 | 19.8 | 0 | | |
| | pSp2 (sea urchin) | 127 | 302 | 21.9 | 0 | | |

of these four highly conserved amino acids may adversely affect the functionality of the encoded H2A protein.

Although the H2B and perhaps also the H2A histone coding sequence of λHHG55 cannot produce a functional histone protein, the functionality of the other histone genes in this cluster (H3 and H4) (see Fig. 1) has not been addressed. There are two possibilities: actively transcribed histone genes may coexist with pseudogenes. This type of arrangement has been described for both the α- and β- globin gene clusters, where pseudogenes are interspersed with functional members of each of these gene families[41],[42]. Alternatively, the entire histone gene cluster represented in λHHG55 may be non-functional. In this regard it is noteworthy that λHHG41[8], an independent isolate analogous to λHHG55 but lacking the H2A and H2B genes, contains H3 and H4 histone genes which, based on DNA sequence analysis[43], are apparently functional. Sequence analysis of the H4 and H3 genes in λHHG55 should clearly distinguish between the above two possibilities.

The origin of the human histone pseudogene is unclear. The multiple types of defects present suggest that more than one mutational event was involved in generating this sequence, perhaps including recombination events with other histone genes. Several recent reports have suggested that pseudogenes can arise from integration of reverse transcripts of mRNAs into the genome[44-50]. It is unlikely that the H2B histone pseudogene is the result of such a mechanism since it lacks the flanking direct repeats characteristic of reverse-transcribed pseudogenes. It is interesting that to date two types of arrangements of non-functional histone genes have been observed. In the lower eucaryotes sea urchin and Drosophila, solitary members of the histone gene family, designated orphons, are found at a frequency of 50 per genome[51]. In contrast, the human histone pseudogenes we have identified are clustered with other human genes whose functionality has yet to be determined. Furthermore, these pseudogenes reside in a genomic segment organized in a manner similar to that of other human histone gene isolates[8].

Examination of the histone nucleotide sequence comparison presented in Table I indicates that there is no more nucleotide divergence between histone genes of different vertebrates than there is between different human histone genes coding for the same (or very similar) proteins. This observation is consistent with the identification of multiple histone H4 mRNAs in HeLa cells[32] and with the presence of multiple size classes for core histone mRNAs in both HeLa[52] and other human cells in culture.

The complete nucleotide sequences presented in Figure 2 indicate the absence of intervening sequences within the protein coding regions of these genes. Similar observations have been made for most histone genes studied so far, with the sole exception of a chicken H3 gene[53]. The S1 nuclease protection experiments of Lichtler, et al.[32] and primer extension analysis carried out by Sierra, et al.[43] provide further evidence that the λHHG41 H4 histone gene contains no intervening sequences.

Data obtained for the H3 and H4 genes in λHHG41 indicate that these two genes are transcribed convergently from opposite strands of DNA while the H2A and H2B genes in λHHG55 are transcribed divergently.

Putative Regulatory Sequences

Regions 3' and 5' to the mRNA coding sequences of genes transcribed by RNA polymerase II have been postulated to be involved in the control of gene expression. To gain insight into the regulation of human histone gene expression, we have focused our attention on the sequences flanking the H4 gene present in λHHG41. The complete nucleotide sequence has been deter-

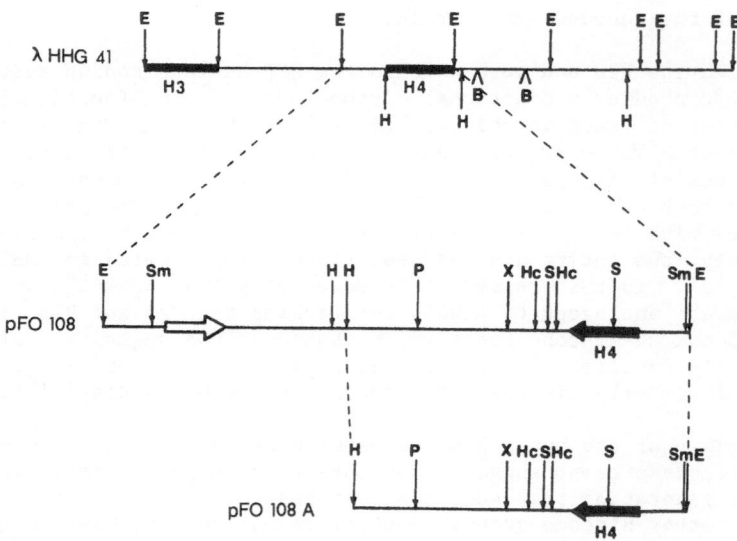

Fig. 3: Restriction maps of HHG41 and subclones pFO108 and pFO108A.
λHHG41 is a λCH4a recombinant clone containing H3 and H4 human
histone DNA sequences; its isolation and characterization have
been described elsewhere[8,43]. pFO108 contains the 3.1 Kb EcoRI
fragment of λHHG41 (containing the H4 histone gene) inserted into
the EcoRI site of pBR322. This 3.1 Kb fragment also contains a
member of the Alu family of repeated DNA sequences, indicated by
the white arrow. The 1.8 Kb EcoRI/HindIII fragment containing
the H4 gene, but not the Alu sequence, has been subcloned into
EcoRI/HindIII-digested pBR322 and is designated pFO108A. E =
EcoRI, H = HindIII, B = BamHI, Sm = SmaI, p = PstI, X = XbaI, Hc =
Hinc II, S = SacII.

mined[43] (and see Fig. 2) and the functional roles of various regions of
the gene have been examined.

The 3.1 Kb EcoRI fragment from λHHG41 containing the H4 histone gene
was subcloned into the EcoRI site of pBR322. Figure 3 shows a detailed restriction map of this clone (pFO108) and of a subclone (pFO108A) containing
only the 1.8 Kb EcoRI/HindIII fragment. pFO108A does not contain the Alu
I sequence found in pFO108 (indicated by the white arrow in Fig. 3A).

The complete nucleotide sequence of the pFO108A H4 gene, including 5'
and 3' flanking regions, is presented in Figure 2. Analysis of the sequences upstream from the ATG translation initiation codon indicates the
presence of several sequences that may be involved in some functional or
regulatory capacity in vivo. For example, the sequence GGTCC which occurs
approximately 10bp upstream from the TATA box is very similar to the GATCC
motif found in an analogous position in several sea urchin histone genes[39].
Further upstream are two tandem CAAT boxes (indicated in Fig. 2 by closed
boxes), remarkably similar to homology blocks found in most other genes
transcribed by RNA polymerase II[54,55], including several histone genes[39].
Although in some cases, for example the H2A histone gene present in the sea
urchin clone h22, two CAAT boxes have been found in tandem arrangement,
this homology block has not been observed in other H4 or H1 histone genes[39].
Despite the apparent conservation of these homology blocks, it must be emphasized that their functional significance is as yet unknown.

Further upstream from the H4 histone coding region are several non-random sequences. Notably, between nucleotides −152 and −174 there is a stretch of 21 nucleotides containing only A and G residues, most usually in the form of the trinucleotide GGA (see Fig. 2). Similar although not identical stretches have been found in the spacer regions of other histone genes[39,56], and a role in recombination has been proposed. Finally, several short direct repeats (indicated by horizontal arrows in Fig. 2) are present in the 5' flanking region of the H4 gene. It is well documented that direct repeats present in the SV40 and retrovirus genomes act as strong promoters of transcription, both in vivo and in vitro[57,58].

The 3' flanking region of the H4 gene present in pF0108A exhibits many features found in histone genes of other species. The 3' end of the mRNA is most likely located at the ACCA motif found a few nucleotides downstream from the hyphenated dyad symmetry which is characteristic of histone mRNA 3' ends[39], although termination of transcription probably occurs even further downstream (M. Birnstiel, personal communication). Interestingly, the hyphenated dyad symmetry region of the RNA can, theoretically at least, form a stem and loop structure similar to that which appears to be involved in transcription termination by RNA polymerase III[59]. Birchmeier et al.[60] found this sequence to be necessary, although not sufficient, for formation of correct mRNA 3' ends from a sea urchin H2A histone gene microinjected into Xenopus oocytes. Deletions of the hyphenated dyad symmetry sequence induced apparent read-through by RNA polymerase II, but reinsertion of the same motif in the middle of an H2B gene did not by itself promote termination of transcription at this point. Twelve nucleotides downstream from the ACCA motif there is another histone gene-related motif, characterized mainly by its high A + G content. No specific function has yet been ascribed to these sequences.

To test the functional relevance of these putative regulatory sequences, we used an in vitro transcription assay based on the whole HeLa cell lysate described by Manley, et al.[61]. Preliminary experiments showed that under the appropriate conditions, in vitro transcription of EcoRI/Hind III-digested pF0108A DNA produced a correct run-off transcript of 1.8 Kb in length[43]. This transcript was sensitive to low concentrations of α-amanitin (2μg/ml), implicating the involvement of RNA polymerase II, which has been reported to transcribe human histone genes in vivo[62]. Primer extension analysis indicated that these transcripts were initiated at the same site used in vivo.

This in vitro transcription system was used to assay a series of deletion mutants constructed from pF0108A, which spanned almost all the 5' flanking region of the H4 gene but did not include the TATA box[43]. The TATA box has been implicated in numerous systems as playing a role in directing the precise site of initiation of transcription by RNA polymerase II[54,63-65]. Deletion mutants of pF0108A were constructed by BAL-31 nuclease digestion of EcoRI-linearized DNA, followed by the addition of EcoRI linkers and cloning into the EcoRI/HindIII sites of pBR322. Figure 4 shows the sequences upstream from the H4 gene and indicates the end points of the deletions determined for several clones.

Several of these deletion mutants were selected for further analysis. They were restricted with either HindIII or with HindIII plus EcoRI, and then transcribed in the in vitro system. All the clones examined gave rise to an in vitro transcript of the expected size (Fig. 5), including clone pF0108A 5'Δ80, which lacks the direct repeats as well as the "CAAT" boxes previously described. The same deletion mutants exhibited a decreased level of this specific transcript when the DNA template was digested only with HindIII. Apparently, EcoRI cleavage (5' to the H4 gene) can provide an artificial site of entry for the RNA polymerase, which then begins transcribing at its normal site. Primer extension experiments have shown that

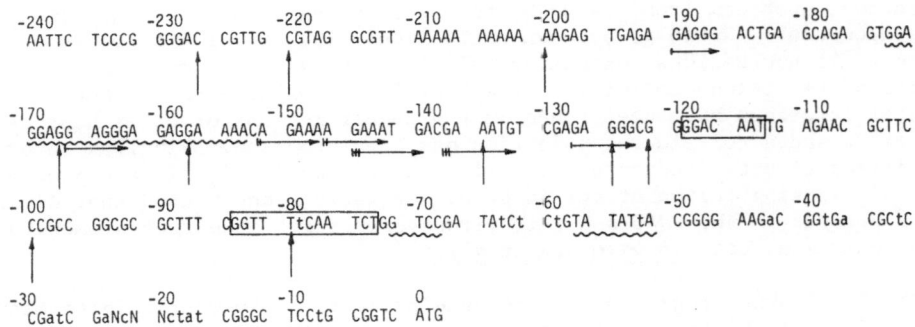

```
-240           -230                -220                  -210           -200              -190          -180
AATTC  TCCCG  GGGAC  CGTTG  CGTAG  GCGTT  AAAAA  AAAAA  AAGAG  TGAGA  GAGGG  ACTGA  GCAGA  GTGGA
                                                                            ─────→

-170           -160                -150           -140                -130              -120          -110
GGAGG  AGGGA  GAGGA  AAACA  GAAAA  GAAAT  GACGA  AATGT  CGAGA  GGGCG  GGGAC  AATTG  AGAAC  GCTTC
─────────→      ↑          ─⊩⊩→   ─⊩⊩─→       ─⊩⊩─→         ↑              ↑     ↑

-100           -90                 -80            -70                 -60               -50           -40
CCGCC  GGCGC  GCTTT  CGGTT  TtCAA  TCTGG  TCCGA  TAtCt  CtGTA  TATtA  CGGGG  AAGaC  GGtGa  CGCtC
         ↑

-30            -20                 -10            0
CGatC  GaNcN  Nctat  CGGGC  TCCtG  CGGTC  ATG
  ↑
```

Fig. 4: Endpoints of 5' deletion mutants of pF0108A.
Sequences upstream from the 5' end of the H4 coding region are
shown. Vertical arrows indicate the end points of the different
deletion mutants. Nucleotide residues are numbered from the AUG
initiation codon, and decrease in the upstream direction. The
deletion clones are designated by the nucleotide at which the end
point of deletion lies. Deletion mutants were constructed by
digestion of EcoRI-linearized pF0108A DNA with BAL-31 nuclease to
remove nucleotides located upstream from the H4 gene. Synthetic
EcoRI linkers were added, and the DNA was exhaustively digested
with EcoRI and HindIII restriction endonucleases and then ligated
to calf intestine alkaline phosphatase-treated, EcoRI/HindIII-
digested pBR322. Ligation mixes were used to transform E. coli
strain HB 101.

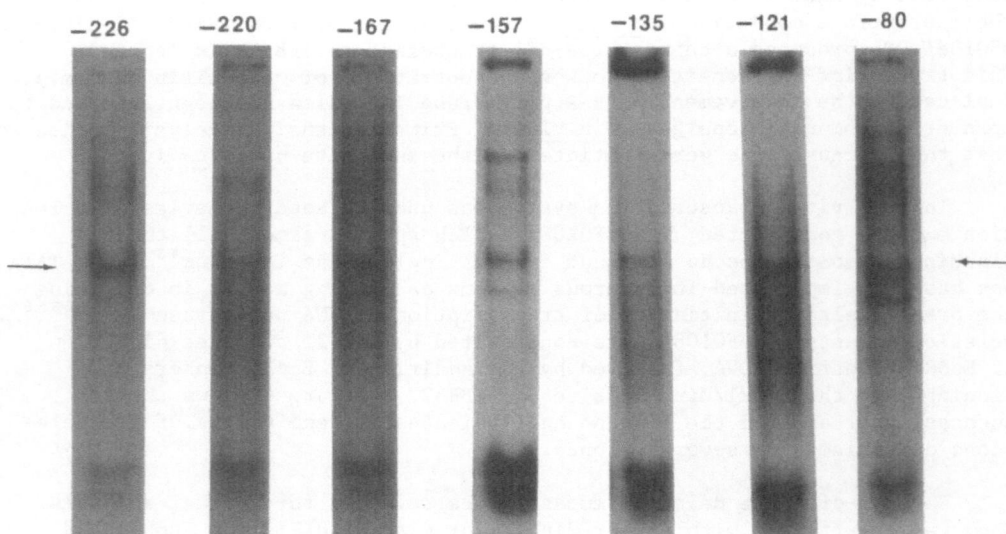

Fig. 5: In vitro transcription of deletion mutants constructed from pF0108A.
Autoradiograms of 1.5% agarose, 3% formaldehyde gels showing the
transcripts obtained from selected deletion mutants. The template
DNA was digested with EcoRI and HindIII restriction endonucleases.
The arrows indicate the position of the expected read-through transcript. Numbers above the lanes refer to the position of the
deletion end point with respect to the AUG initiation codon.

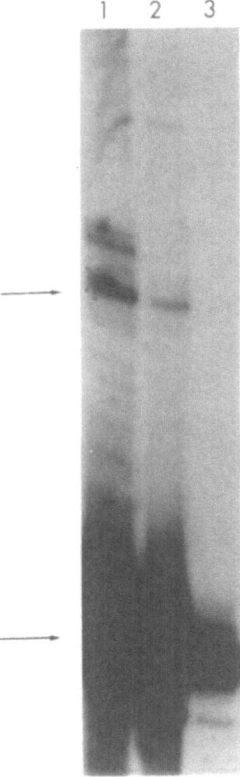

Fig. 6:  Primer extension analysis of transcripts generated using pFO108A
         5'Δ80 as a template.
         Autoradiogram of a 10% polyacrylamide/8.3 M urea gel showing the
         DNA fragments obtained after extension of the 64 bp primer by AMV
         reverse transcriptase, using different RNA samples as templates.
         Lane 1:  HeLa polysomal RNA.  Lane 2:  in vitro transcripts from
         pFO108A 5'Δ80.  Lane 3:  unhybridized primer.  The positions of
         the unextended and the extended primers are indicated by arrows.


the in vitro transcripts from clone pFO108A 5'Δ80 are initiated at the in
vivo 5' initiation site, as demonstrated by comparison with HeLa cell polysomal RNA (Fig. 6).  We can therefore conclude that no sequences upstream
from the TATA box are required for site-specific initiation of in vitro
transcription of the H4 histone gene present in pFO108A.

     To determine if sequences downstream from the 3' end of the H4 histone
gene are required for in vitro transcription, our initial approach was to
use pFO108 DNA that had been truncated by digestion with several different
restriction endonucleases[43].  These experiments were performed using double
digestions of pFO108 DNA.  DNA was first digested to completion with EcoRI
restriction endonuclease, thus separating the insert containing the H4
histone gene from vector sequences and eliminating the possibility of inter-
ference due to the presence of promoters in the pBR322 vector.  The DNA was
then cleaved with each of the other restriction endonucleases indicated in
Figure 3.  Transcriptions were performed in parallel in the presence or
absence of 2µg/ml of α-amanitin to identify transcripts produced by RNA
polymerase II, the enzyme responsible for transcription of the histone genes
in vivo.

     Figure 7A shows an example of the type of results obtained when pFO108

135

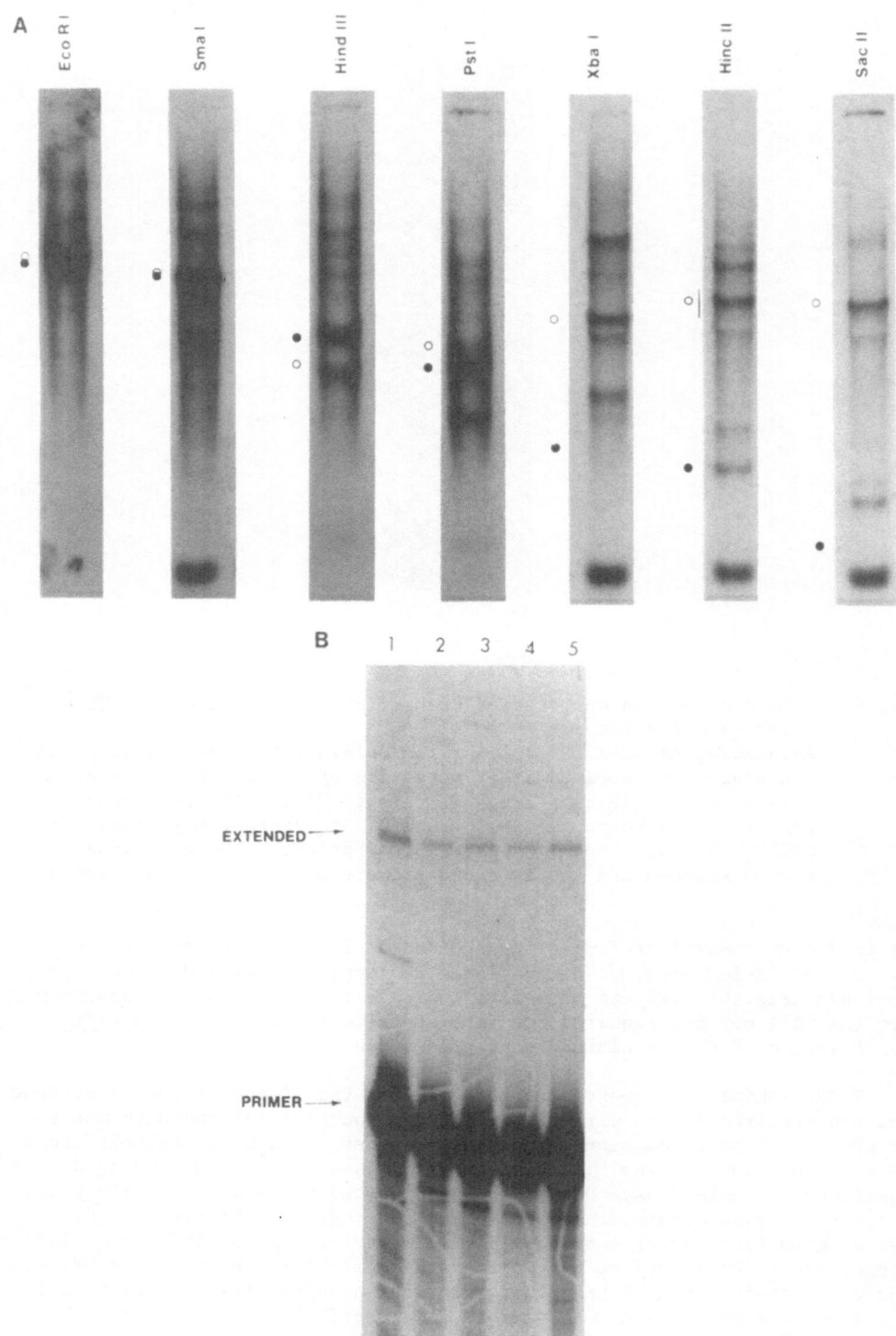

DNA digested with a series of different restriction endonucleases was transcribed in vitro and the resulting transcripts were analyzed on a 1.5% agarose/formaldehyde gel. The black dots at the left of lanes 1, 3, 5, 7, 9, 10 and 12 indicate the positions expected for the migration of transcripts initiated at the correct 5' terminus of the H4 gene and terminated at the point of truncation. It can be observed that in vitro transcription of pFO108 DNA that had been digested with EcoRI, either alone or in combination with SmaI, Hind III or PstI restriction endonucleases gives rise to an α-amanitin sensitive run-off transcript of the predicted size. However, when the template was truncated closer to the 3' end of the gene (with XbaI, HincII or SacII), no run-off transcript of the appropriate size was observed. A transcript of the predicted size is present among the in vitro transcripts obtained using EcoRI/HincII-digested pFO108 as template; however, this transcript is not sensitive to low concentrations of α-amanitin (Fig. 7) and is also produced when EcoRI/HincII-digested pBR322 DNA is used as a template.

The transcripts indicated by the open circles in Figure 7A are most likely products of in vitro transcription initiated at the Alu DNA sequence present in pFO108, since they are not sensitive to low concentrations of α-amanitin (Alu DNA is transcribed in vitro by RNA polymerase III[66,67]) and are not produced when pFO108A DNA is used as a template.

The in vitro transcription of truncated pFO108 and pFO108A DNA templates shows that, under appropriate conditions, specific RNA polymerase II transcripts as long as 2.8Kb can be produced. However, removal of sequences within or downstream from the 3' end of the H4 histone gene abolished the production of transcripts of the expected size. Analysis of these transcription products on 5% polyacrylamide gels containing 8.3M urea failed to resolve smaller, specifically terminated transcripts. These results suggested that sequences located at the 3' end of the gene might enhance in vitro initiation and/or elongation of transcription of the H4 histone gene present in pFO108.

To explore these possibilities further, a series of primer extension experiments[68,69] was designed to determine if initiation of transcription had indeed occurred in cases where no run-off transcript was detected. A 64 bp AluI/HhaI fragment, containing those nucleotides coding for amino acids 17 through 38 (see Fig. 2), was used as a primer to assay for specific

---

Fig. 7A: In vitro transcription of pFO108 DNA digested with different restriction enzymes.
Autoradiograms of 1.5% agarose, 3% formaldehyde gels showing in vitro transcripts obtained when using as a template pFO108 DNA that had been previously digested with EcoRI, as well as with one other restriction enzyme (indicated at the top of each lane), both in the presence and absence of 2μg/ml of α-amanitin (+ and -). The black dot at the left of each lane indicates the position of the expected read-through transcript. The open circle at the left of each lane indicates the position of the α-amanitin insensitive, insert-dependent transcript discussed in the text.

Fig. 7B: Primer extension analysis of in vitro transcripts.
Autoradiogram of a 10% polyacrylamide/8.3 M urea gel showing the DNA fragments obtained after extension of the 64 bp primer by AMV reverse transcriptase, using different RNA samples as templates. Lane 1: HeLa polysomal RNA. Lanes 2 through 5: In vitro transcripts obtained using as a template pFO108A DNA digested with EcoRI restriction endonuclease, as well as: Lane 2: HindIII, Lane 3: PstI, Lane 4: XbaI, Lane 5: HincII.
The positions of the unextended and the extended primers are indicated by arrows.

initiation of transcription. If accurate initiation occurred, this DNA primer would be elongated to a molecule of approximately 160 nucleotides in length. Figure 7B, lane 1 shows the extended primers obtained with HeLa polysomal RNA. Two bands are resolved, indicating that more than one of the multiple HeLa H4 histone mRNAs[32] has sufficient sequence homology with the 64bp fragment from pF0108A to form stable hybrids; differences in the 5' leader probably account for the size heterogeneity observed in the extended primer molecules. Lanes 2-5 show the extended primers obtained with RNAs transcribed in vitro from pF0108A DNA-digested with both EcoRI and either HindIII (lane 2), PstI (lane 3), XbaI (lane 4) or HincII (lane 5). In all cases, a single band, comigrating with one of the two extended primers observed with HeLa polysomal RNA was resolved.

These results confirmed the previous finding that specific and accurate initiation of transcription of the H4 histone gene in pF0108A does occur in vitro. Furthermore, specific initiation of transcription was observed with all templates analyzed, despite the fact that two of these truncated templates (pF0108A DNA digested with restriction endonucleases EcoRI and either XbaI or HincII) gave no detectable α-amanitin sensitive run-off transcript. Although this assay is only semi-quantitative, the apparent rate of initiation of transcription was similar in all cases.

In summary, our results seem to indicate that truncating the pF0108A template closer than approximately 800 nucleotides from the 3' end of the H4 gene either inhibits elongation of transcription or affects transcript stability, since site-specific initiation still occurs at approximately normal rates even though no full-size transcripts are produced.


THE REGULATION OF HISTONE GENE EXPRESSION

The analysis of gene expression in vivo requires an understanding of the relationship between at least five intracellular processes which may modulate the activity of the functional gene product. These potential regulatory events may be simplistically summarized as follows: i) Transcription; ii) Transcript processing (splicing, 5'-capping and 3'-polyadenylation; iii) Transcript translocation to the cytoplasm; iv) Translation and post-translation modifications; and v) Transcript turnover. Analysis of the cell cycle specific regulation of histone gene expression has therefore necessitated the study of the temporal relationship between these intracelcellular events as applied to histone genes in synchronized cells.

## Are Histone Proteins Synthesized in a Cell Cycle Specific Manner?

Histone protein synthesis must be considered in the context of the function of these proteins, so it is worth re-emphasizing several properties which are relevant to an understanding of the regulation of their synthesis: i) Histone proteins are largely responsible for the organization and structure of the cellular genome. ii) Histone proteins are found complexed to DNA in a relatively invariant molar ratio and there is reason to believe that a change in this stoichiometry would severely affect a cell's viability. iii) No free histone pools have been identified in higher eucaryotes, indicating that newly synthesized histones are rapidly sequestered by the nucleus; and iv) There is no evidence that histone proteins are derived from precursor translation products. These properties in themselves strongly argue for a coupling between histone protein synthesis and DNA replication.

It has now been well documented that in most eucaryotic cells, the bulk synthesis of histones (that which is required during DNA replication) occurs in the S phase of the cell cycle[70-72]. Exceptions include the recent identification of "basal levels" of core histone protein systhesis in G1 and $G1_0$

in several mammalian cell lines; these basal levels correspond to approximately 8% of the rate of synthesis observed in S phase     Similarly, histone H1 synthesis may occur outside cell cycle control under special circumstances[75],[76], and a constant rate of histone synthesis during the cell cycle has been reported in S49 mouse lymphoma cells[77].  Core and H1 histone proteins and/or mRNAs are also synthesized and stored during oocyte maturation in some organisms[56].

Early studies with synchronized HeLa cells and with nondividing human diploid fibroblasts stimulated to proliferate indicated that the specific activity of nuclear histones was highest when cells were pulse-labeled with $^3$H- or $^{14}$C-labeled amino acids during S phase[71],[78].  To eliminate the possibility of cell cycle specific compartmentalization of newly synthesized histone proteins, we have pulse-labeled G1 and S phase HeLa cells with $^{35}$S methionine, and analyzed total cellular proteins (Fig. 8A) or 0.4N $H_2SO_4$ soluble cellular proteins (Fig. 8B) for the presence of radiolabeled histones.  As shown in Figure 8, S phase total cellular histone proteins have a considerably higher specific activity than those isolated from G1 cells[70], an observation consistent with S phase-specific histone protein synthesis.  The synthesis of histone proteins primarily during S phase is also suggested by the very low levels of histone protein synthesis and cytoplasmic histone mRNAs at nonpermissive temperatures in temperature-sensitive cell cycle mutants[79] (see also Hirschhorn et al., Biochemistry 23:3731 (1984)).

Is the Cellular Abundance of Histone mRNA Under Cell Cycle Control?

The S-phase-specific synthesis of histone proteins poses the question of whether regulation occurs at the level of translation or whether translation is governed by the availability of histone mRNA.  Within this context, several properties of histone gene transcripts must be borne in mind:  i) With the exception of a chicken H3 gene[53] there is no evidence that histone genes contain intervening sequences.  As histone mRNAs are generally not polyadenylated, the only documented post-transcriptional processing prior to translocation and translation is 5'-capping[80],[81] and a 3'-trimming (M. Birnstiel, personal communication).  ii) Possibly because of the minimal post-transcriptional processing required, histone mRNAs are found only transiently in the nucleus, the bulk of the cellular histone mRNAs being found associated with the polysomes.  iii) As alluded to above, histone mRNAs are a heterologous population of macromolecules derived from a polymorphic, middle repetitive family of genes.

We have used the cloned genomic human histone sequences (Figs. 1A and 9) to examine the representation and synthesis of histone mRNA in synchronized, continuously dividing HeLa S3 cells[52],[82] and in quiescent human diploid fibroblasts stimulated to proliferate[83].  This problem necessitated the analysis of multiple histone mRNAs of variable sequence homology to our cloned genomic probes in order to determine whether or not members of this repetitive family of genes are differentially regulated.  We therefore employed an experimental approach which permits the resolution of more than 15 different histone mRNAs.  Our results are consistent with the cellular abundance of human histone mRNAs being coordinately regulated at both the transcriptional and post-transcriptional levels during the cell cycle.  In agreement with earlier observations from this laboratory and with findings of others[84],[89] in which histone mRNAs were analyzed by RNA excess hybridization with homologous histone cDNA, histone mRNA sequences are predominately synthesized and present during S phase when DNA replication and histone protein synthesis occur.  Recently similar results have also been obtained by Heintz, et al. using cloned histone gene probes[90].

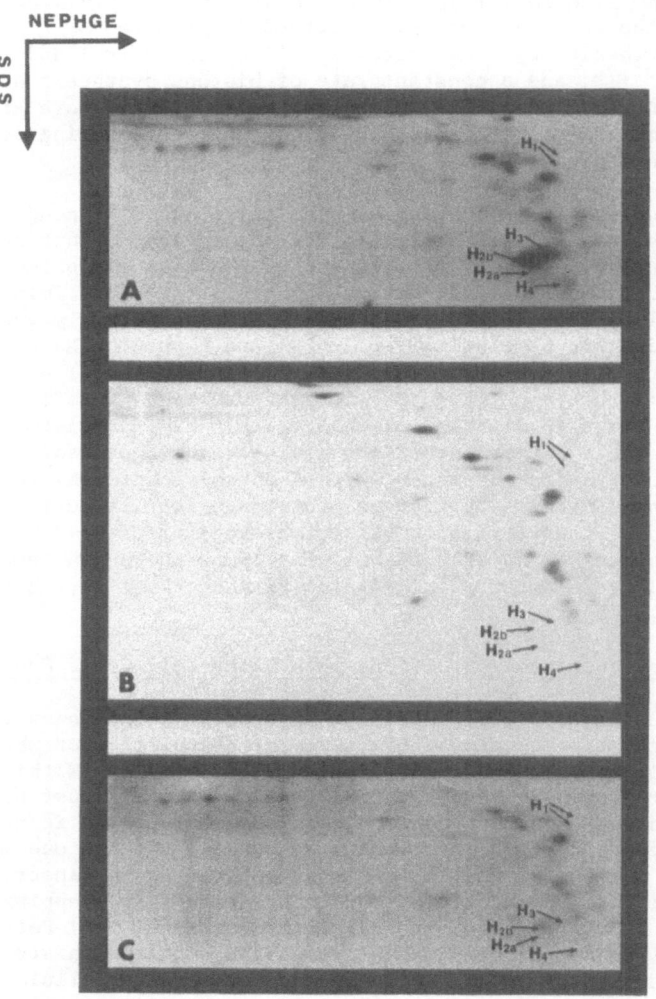

Fig. 8: Two-dimensional NEPHGE/SDS electrophoresis of acid-extracted
nuclear proteins of (A) S-phase, (B) $G_1$ and (C) cytosine-arabino-
side-treated S phase cells. $^{35}$S-methionine-labeled cells were
lysed in 10mM KC1-10mM Tris-1.3mM $MgCl_2$ (pH 7.4) containing 0.65%
(v/v) Triton X-100, and nuclei were pelleted by centrifugation at
800 x g. Nuclear pellets were extracted with 0.4M $H_2SO_4$ for 30
min and the acid soluble nuclear proteins were precipitated from
the supernatant at -20° overnight after addition of three volumes
of 95% ethanol.

Is the Abundance of Histone mRNA Temporally Coupled to DNA Replication?

The relationship between histone mRNA levels and DNA replication can
only be considered within the limits of the assay used to detect cellular
histone mRNA levels. Sequence data presented above (Fig. 2 and Table 1) indicate that within the same cell, a sequence divergence of 15-20% between
gene transcripts coding for the same or very similar histone proteins is to
be expected. Hybridization r-sults emphasize the complexity of the problem.
For example, when in vivo $^3$H-uridine-labeled total cellular RNA was hybridized to filter-immobilized plasmid NDAs containing human histone gene
sequences and the eluted RNAs were resolved by denaturing polyacrylamide
gel electrophoresis and visualized by fluorography, several distince mRNA
size classes were selected by each probe (Fig. 10). As shown for the

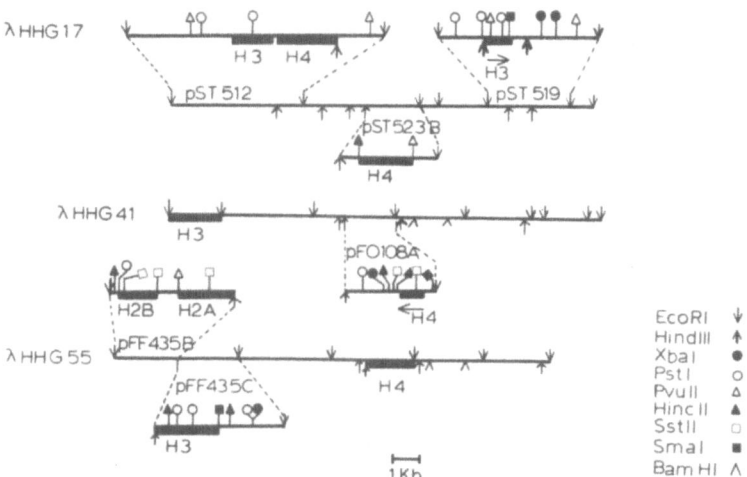

Fig. 9: Restriction endonuclease maps of λCh4A recombinants containing
human histone gene clusters isolated and characterized as described[8] and fine restriction mapping of fragments subcloned into
pBR322. Histone coding sequences were identified by hybrid
selection-in vitro translation, hybridization to homologous and
heterologous probes and partial sequencing.

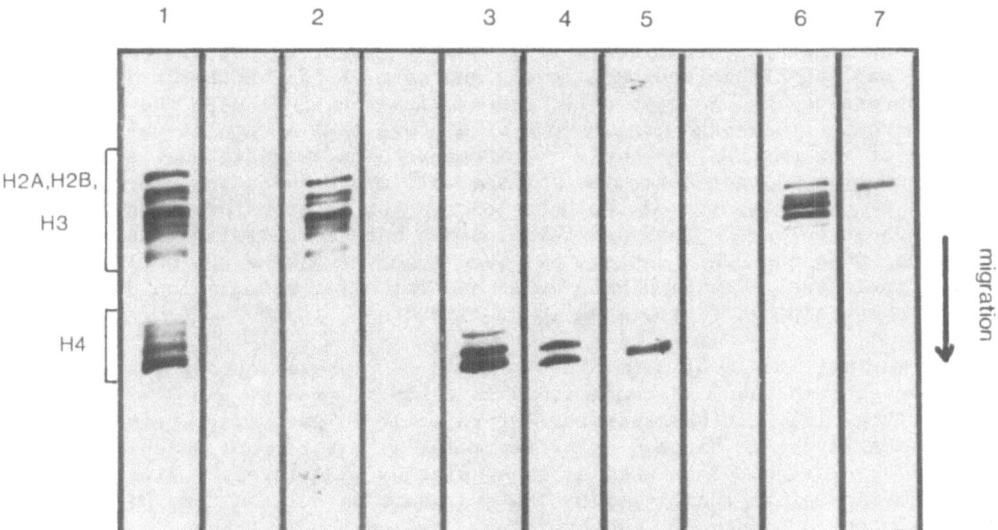

Fig. 10: The effect of temperature on hybrid-selection of histone mRNA
variants. One hundred fifty μg of in vivo $^3$H-uridine pulse-
labeled total cellular RNA was hybridized with 50μg of filter-
immobilized cloned human histone sequences. Hybridized RNAs were
eluted and resolved by denaturing 6% (w/v) polyacrylamide, 50%
(w/v) urea gel electrophoresis and visualized by fluorography.
Lane 1) pF0108A (H4), pFF435B (H2A + H2B) and pFF435C (H3)
hybridized at 43°C, Lane 2) pFF435B (H2A + H2B) hybridized at
45°C; Lanes 3) and 4) and 5) pF0108A (H4) hybridized at 43°C,
45°C and 48°C respectively; and Lanes 6) and 7) pFF435C hybridized
at 45°C and 48°C respectively.

141

histone H3 and H4 probes, the complexity of the resolved mRNAs is dependent on the temperature of hybridization (43-48°C in 50% [w/v] formamide). At an intermediate temperature of hybridization (45°C) we detect over 15 mRNA size classes which code for core histone proteins.

To compensate for the variable sequence homology between different histone mRNAs, we adopted the following approach to analyze total histone mRNA levels during the cell cycle: HeLa cells were synchronized at the G1/S phase boundary by two cycles of 2mM thymidine treatment, and total cellular RNA was isolated at various times as the cells progressed through S phase after release. Northern blot analysis of this RNA was then performed with four different cloned human histone gene probes and a heterologous chicken histone (H3 and H4) gene fragment (p2.6H)[11]. The temperature of hybridization was varied (45-50°C) to alter the complexity of the histone mRNAs detected. Three northern blot analyses are shown in Figure 11A and the data from three experiments are quantitatively summarized in Figure 11B. The relative abundance of the four core histone mRNAs varied only within limits of experimental error, indicating that their relative cellular levels are coordinately regulated. The in vivo rates of DNA synthesis were monitored in parallel, and as shown in Figure 11, the relative abundance of histone mRNAs is temporally coupled with the relative rate of DNA synthesis[52].

To eliminate the possibility that temporal coupling was an artifact of either the synchronization technique or the cell line, two analogous experiments were performed. We found that the relative abundance of core histone mRNAs in HeLa cells progressing from G1 to S (synchronized by mitotic selective detachment) paralleled the relative rates of DNA synthesis (Fig. 12). A similar coupling of core histone mRNA levels and the rate of DNA synthesis was observed following the stimulation of quiescent WI-38 human diploid fibroblasts to proliferate (Fig. 13)[83]. Hereford et al. have also detected coupling of histone mRNA levels and rate of DNA synthesis in yeast cells progressing into S phase after synchronization in G1 with the yeast mating pheromone, although the maximum of histone mRNA accumulation preceded the point of maximal DNA synthesis[91]. These results indicate that the temporal coupling is not determined by the cell synchronization protocol, nor is it a characteristic of the HeLa genotype or of transformed human cells grown in culture. The same relationship between cellular levels of H1 histone mRNAs and DNA synthesis has been observed during the cell cycle both in continuously dividing HeLa cells and following stimulation of nondividing human diploid fibroblasts to proliferate[92].

The maximal levels of HeLa histone mRNAs in S phase represent a 6-7 fold increase compared with those found in cells blocked at the G1/S boundary (Fig. 11). It was therefore of interest to determine whether the histone mRNA levels in blocked cells represent a "basal" pool which is not under cell cycle control or whether these histone mRNA levels reflect a "leaky" or incomplete inhibition of DNA synthesis in cells at the G1/S boundary in the presence of 2mM thymidine. Wu and Bonner[73] have defined cellular "basal" levels of histone protein synthesis as those which are insensitive to the DNA synthesis inhibitor hydroxyurea. We therefore used the same approach to determine the origins of histone mRNAs present in thymidine blocked cells. Synchronized cells at 0, 2, 6 or 11 hours after release from the second thymidine treatment were exposed to 1mM hydroxyurea for 30 minutes, total cellular RNA was isolated, and histone mRNA levels were determined by Northern blot analysis. We found that the relative abundance of histone mRNAs decreased to 30-60% of the levels found in cells blocked at the G1/S boundary with thymidine, irrespective of the levels observed in the appropriate S phase control cells[52]. Thus, only 50% of the total histone mRNAs found in cells arrested at the G1/S boundary by synchronization with double thymidine blocks represents a "basal" pool which,

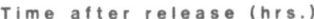

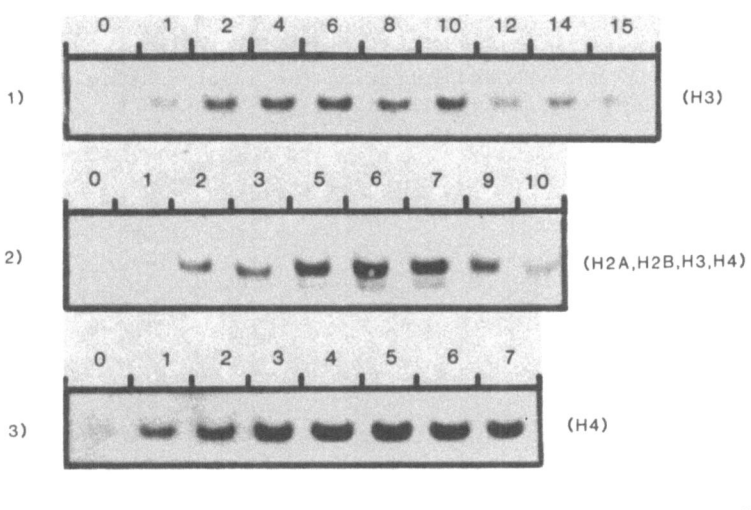

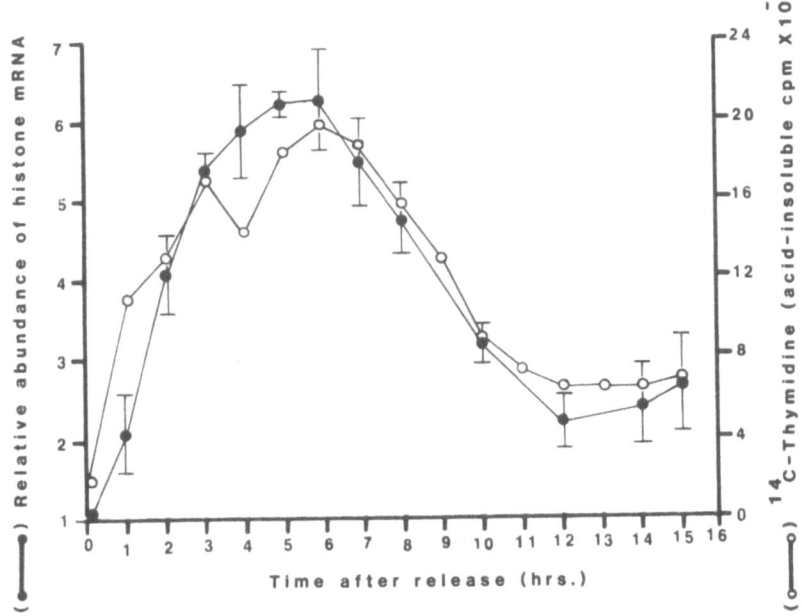

Fig. 11:   Northern blot analysis of total cellular histone mRNA in HeLa
cells after synchronization by two cycles of 2mM thymidine treatment.  At various times after release from the second thymidine
block, total cellular RNA was isolated, 50µg of RNA from each
preparation were resolved by 1.5% (w/v) agarose, 6% (w/v) formaldehyde gel electrophoresis, and the RNAs were transferred to
nitrocellulose.  Filters were hybridized at 48°C in 50% (w/v)
formamide to one of each nick-translated probes:  1) pFF435C (H3);
2) pFF435 (B + C) (H2A, H2B and H3) and p2.6H (chicken H3 + H4);
3) pF0108A (H4) and hybrids were visualized by autoradiography.
B.   The relative abundance of histone mRNAs (●——●, S.E.M.) in
cells released into S phase after synchronization by two cycles
of thymidine treatment, and assayed by Northern Blot analysis.
Hybrids were quantitated for 9 Northern blots by densitometry
and/or liquid scintillation spectrometry, after hybridization

with the five histone gene probes as described above and in the text. Values represent the mean relative abundances of histone H4, H3 and H2A + H2B mRNAs. The rate of DNA synthesis (o——o) was monitored by pulse labeling $10^6$ cells with 0.2μCi of $^{14}$C-thymidine for 20 minutes and measuring the incorporation of radiolabel into acid-precipitable material.

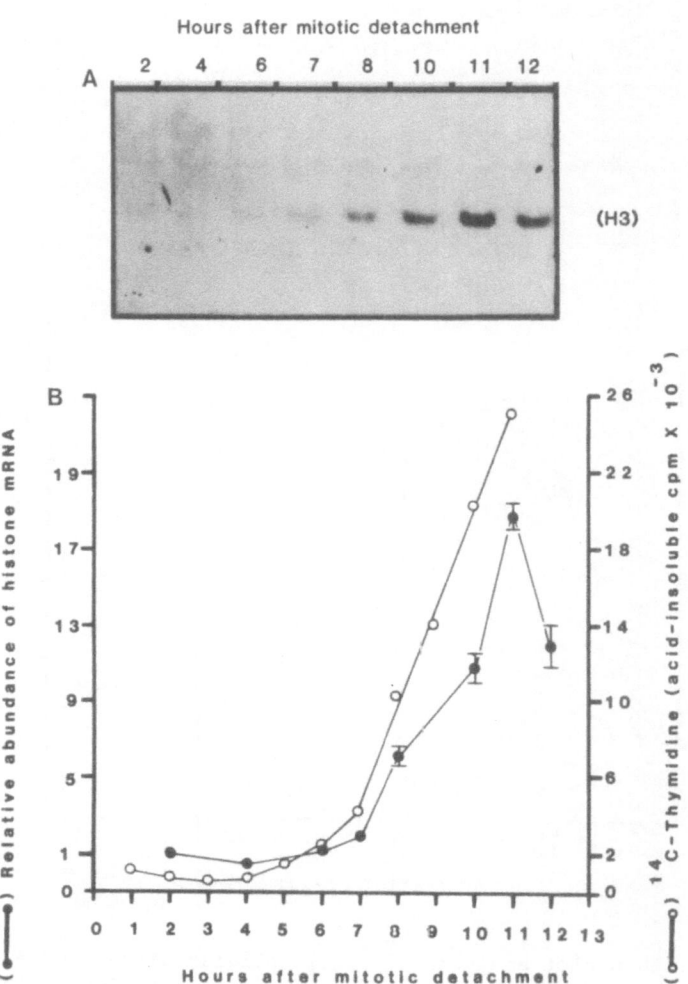

Fig. 12: Northern blot analysis of total cellular histone mRNA in HeLa cells synchronized by selective mitotic detachment. At various times after mitotic detachment, total cellular RNA was isolated, 50μg of each were resolved by 1.5% (w/v) agarose, 6% formaldehyde gel electrophoresis, and the RNAs transferred to nitrocellulose. The filter was hybridized to nick-translated pST519 (H3) probe, and visualized by autoradiography. B. Histone mRNA accumulation (•——•, ±, S.E.M.) assayed for three Northern blots probed with pST519 (H3), pF0108A (H4), or pFF435B (H2A + H2B), quantitated as described in Figure 8B. DNA synthesis rates (o——o) were monitored by measuring the incorporation of $^{14}$C-thymidine into acid-precipitable material in a 20 minute pulse.

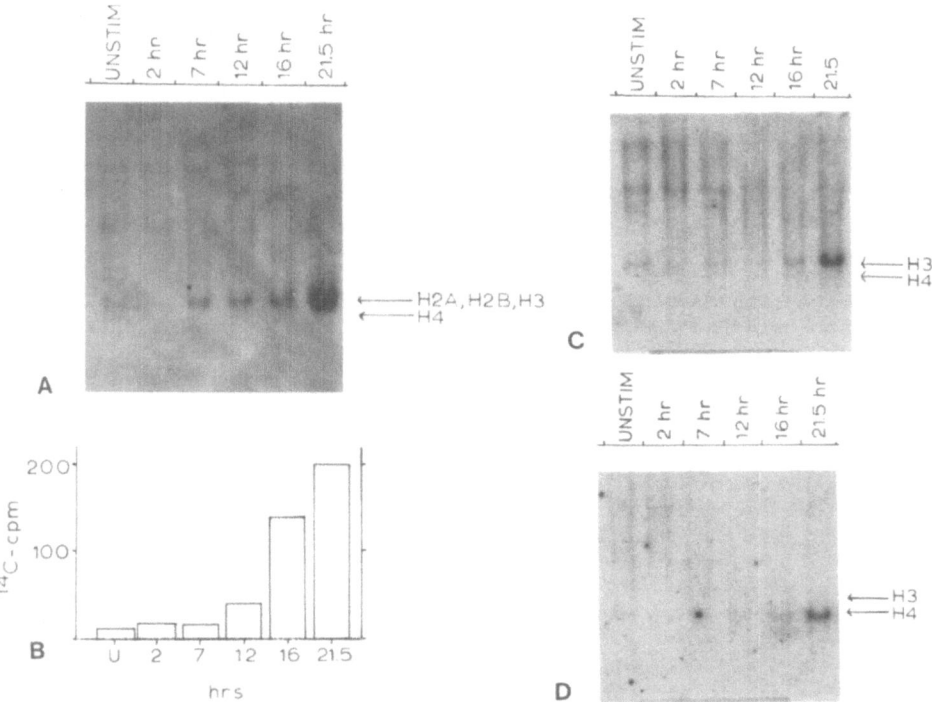

Fig. 13:  A) Hybridization of total cellular RNAs from WI38 human diploid
fibroblasts with a cloned human histone DNA sequence (pFF435)
encoding histones H2A, H2B, and H3.  The signals shown were
obtained using 50μg of electrophoretically fractionated, nitrocellulose-immobilized total cellular RNAs from quiescent WI38
human diploid fibroblasts isolated at various times after serum
stimulation (2 hours, 7 hours, 12 hours and 21.5 hours) and from
unstimulated cells.  The lower bar graph depicts the levels of
DNA synthesis at various times after serum stimulation (2 hours,
7 hours, 12 hours, 16 hours, and 21.5 hours) and in unstimulated
cells.  The levels are expressed as $^{14}$C-cpm incorporated into
DNA, determined by pulse-labeling duplicate cultures with
$^{14}$C-thymidine for 30 minutes followed by assaying TCA-precipitable
radioactivity.  B)  Histone mRNA levels and DNA synthesis at
various times after serum stimulation of quiescent WI38 human
diploid fibroblasts.  The histone mRNA levels were determined by
densitometric analysis of hybridization signals obtained when
50μg of electrophoretically fractionated, nitrocellulose-
immobilized WI38 total cellular RNAs were hybridized with cloned
human histone DNA sequences ⋆—⋆, H3 (pF0422);▫—▫ , H4 (pF0108A);
●—●, H2A, H2B, H3 (pFF435).  The DNA synthesis levels are expressed as $^{14}$C-cpm incorporated into DNA by pulse-labeling with
$^{14}$C-thymidine for 30 minutes followed by assaying TCA precipitable
radioactivity, [o—o].  C) and D)  Hybridization of total cellular
RNAs from WI38 human diploid fibroblasts to cloned human histone
DNA sequences (pF0535 and pF0108A) encoding histones H3 and H4
respectively.  The signals shown were obtained using 50μg of
electrophoretically fractionated, nitrocellulose-immobilized
total cellular RNA from WI38 cells isolated at various times after
stimulation (2 hours, 7 hours, 12 hours, 21.5 hours)
and from unstimulated cells C) H3; D) H4.

by these criteria, is not S-phase specific (∿5% of maximal levels).

Are Histone mRNAs Periodically Synthesized During the Cell Cycle? The evidence discussed above indicates that histone protein synthesis is regulated primarily by modulating the cellular levels of histone mRNAs available for translation during S phase. Three possible regulatory mechanisms are invoked by this observation: i) Histone mRNA synthesis is constitutive in the presence of a variable turnover rate; ii) The rate of histone gene transcription varies in the presence of a constant turnover rate; and iii) Both the rates of histone mRNA synthesis and turnover are under cell cycle control. Experiments designed to distinguish among the three are severely complicated, in the case of histone mRNAs, by the fact that histone mRNAs are only transiently present in the nucleus, and by the assumption that histone mRNA turnover occurs predominantly in the cytoplasm. As histone mRNA transport to the cytoplasm occurs within minutes, in vivo pulse labeling experiments are unlikely to yield a definitive indication of transcription rates. Despite these limitations, we have measured the specific activity of histone mRNAs labeled in vivo with $^3$H-uridine for one hour at various times in synchronized HeLa cells. Our choice of a one hour labeling interval was influenced primarily by the specific activity of the total cellular RNA thus produced. The high specific activity (2-3 x 10$^5$ cpm/µg of RNA) permitted the detection of radiolabel incorporation into distinct histone mRNA size classes, and therefore we might detect the differential regulation of member(s) of the heterologous histone mRNA population. It must be emphasized however, that these results reflect both transcriptional and post-transcriptional events.

Radiolabeled total cellular RNA was hybridized to filter-immobilized plasmid DNAs containing cloned human histone gene sequences, and the eluted RNAs were resolved by denaturing polyacrylamide gel electrophoresis. To maximize the complexity of mRNAs hybridizing to the immobilized probe, the temperature of hybridization was kept at 45°C (in 50% [w/v] formamide, see Fig. 10). At this temperature we have observed some cross hybridization with ribosomal RNAs, probably due to the high G:C content of both ribosomal RNA and histone mRNAs. This cross hybridization can be eliminated by increasing the temperature of hybridization to above 48°C, but as shown in Figure 9, this reduces the complexity of detected histone mRNAs. For quantitation therefore, either RNA was hybridized at a higher temperature and radioactivity bound to a pBR322 control was subtracted, or, radioactivity was monitored in specific areas of the polyacrylamide gel after electrophoretic resolution and fluorography of RNAs.

As shown in Figure 14A, there are no obvious qualitative differences in the histone mRNAs synthesized at different times during S phase, either for H4 (pFO108A), H2A + H2B (pFF435B) or H3 (pFF435C). Moreover, the specific activity of any one mRNA size class relative to another in the same sample does not change appreciably as cells traverse S phase. In total, five histone clones (pST512 [H3 + H4], pST519 [H3], pFO108A [H4], pFF435B [H2A + H2B] and pFF435C [H3], see Fig. 9) were used to hybridize total cellular RNA, and the same pattern was observed at two hybridization temperatures (45°C and 48°C) and over a three-fold range of RNA concentration (50-150µg of total cellular RNA/50µg of filter-immobilized plasmid DNA).

The results are quantitatively summarized in Figure 14B along with the observed rates of DNA synthesis and the total histone mRNA levels detected by Northern blot analysis. The maximal incorporation of $^3$H-uridine into histone mRNAs of all size classes occurs between the first and second hour of S phase. As histone mRNA accumulation and DNA synthesis rates have only reached 50-60% of maximal levels after two hours, we conclude that transcription is the predominant regulatory mechanism modulating the concentration of cellular core histone mRNAs in the first half of S phase. We have

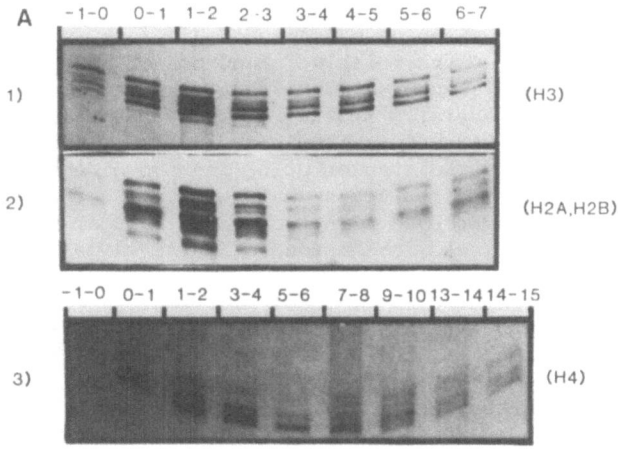

$^3$H-uridine labelling interval (hours after release)

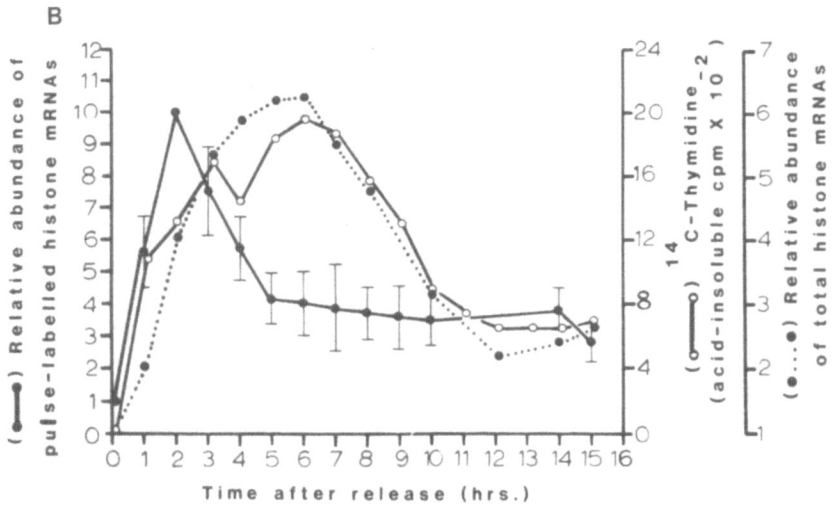

Fig. 14: A. Electrophoretic resolution of histone mRNAs pulse-labeled in vivo for one hour (for the times indicated) after synchronization of HeLa cells by double thymidine blocks. One hundred fifty μg of one hour $^3$H-uridine pulse labeled total cellular RNA was hybrid selected at 45°C with 50μg of filter-immobilized plasmid DNA. Eluted RNAs were electrophoretically resolved on denaturing 6% (w/v) polyacrylamide, 50% urea gels and visualized by fluorography. Histone mRNA selected by 1) pFF435C (H3); 2) by pFF435B (H2A + H2B) and 3) by pF0108A (H4). B. (●──●, ±, S.E.M.) Quantitation for 3 hybrid selections using three probes (pFF435B [H2A + H2B], pFF435C [H3] and pF0108A [H4]). Values were plotted at the end of the hour pulse label, and represent the mean relative abundances of pulse labeled histone H4, H3, or H2A + H2B mRNAs. The DNA synthesis rates (o──o) and the relative abundance of total histone mRNAs (●──●) are reproduced from Figure 11B.

147

observed a 2-3 fold stimulation of total cellular transcription in the first 2-3 hours of S phase, but as this is significantly less than the apparent increase in $^3$H-uridine incorporation into histone mRNAs (Fig. 14B), we conclude that there is a preferential stimulation of histone gene transcription as cells enter S phase. Five to six hours into S phase, a transition point is reached at which both DNA synthesis rates and total histone mRNA levels are maximal, but the relative abundance of pulse-labeled mRNAs is reduced (Fig. 14). Thereafter total histone mRNA levels decrease with an apparent half-life of about 2.0 hours. As the apparent incorporation of $^3$H-uridine into histone mRNAs remains low but relatively constant at this time, we conclude that both the transcription and the mRNA turnover rates are approximately constant in the second half of S phase, but the turnover rate exceeds the rate of synthesis. In the second half of S phase, therefore, the concentration of cellular histone mRNAs is largely regulated at the post-transcriptional level.

It is unclear whether the reduced concentration of pulse-labeled histone mRNAs in the second half of S phase (Fig. 14) represents an S phase-specific "maintenance level" of transcription, or whether it reflects synchrony decay. We therefore examined $^3$H-uridine incorporation into histone mRNA over one hour labeling intervals in cells progressing from G1 to S phase after synchronization by selective mitotic detachment. HeLa cells were pulse labeled at various times after mitotic detachment, and total cellular RNA was hybrid-selected for histone mRNAs, which were then electrophoretically resolved as shown in Figure 15. We observed no obvious qualitative differences in the histone mRNA size classes as cells progressed from G1 to S phase, nor was there a significant change in the specific activity of one mRNA size class relative to another in the sample. As these histone mRNAs are qualitatively equivalent to those from cells synchronized by double thymidine treatment (Fig. 14), we conclude that all the detected histone mRNA size classes are coordinately regulated in the HeLa cell cycle.

The in vivo incorporation of $^3$H-uridine during one hour labeling intervals into histone mRNAs in cells progressing from G1 to S phase is quantitatively summarized in Figure 15B. $^3$H-labeled histone mRNAs are detected in G1 (0-7 hours after mitosis) but these have a significantly lower radiolabel content than those found in S phase (8-12 hours after mitosis) (Fig. 15). There is therefore a detectable but reduced apparent level of transcription in G1 cells. It is not yet clear whether this represents a G1 basal level of transcription, or whether it reflects contamination with a small proportion of S phase cells after mitotic shake-off. As there is not a significant accumulation of histone mRNAs until 8 hours after mitosis (Fig. 15), we infer that the reduced apparent transcription in G1 is insufficient to permit accumulation above the putative G1-specific "basal" histone mRNAs which are translated in the presence of hydroxyurea as described by Wu and Bonner[73].

There is a sharp increase in the relative abundance of pulse-labeled histone mRNAs 7-8 hours after mitosis, and this level does not change significantly over the next four hours (Fig. 15). As maximal histone mRNA levels are not reached until 11 hours after mitosis, we conclude that these data are consistent with maximal histone mRNA synthesis in early S phase, as was observed in cells synchronized by double thymidine treatment (Fig. 14). The relatively constant abundance of pulse-labeled histone mRNAs in early- and mid-S phase after selective mitotic detachment is attributed to the synchrony decay which occurs as cells in G1 enter S phase[93]. These cells therefore probably represent a semisynchronous population which initiates DNA synthesis over a 3-4 hour period.

148

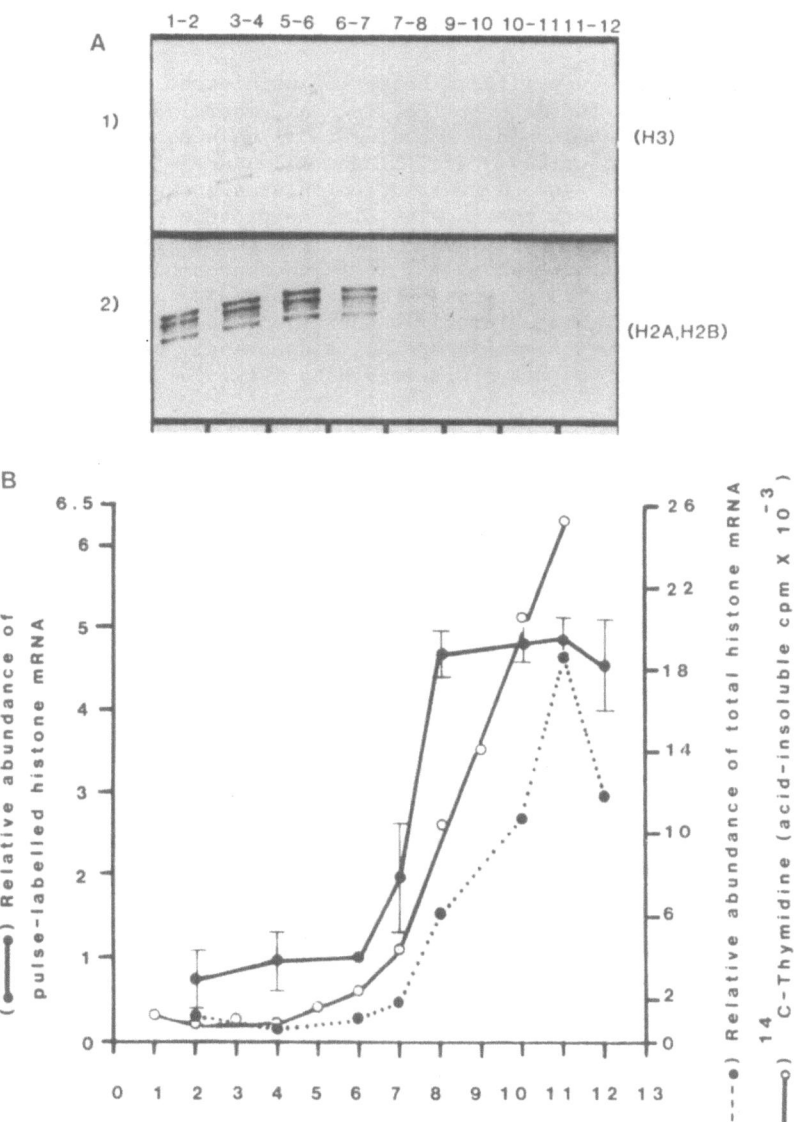

Fig. 15: A. Electrophoretic resolution of histone mRNAs pulse labeled in vivo for one hour (at the times indicated) after synchronization of HeLa cells by selective mitotic detachment. One hundred fifty μg of $^3$H-uridine pulse labeled total cellular RNA was hybridized at 45°C with 50μg of filter-immobilized plasmid DNA. Bound RNAs were eluted and electrophoretically resolved on denaturing 6% (w/v) polyacrylamide, 50% urea gels and visualized by fluorography. RNA selected by 1) pFF435C (H3) and 2) pFF435B (H2A + HB). B. (●—●, ± S.E.M.) Quantitation for 3 hybrid selections using three probes (pFF435B [H2A + H2B], pFF435C [H3] and pFO108A [H4]). Values are plotted at the end of the hour pulse label, and represent the mean relative abundances of pulse-labeled histone H4, H3 or H2A + H2B mRNAs. The DNA synthesis rates (o—o) and the

relative abundance of total histone mRNAs (o---o) are reproduced
from Figure 12B.

## Is There More Than One Type of Regulation of Histone Gene Expression?

We have shown that over fifteen heterologous histone mRNAs are coordinately regulated during the HeLa cell cycle. A temporal coupling between
cellular histone mRNA levels and DNA synthesis rates has now been demonstrated for both HeLa S3 cells[52] (Figs. 11 and 12) and WI-38 human diploid
fibroblasts[83] (Fig. 13). As the relative cellular abundance of histone
mRNAs closely parallels both the in vivo histone protein synthesis reported
for cells under equivalent conditions[70],[71],[78] and the in vitro translata-
bility of polysomal histone mRNAs[94]-[96], it is not unreasonable to propose
that histone gene expression (histone protein synthesis) is regulated
primarily by modulating the cellular concentration of histone mRNAs available for translation. Histone mRNA synthesis apparently precedes maximal
accumulation of mRNAs in both synchronized HeLa (Fig. 16) and yeast[97]

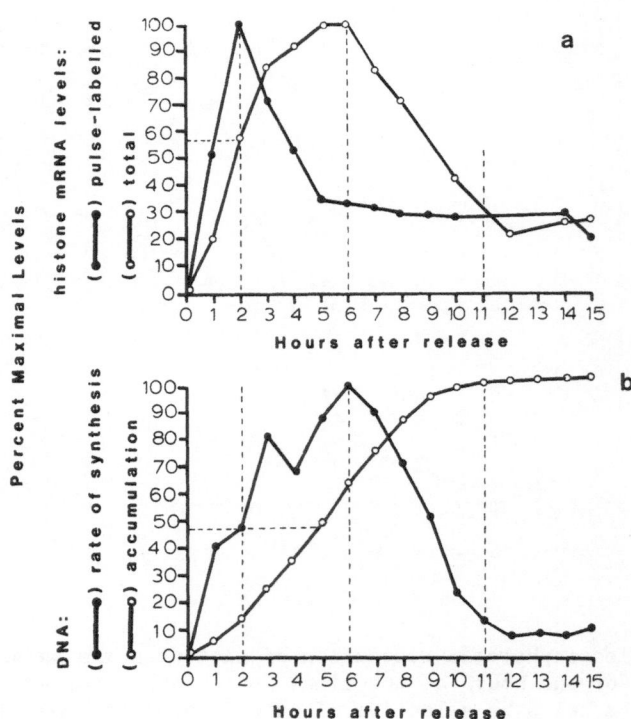

Fig. 16: Summaries for the data obtained for cells synchronized by double
thymidine blocks. Data are expressed as the percentage maximal
levels detected above those observed in cells just before release
from the second thymidine block. a): (o—o) The relative abundance
of total histone mRNA. (●—●) The relative incorporation of $^3$H-
uridine into histone mRNA in one hour labeling intervals, plotted
at the end of the pulse. b): (●—●) Relative rates of DNA synthesis monitored by pulse labeling with $^{14}$C-thymidine; (o—o)
Accumulation of DNA calculated from the rates of DNA.

cells, indicating that the cellular abundance of histone mRNAs in early S phase is predominantly under transcriptional control. For the moment, we cannot determine whether the onset of histone gene transcription in HeLa cells precedes the initiation of DNA synthesis, as is apparently the case in yeast[97], although our data (Fig. 15) would suggest that the two occur within 30 minutes of each other ( ∿6% of the HeLa S phase).

In the second half of the HeLa S phase, cellular histone mRNA levels are regulated predominantly at the post-transcriptional level as suggested by the decay of cellular histone mRNAs with apparent half-lives of 2.0 hours, and by the reduced and relatively constant incorporation of $^3$H-uridine into histone mRNAs. These data are compatible with constant rates of both synthesis and turnover of histone mRNAs in the second half of S phase, but with the turnover rate exceeding the rate of synthesis. As studies in HeLa and yeast cells[52,97] suggest that histone gene transcription rates vary during S phase, it is now of interest to determine whether the turnover of histone mRNAs varies during the cell cycle, in order to determine whether only one level of regulation (regulated transcription) or two (regulated synthesis and turnover) is responsible for the control of histone gene expression.

As a working model, we propose that the turnover of histone mRNAs remains constant throughout the cell cycle of HeLa cells. This model is consistent with Perry and Kelley's observation[98] that the mean lifetime of polysomal histone mRNAs in exponentially growing mouse L cells is equal to the length of S phase. As will be discussed below, however, histone mRNA destabilization can be induced, but this may reflect a secondary regulatory mechanism which is only applied under extreme biological circumstances. Our working model therefore relies predominantly on the regulation of histone mRNA synthesis. In early S phase an elevated transcription rate permits the accumulation of histone mRNAs, and histone mRNA levels decrease in late S phase after the reduction of transcription allows the decay of histone mRNA in the presence of a constant turnover rate. Furthermore, the abundance of pulse-labeled histone mRNAs and the kinetics of accumulation of histone mRNAs in early S phase are suggestive of a feedback regulatory mechanism. One possibility currently being investigated is that histone gene replication is temporally and functionally related to transcription of the histone genes.

## Can Histone Gene Expression Be Uncoupled From DNA Replication?

Other potential regulatory aspects of human histone gene expression are suggested by observations reported for other biological systems. For example, the differential expression of "early" and "late" histone gene clusters in developing sea urchin embryos[99-101] has stimulated the search for an analogous situation in higher eucaryotes. It is becoming evident that differential translation of variant histone proteins occurs during the cell cycle[73,74] and differential expression of histones during development of higher eucaryotes has also been observed[102,103]. In lower eucaryotes, histone gene expression immediately prior to and shortly after fertilization is regulated almost exclusively at post-transcriptional levels. During the extremely rapid rate of cell division just after fertilization, it appears that developing Xenopus oocytes rely predominantly on a maternal store of histone proteins[104] and sea urchin embryos rely predominantly on a maternal store of histone mRNAs[101,105-107], to provide the histone proteins required for packaging the rapidly replicating DNA. Although the rate of cell division of embryos in higher eucaryotes is significantly slower, it is of some interest to determine whether such post-transcriptional regulation occurs during early development and whether there are equivalants of the "early" and "late" histone genes of lower eucaryotes.

As has been described above, there is a plethora of information which supports temporal coupling of histone gene expression and DNA replication. Although the molecular basis for the coupling remains to be elucidated, it is becoming clear that the inhibition of DNA synthesis by a variety of un-related exogenous cellular perturbations results in a parallel decrease in cellular histone mRNA levels, and an equivalent decrease in histone protein synthesis. Early studies, for example, established that the inhibition of DNA replication by metabolic inhibitors (hydroxyurea[73,74,95,96,108-113], cytosine arabinoside[70,71,94,96,98,113-115] and actinomycin D[109,110,112,114,116]) resulted in the rapid reduction of histone protein synthesis and the loss of polysomal histone mRNAs. More recently we have monitored total cellular levels of histone mRNAs following the inhibition of DNA replication by: a) Metabolic inhibitors[117,118] and b) after shifting temperature-sensitive cell cycle mutants to the nonpermissive temperature (Hirshhorn et al., Biochem. 23:3731 (1984)). In these cases, the perturbation of distinct cellular processes resulted in both the inhibition of DNA re-plication and an equivalent reduction in total cellular histone mRNA levels.

When DNA replication is completely (~ 95%) inhibited by compounds which disrupt the metabolism of deoxynucleotide precursors (100 $\mu$M cytosine arabinoside or 1mM hydroxyurea, see Fig. 17) or which inhibit DNA polymerase $\alpha$ (2$\mu$g/ml aphidicolin[90,118,119]; see Fig. 17), the cellular representation of histone mRNAs is reduced to an inhibitor-resistant "basal level" cor-responding to approximately 10% of the levels observed in exponentially growing cells, and reduced to approximately 6% of the peak levels observed in synchronized S phase HeLa cells. These estimates for "basal levels" of histone mRNAs are quantitatively consistent with the basal levels of histone protein synthesis observed in G1 and S phase cells in the presence of 1mM hydroxyurea[73,74,117,118]. Both the inhibition of DNA synthesis and the decay of histone mRNA occurred with apparent half-lives of less than 10 minutes. These kinetics differ significantly from the reported mean life-time of 9 hours for polysomal histone mRNAs in exponentially growing L cells[98], and also differ from the estimated apparent histone mRNA half-lives of 2.0 hours described above for the latter part of S phase in synchronized HeLa cells[52,117,118] (See Fig. 16). The inhibitors therefore apparently cause the rapid destabilization of histone mRNAs. Such a post-transcrip-tional coupling is supported by the observation that after transcriptional inhibition with 5$\mu$g/ml actinomycin D, cellular histone mRNA levels decay in parallel with inhibition of DNA synthesis (85% inhibition after 2 hours[117,118] despite complete inhibition of transcription with 6 minutes. Additional support for the coupling of histone gene expression and DNA replication being mediated at a post-transcriptional level comes from ex-perimental results showing that: 1) Inhibition of RNA synthesis does not affect either the kinetics or extent of the hydroxyurea-induced destabiliz-ation of cellular histone mRNAs[118] and 2) Protein synthesis is required for histone mRNA turnover -- in untreated cells or following inhibition of DNA replication[118].

We are presently examining the coupling of DNA synthesis and histone mRNA levels under conditions which result in the incomplete inhibition of DNA synthesis - using reduced concentrations of the metabolic inhibitors hydroxyurea (10$\mu$M - 1mM), cytosine arabinoside (7nm - 100$\mu$M) and aphidicolin (10ng/L-2mg/L). As shown in Figure 17, partial inhibition of DNA synthesis results in the stoichiometric reduction of total cellular histone mRNAs ir-respective of the inhibitor or its concentration. Time course experiments have indicated that both the rate of DNA synthesis and level of histone mRNAs equilibrate within 30 minutes of the metabolic perturbation, implying that the primary coupling mechanism occurs at the post-transcriptional level. The tightness and functionality of this relationship between DNA replication and cellular histone mRNA levels are indicated by the rapid and

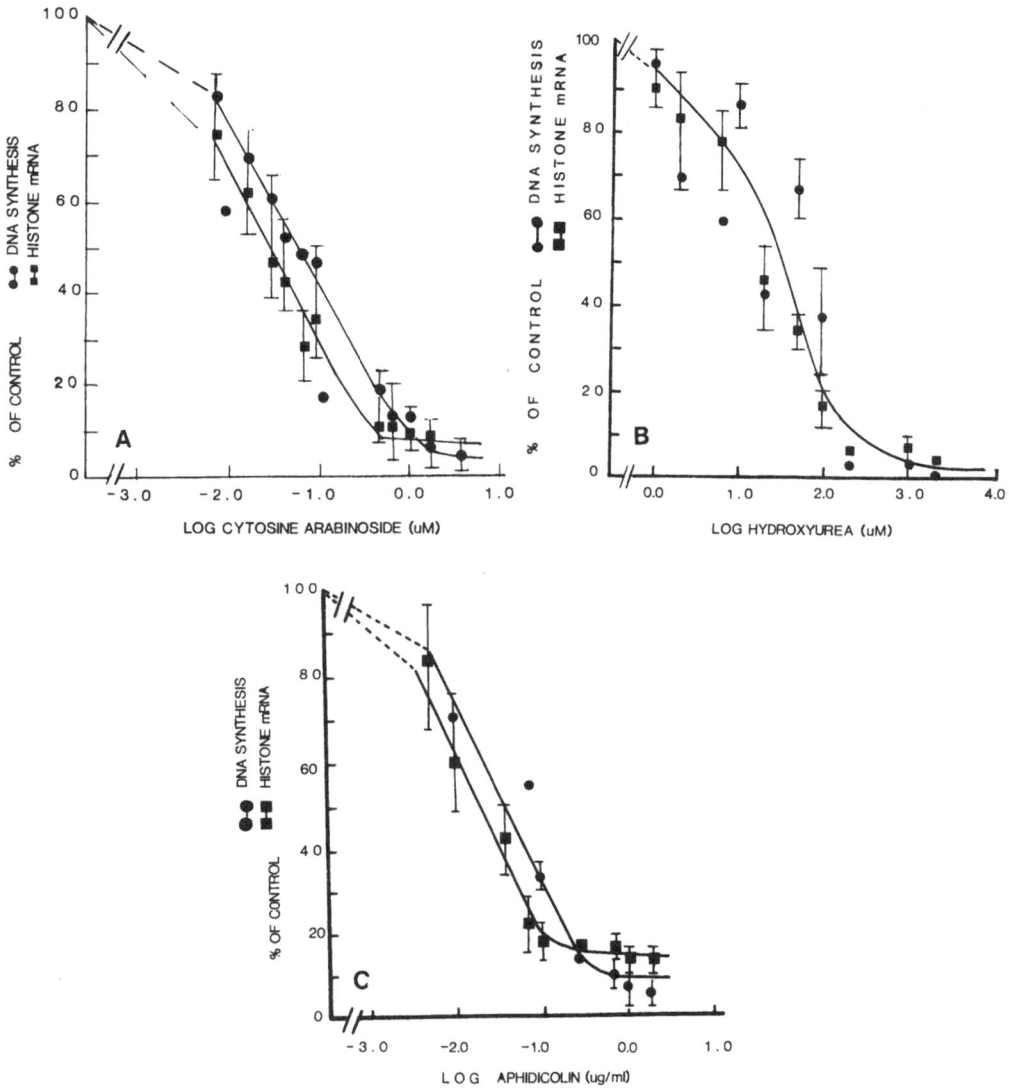

Fig. 17: The effects of A) cytosine arabinoside, B) hydroxyurea and C) aphidicolin on histone mRNA levels and DNA synthesis in exponentially growing HeLa cells. DNA synthesis was monitored by incorporation of [3]H-thymidine ($2\mu$Ci/ml and $4 \times 10^5$ cells/ml) into 10% TCA precipitable material. Cells were pretreated for 30 minutes with each of the various inhibitors and then pulse-labeled for 30 minutes. Total cellular RNA was prepared and histone mRNA steady-state levels determined as described in Figure 11. Each value represents the mean of five Northern blots using various histone gene probes: pF0108A (H4), pFF435B (H2A + H2B), pFF435C (H3), pST519D (H3) and pF0535 (H3).

parallel restoration of both processes following release from DNA synthesis inhibition[117].

As our studies on the effects of metabolic inhibitors discussed above only yielded a generalized indication of the fate of the core histone mRNAs

after complete or partial inhibition of DNA synthesis, it was of interest
to determine whether coordinate regulation of the expression of the polymorphic histone gene family was operative. This question was also relevant
to the observations that specific histone variant proteins are differentially
synthesized in G1, $G1_0$ and S phase cells exposed to 1mM hydroxyurea[73],[74].
We have initially approached this problem by posing three questions: i) Are
S phase newly synthesized multiple histone mRNAs differentially turned over
in the presence of 1mM hydroxyurea? ii) Are specific histone mRNA subspecies
differentially transcribed in S phase cells exposed to 1mM hydroxyurea? and
iii) Are specific histone mRNAs differentially sensitive to destabilization
by 1mM hydroxyurea at different times in the cell cycle? Using the hybrid
selection of $^3$H-uridine pulse-labeled histone mRNAs to visualize the incorporation of radiolabel into more than 15 distinct histone mRNA size
classes, we have found: a) that the levels of these multiple histone mRNA
species are apparently coordinately controlled at the post-transcriptional
level when HeLa cells with pre-labeled histone mRNAs are exposed to hydroxyurea either before, during or after S phase (see Fig. 18 A), and b) that the
incorporation of $^3$H-uridine into the multiple histone mRNA species is
reduced, but both qualitatively and quantitatively similar, after cells at
various times in the cell cycle have been pre-treated with 1mM hydroxyurea
for 30 minutes (see Fig. 18B).

Several cautionary provisos must be maintained when interpreting these
results. As alluded to earlier (Fig. 10), the detection of $^3$H-uridine
pulse-labeled histone mRNAs is largely governed by the choice of probe and
the hybridization conditions used. It is therefore possible that, with the
probes we have used, we are not detecting all histone mRNA species and that
those not detected may be regulated by a distinct mechanism. Similarly,
we have relied to a greater or lesser degree on the assumption that the
turnover of all histone mRNA species is sufficiently high to detect incorporation of $^3$H-uridine in one hour pulse periods, but this assumption
may not be valid. Finally, it must be emphasized that the interpretation
of data obtained from perturbed cells may in fact reflect a secondary
(fail-safe) regulatory mechanism which is not normally operative during the
G1-S-G2 transitions. It is also possible that histone gene expression is
functionally coupled to DNA replication by means of the histone gene products themselves, as it is not unreasonable to predict that the constitutive synthesis of histone proteins would severely affect cell viability.

Fig. 18: A. The effect of hydroxyurea on S-phase HeLa histone mRNA species
prelabeled with $^3$H-uridine at various times after release from
double thymidine block synchronization. At -1.5, 1, 4.5 and 9.5
hours after release from thymidine, cells were labeled with $^3$H-
uridine (0.1mCi/ml and 2.5 x $10^6$ cells /ml) for one hour and then
exposed to 1mM hydroxyurea for 30 minutes in the presence of
radiolabel. Control cells (not treated with hydroxyurea) were
labeled for 90 minutes over the same time intervals. Total cellular RNA was prepared and 300µg hybridized at 43°C to filter-immobilized plasmid DNA as described in Figure 7. Bound RNAs were
eluted, resolved electrophoretically and visualized by fluorography. B. The incorporation of $^3$H-uridine into S phase HeLa
histone mRNA species after 30 minutes pretreatment with hydroxyurea
at various times after release from double thymidine block synchronization. At -1.5, 1, 4.5 and 9.5 hours after release, cells
were treated for 30 minutes with 1mM hydroxyurea, and then labeled
for one hour with $^3$H-uridine (0.1mCi/ml and 2.5 x $10^6$ cells/ml)
in the presence of hydroxyurea. Control cells were labeled for
one hour of the 1.5 hour time interval. Total cellular RNA was
prepared and 300µg hybridized at 43°C to filter-immobilized
plasmid DNA as described in Figure 7. Bound RNAs were eluted,
resolved electrophoretically and visualized by fluorography.

Hours after release

| ³H-uridine labelling intervals | (prerelease) −1.5−0 | | 1−2.5 | | 5−6.5 | | 10−11.5 | |
|---|---|---|---|---|---|---|---|---|
| 1mM hydroxyurea treatments | − | −0.5−0 | − | 2−2.5 | − | 6−6.5 | − | 11−11.5 |

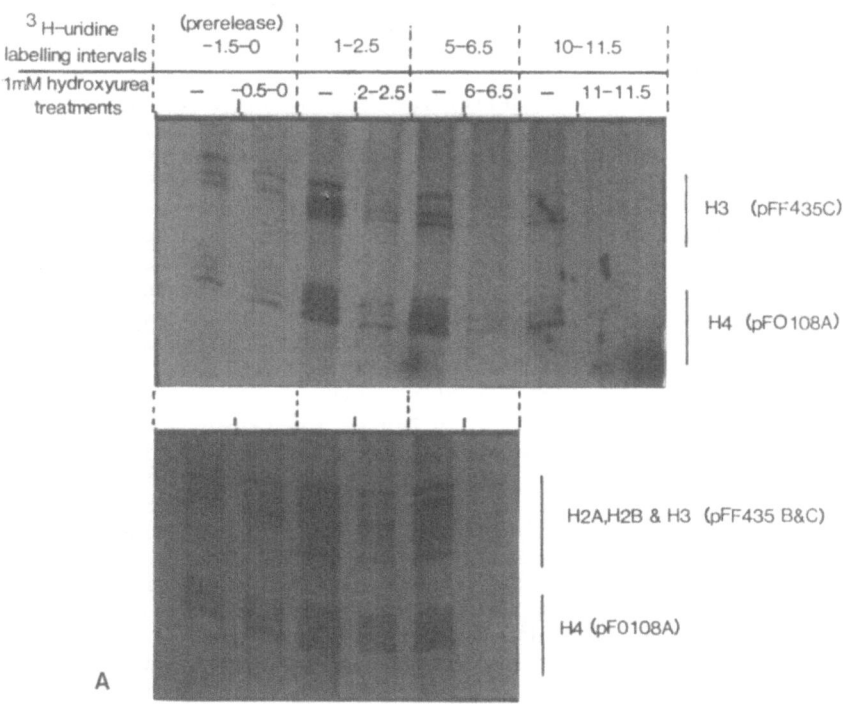

H3 (pFF435C)

H4 (pFO108A)

H2A,H2B & H3 (pFF435 B&C)

H4 (pFO108A)

A

Hours after release

| ³H-uridine labelling intervals | (prerelease) −1−0 | | 1.5−2.5 | | 5.5−6.5 | | 10.5−11.5 | |
|---|---|---|---|---|---|---|---|---|
| 1mM hydroxyurea treatments | − | −1.5−0 | 1−2.5 | − | − | 5−6.5 | − | 10−11.5 |

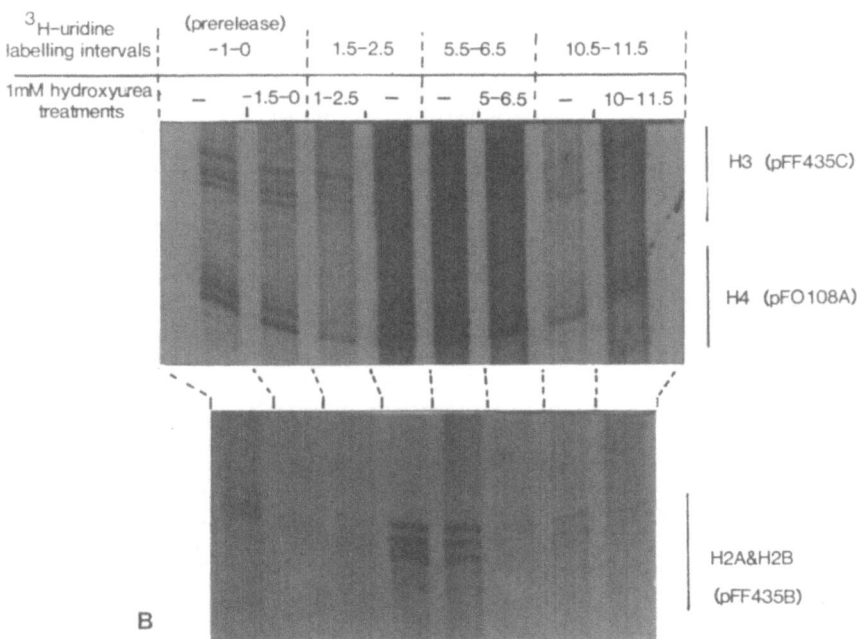

H3 (pFF435C)

H4 (pFO108A)

H2A&H2B (pFF435B)

B

## CONCLUSIONS AND SPECULATION

Specific mechanisms which are operative in the regulation of human histone gene expression and the molecular events responsible for the functional coupling of DNA synthesis with cellular histone mRNA levels remain to be established. Yet, it appears that a viable model must account for a) the onset of histone gene transcription and accumulation of histone mRNAs at the beginning of S phase; b) the decline in transcription of histone mRNAs early in S phase; and c) the rapid destabilization of histone mRNAs concomitant with the termination of DNA replication at the natural end of S phase or following inhibition of DNA synthesis. One possibility we have been considering which would be compatible with these cellular events is autogenous control of histone gene expression. Termination of DNA replication results in an immediate loss of binding sites for newly synthesized histone proteins which might bring about a transient accumulation of "unbound histones". These unbound histones could modify the histone translation complex, via interactions with polysomal histone mRNAs, in such a manner as to render histone mRNAs susceptible to cellular ribonucleases. This type of mechanism could be operative solely at the post-transcriptional level and would be compatible with the rapid, RNA synthesis-independent destabilization of histone mRNAs which occurs following inhibition of DNA replication as well as with the requirement for protein synthesis (in this case we are postulating synthesis of histones) for the histone mRNA destabilization to be initiated. It is unnecessary to invoke regulation of cellular nucleases, which could be expressed constitutively. The onset and/or termination of histone gene transcription could be functionally related to the initiation of DNA synthesis. At that time availability of newly replicated DNA could provide "high affinity" binding sites for newly synthesized histone proteins which would be actively involved in packaging DNA into nucleosomes and thereby unavailable for "feedback" to the histone translation complex.

Initiation of DNA synthesis may itself be sufficient to account for the onset and termination of histone gene transcription if one postulates that conformational modifications in the histone genes render them accessible to RNA polymerase and other molecules required for expression. The credibility of this line of reasoning is supported by the recent observations that human histone genes replicate early in S phase at approximately the time they are transcribed (Plumb, Schildkraut, Stein and Stein, unpublished observations) and that deletion of a functional origin of replication (ars element) associated with yeast histone gene uncouples the expression of the genes and DNA synthesis. Whether or not this model we are proposing reflects the regulatory processes which are occurring in intact cells, remains to be established. But the model is attractive because it circumvents the need to postulate a complex array of regulatory macromolecules which recognize specific genetic loci, the levels of each such putative regulatory macromolecule itself requiring control. Moreover, while perhaps an oversimplification of the molecular events related to genome replication in living cells, the various elements of our model are biologically rational and most important are amenable to experimental verification.

In this chapter we have restricted our considerations to the regulation of histone genes, a specific set of repetitive genetic sequences which are differentially expressed during the cell cycle. Of broader biological relevance is the relationship between expression of histone genes and of other genetic sequences required for execution of the proliferative process. While it is well documented that cell proliferation involves a complex and

interdependent series of biochemical events, the molecular basis for the
control of these events or for their interrelationship remains to be
resolved. An intriguing possibility is that genetic sequences whose expression is related to specific cell cycle processes are coordinately controlled. Within this context it is tempting to postulate that genes
functionally related to DNA replication share common structural and/or
regulatory elements. Do histone genes and other S phase-specific sequences
respond to similar cellular signals or regulatory molecules? These questions are being approached experimentally and will establish the credibility
of such speculation.

ACKNOWLEDGEMENT:

Studies described in this chapter were supported by grants PCM80-18075
and PCM81-18951 from the National Science Foundation 1-813 from the March
of Dimes Birth Defects Foundation and GM32010 from the National Institutes
of Health.

REFERENCES

1. R. M. Lawn, E. F. Fritsch, R. C. Parker, G. Blake, and T. Maniatis,
   The isolation and characterization of linked δ- and β-globin genes
   from a cloned library of human DNA, Cell 15:1157-1174 (1978).

2. R. P. Lifton, M. L. Goldberg, R. W. Karp, and D. S. Hogness, The
   organization of the histone genes in Drosophila melanogaster:
   functional and evolutionary implications, Cold Spring Harbor Symp.
   Quant. Biol. 42:1047-1051 (1977).

3. K. Gross, W. Schaffner, J. Telford, and M. Birnstiel, Molecular analysis
   of the histone gene cluster of Psammechinus miliaris: III. Polarity
   and asymmetry of the histone-coding sequences, Cell 8:479-484 (1976).

4. M. Wu, D. S. Holmes, N. Davidson, R. H. Cohn, and L. H. Kedes, The
   relative positions of sea urchin histone genes on the chimeric
   plasmids pSp2 and pSp17 as studied by electron microscopy, Cell
   9:163-169 (1976).

5. M. C. Wilson and M. Melli, Determination of the number of histone genes
   in human DNA, J. Mol. Biol. 110:511-535 (1977).

6. L. C. Yu, P. Szabo, T. W. Borun, and W. Prensky, The localization of
   the genes coding for histone H4 in human chromosomes, Cold Spring
   Harbor Symp. Quant. Biol. 42:1101-1105 (1977).

7. M. E. Chandler, L. H. Kedes, R. H. Cohn, and J. J. Yunis, Genes coding
   for histone proteins in man are located on the distal end of the
   long arm of chromosome 7, Science 205:908-910 (1979).

8. F. Sierra, A. Lichtler, F. Marashi, R. Rickles, T. Van Dyke, S. Clark,
   J. Wells, G. Stein, and J. Stein, Organization of hyman histone
   genes, Proc. Natl. Acad. Sci. USA 79:1795-1799 (1982).

9. N. Carozzi, F. Marashi, M. Plumb, S. Zimmerman, A. Zimmerman, J. R. E.
   Wells, G. Stein, and J. Stein, Clustering of human H1 and core
   histone genes, Science 22:41115 (1984).

10. N. Heintz, M. Zernik, and R. G. Roeder, The structure of the human histone genes: clustered but not tandemly repeated, Cell 24:661-668 (1981).

11. S. J. Clark, Chicken and human histone genes, Ph.D. Thesis, University of Adelaide, Adelaide, Australia (1982).

12. L. M. Hereford, K. Fahrner, J. Woolford, and M. Rosbash, Isolation of yeast histone genes H2A and H2B, Cell 18:1261-1271 (1979).

13. J. W. Wallis, L. Hereford, and M. Grunstein, Histone H2B genes of yeast encode two different proteins, Cell 22:799-805 (1980).

14. M. M. Smith, The organization of the yeast histone gene, in: "Histone Genes," G. S. Stein, J. L. Stein, and W. F. Marzluff, eds. John Wiley and Sons, New York, (1984).

15. M. Zernik, N. Heintz, I. Boime, and R. G. Roeder, Xenopus laevis histone genes: variant H1 genes are present in different clusters, Cell 22:807-815 (1980).

16. A. F. Moorman, R. T. de Laaf, O. H. Destree, J. Telford, and M. L. Birnstiel, Histone genes from Xenopus laevis: molecular cloning and initial characterization, Gene 10:185-193 (1980).

17. W. Van Dongen, L. deLaaf, R. Zaal, A. Moorman, and O. Destree, The organization of the histone genes in the genome of Xenopus laevis, Nucl. Acids Res. 9:2297-2311 (1981).

18. E. C. Stephenson, H. P. Erba, and J. G. Gall, Histone gene clusters of the Newt Notophthalmus are separated by long tracts of satellite DNA, Cell 24:639-647 (1981).

19. J. G. Gall, E. C. Stephenson, H. P. Erba, M. O. Diaz, and G. Barsacchi-Pilone, Histone genes are located at the sphere loci of Newt Lampbrush chromosomes, Chromosoma 84:159-171 (1981).

20. E. C. Stephenson, Organization and expression of Newt histone genes, in: "Histone Genes," G. S. Stein, J. L. Stein, and W. F. Marzluff, eds. John Wiley and Sons, New York (1984).

21. R. P. Harvey, J. R. E. Wells, Chicken histones and their variants, in: "Histone Genes," G. S. Stein, J. L. Stein,aand W. F. Marzluff, eds. John Wiley and Sons, New York (1984).

22. J. C. Engel,Organization and expression of chicken histone genes, in: "Histone Genes," G. S. Stein, J. L. Stein, and W. F. Marzluff, eds., John Wiley and Sons, New York (1984).

23. A. Seiler-Tuyns and M. L. Birnstiel, Structure and expression in L-cells of a cloned H4 histone gene of the mouse, J. Mol. Biol. 151:607-625 (1981).

24. W. F. Marzluff, Organization and expression of mouse histone genes, in: "Histone Genes," G. S. Stein, J. L. Stein, and W. F. Marzluff, eds., John Wiley and Sons, New York (1984).

25. R. J. Britten and E. H. Davidson, Gene regulation for higher cells. A Theory, Science 165:349-357 (1969).

26. R. Britten and D. E. Kohne, Repeated sequences in DNA, Science 161: 529-540 (1968).

27. E. H. Davidson, G. A. Galau, R. C. Angerer, and R. J. Britten, Comparative aspects of DNA organization in metazoa, Chromosoma 51:253-259 (1975).

28. W. R. Jelinek and C. W. Schmid, Repetitive sequences in eukaryotic DNA and their expression, Ann. Rev. Biochem. 51:813-844 (1982).

29. C. M. Houck, F. P. Rinehart, and C. W. Schmid, A ubiquitous family of repeated DNA sequences in the human genome, J. Mol. Biol. 132: 289-306 (1979).

30. F. Sierra, A. Leza, F. Marashi, M. Plumb, R. Rickles, T. Van Dyke, S. Clark, J. R. E. Wells, G. S. Stein, and J. L. Stein, Human histone genes are interspersed with members of the Alu family and with other transcribed sequences. Biochem. Biophys. Res. Comm. 104:785-792 (1982).

31. I. Isenberg, Histones, Ann. Rev. Biochem. 48:159-191 (1979).

32. A. C. Lichtler, F. Sierra, S. Clark, J. R. E. Wells, J. L. Stein, and G. S. Stein, Multiple H4 histone mRNAs of HeLa cells are encoded in different genes, Nature 298:195-198 (1982).

33. A. C. Lichtler, S. Detke, I. R. Phillips, G. S. Stein, and J. L. Stein, Multiple forms of H4 histone mRNA in human cells, Proc. Natl. Acad. Sci, USA 77:1942-1946 (1980).

34. M. Grunstein, S. Levy, P. Schedl, and L. Kedes, Messenger RNAs for individual histone proteins: fingerprint analysis and in vitro translation, Cold Spring Harbor Symp. on Quant. Biol. 38:717-724 (1973).

35. W. Schaffner, G. Kunz, H. Daetwyler, J. Telford, H. O. Smith, and M. L. Birnstiel, Genes and spacers of cloned sea urchin histone DNA analyzed by sequencing, Cell 14:655-671 (1978).

36. M. Busslinger, R. Portmann, J. C. Irminger, and M. L. Birnstiel, Ubiquitous and gene-specific regulatory 5' sequences in a sea urchin histone DNA clone coding for histone protein variants, Nucl. Acids Res. 8:957-977 (1980).

37. Y. Ohe, H. Hayashi, and K. Iwai, Human spleen histone H2B, J. Biochem. 85:615-624 (1979).

38. F. Marashi, K. Prokopp, J. Stein, and G. Stein, Evidence for a human histone gene cluster containing H2B and H2A pseudogene, Proc. Natl. Acad. Sci. USA, 81:1936 (1984).

39. C. C. Hentschel and M. L. Birnstiel, The organization and expression of histone gene families, Cell 25:301-313 (1981).

40. R. P. Harvey, A. J. Robins, and J. R. E. Wells, Independently evolving chicken H2B genes: identification of a ubiquitous H2B-specific 5' element, Nucl. Acids Res. 10:7851-7863 (1982).

41. E. F. Fritsch, R. M. Lawn, and T. Maniatis, Molecular cloning and characterization of the human β-like globin gene cluster, Cell 19:959-972 (1980).

42. J. Lauer, C. K. J. Shen, and T. Maniatis, The chromosomal arrangement of human α-like globin genes: sequence homology and α-globin gene deletions, Cell 20:119-130 (1980).

43. F. Sierra, G. Stein, and J. Stein, Structure and in vitro transcription of a human H4 histone gene, Nucl. Acids. Res. 11:7069-7086 (1983).

44. R. Lewin, How mammalian RNA returns to its genome, Science 219:1052-1054 (1983).

45. C. D. Wilde, C. E. Crowther, T. P. Cripe, M. Gwo-Shu Lee, and N. J. Cowan, Evidence that a human α-tubulin pseudogene is derived from its corresponding mRNA, Nature 297:83-84 (1982).

46. Y. Nishioka, A. Leder, and P. Leder, Unusual α-globin-like gene that has cleanly lost both globin intervening sequences, Proc. Natl. Acad. Sci. USA 77:2806-2809 (1980).

47. G. F. Hollis, P. A. Hieter, O. W. McBride, D. Swan, and P. Leder, Processed genes: a dispersed human immunoglobin gene bearing evidence of RNA-type processing, Nature 296:321-325 (1982).

48. P. Jagadeeswaran, B. G. Forget, and S. M. Weissman, Short interspersed repetitive DNA elements in eucaryotes: transposable DNA elements generated by reverse transcription of RNA Pol III transcripts? Cell 26:141-142 (1981).

49. N. J. Proudfoot and T. Maniatis, The structure of a human α-globin pseudogene and its relationship to α-globin gene duplication, Cell 21:537-544 (1980).

50. E. Lacy and T. Maniatis, The nucleotide sequence of a rabbit β-globin pseudogene. Cell 21:545-553 (1980).

51. G. Childs, R. Maxson, R. H. Cohn, and L. Kedes, Orphons: dispersed genetic elements derived from tandem repetitive genes of eucaryotes, Cell 23:651-663 (1981).

52. M. Plumb, J. Stein, and G. Stein, Coordinate regulation of multiple histone mRNAs during the cell cycle in HeLa cells, Nucl. Acids. Res. 11:2391-2410 (1983).

53. J. A. Engle, B. J. Sugarman, and J. B. Dodgson, A chicken histone H3 gene contains intervening sequences, Nature 297:434-436 (1982).

54. A. Efstratiadis, J. W. Posakony, T. Maniatis, R. M. Lawn, C. O'Connell, R. A. Spritz, J. K. de Riel, B. G. Forget, S. M. Weissman, J. L. Slightom, A. E. Blechl, O. Smithies, F. E. Baralle, C. C. Shoulders, and N. J. Proudfoot, The structure and evolution of the human β-globin gene family, Cell 21:653-668 (1980).

55. C. Benoist, K. O'Hare, R. Breathnach, and P. Chambon, The ovalbumin gene sequence of putative control regions, Nucl. Acids Res. 8:127-142 (1980).

56. L. H. Kedes, Histone genes and histone messengers, Ann. Rev. Biochem. 48:837-870 (1979).

57. R. Tjian, T antigen binding and the control of SV40 gene expression, Cell 26:1-2 (1981).

58. J. Banerji, S. Rusconi, and W. Schaffner, Expression of a β-globin

gene is enhanced by remote SV40 DNA sequences, <u>Cell</u> 27:299-308 (1981).

59. L. J. Korn and D. D. Brown, Nucleotide sequence of <u>Xenopus</u> <u>borealis</u> oocyte 5S DNA: Comparison of sequences that flank several related eucaryotic genes, <u>Cell</u> 15:1145-1156 (1978).

60. C. Birchmeier, R. Grosschedl, and M. L. Birnstiel, Generation of authentic 3' termini of an H2B mRNA <u>in</u> <u>vivo</u> is dependent on a short inverted DNA repeat and on spacer sequence, <u>Cell</u> 28:739-745 (1982).

61. J. L. Manley, A. Fire, A. Cano, P. A. Sharp, and M. L. Geftner, DNA-dependent transcription of adenovirus genes in a soluble whole-cell extract, <u>Proc. Natl. Acad. Sci USA</u> 77:3855-3859 (1980).

62. S. Detke, J. L. Stein, and G. S. Stein, Synthesis of histone messenger RNAs by RNA polymerase II in nuclei from S phase HeLa S3 cells, <u>Nucl. Acids Res.</u> 5:1515-1528 (1978).

63. R. Grosschedl and M. L. Birnstiel, Spacer DNA sequences upstream of the T-A-T-A-A-A-T-A sequence are essential for promotion of H2A histone gene transcription <u>in</u> <u>vivo</u>, Proc. Natl. Acad. Sci. <u>USA</u> 77:7102-7106 (1980).

64. G. C. Grosveld, C. K. Shewmaker, P. Jat, and R. A. Flavell, Localization of DNA sequences necessary for transcription of the rabbit β-globin gene <u>in</u> <u>vitro</u>, <u>Cell</u> 25:215-226 (1981).

65. R. Grosschedl and M. L. Birnstiel, Delimitation of far upstream sequences required for maximal <u>in</u> <u>vitro</u> transcription of an H2A histone gene, <u>Proc. Natl. Acad. Sci. USA</u> 79:297-301 (1982).

66. J. Pan, J. T. Elder, C. H. Duncan, and S. M. Weissman, Structural analysis of interspersed repetitive polymerase III transcription units in human DNA, <u>Nucl. Acids Res.</u> 9:1151-1170 (1981).

67. J. L. Manley and M. T. Colozzo, Synthesis <u>in</u> <u>vitro</u> of an exceptionally long RNA transcript promoted by an AluI sequence, <u>Nature</u> 300:376-379 (1982).

68. P. K. Ghosh, V. B. Reddy, J. Swinscoe, P. Lebowitz, and S. M. Weissman, Heterogeneity and 5'-terminal structures of the late DNAs of Simian Virus 40, <u>J. Mol. Biol.</u> 126:813-846 (1978).

69. N. J. Proudfoot, M. H. M. Shander, J. L. Manley, M. L. Gefter, and T. Maniatis, Structure and <u>in</u> <u>vitro</u> transcription of human globin genes, <u>Science</u> 209:1329-1336 (1980).

70. F. Marashi, L. Baumbach, R. Rickles, F. Sierra, J. L. Stein, and G. S. Stein, Histone proteins in HeLa S3 cells are synthesized in a cell cycle stage specific manner. <u>Science</u> 215:683-685 (1982).

71. J. Spalding, K. Kajiwara, and G. C. Mueller, The metabolism of basic proteins in HeLa cell nuclei, <u>Proc. Natl. Acad. Sci. USA</u> 56:1535-1542 (1966).

72. G. Stein and T. W. Borun. The synthesis of acidic chromosomal proteins during the cell cycle of HeLa S3 cells, <u>J. Cell Biol.</u> 52:292-307 (1972).

73. R. S. Wu and W. M. Bonner, Separation of basal histone synthesis from S phase histone synthesis in dividing cells, <u>Cell</u> 27:321-330 (1981).

74.  R. S. Wu, S. Tsai, and W. M. Bonner, Patterns of histone variant synthesis can distinguish G0 from G1 cells, <u>Cell</u> 31:367-374 (1982).

75.  M. A. Tarnowka, C. Baglioni, and C. Basilico, Synthesis of H1 histone by BHK cells in G1, <u>Cell</u> 15:163-171 (1978).

76.  I-M. Chiu and W. F. Marzluff, Uncoordinate synthesis of histone H1 in cells arrested in the G1 phase, <u>Biochem. Biophys. Acta</u> 699:173-182 (1982).

77.  V. E. Groppi and P. Coffino. G1 and S phase mammalian cells synthesize histones at equivalent rates, <u>Cell</u> 21:195-204 (1980).

78.  E. Robbins and T. W. Borun, The cytoplasmic synthesis of histones in HeLa cells and its temporal relationship to DNA replication, <u>Proc. Natl. Acad. Sci. USA</u> 57:409-416 (1967).

79.  A. M. Delegeane and A. L. Lee, Coupling of histone and DNA synthesis in the somatic cell cycle, <u>Science</u> 215:79-81 (1982).

80.  J. L. Stein, G. S. Stein, and P. McGuire, Histone messenger RNA from HeLa cells:  Evidence for modified 5' termini, <u>Biochemistry</u> 16: 2207-2213 (1977).

81.  B. Moss, A. Gershowitz, L. A. Weber, and C. Baglioni, Histone mRNAs contain blocked and methylated 5' terminal sequences but lack methylated nucleosides at internal positions, <u>Cell</u> 10:113-120 (1977).

82.  R. Rickles, F. Marashi, F. Sierra, S. Clark, J. Wells, J. Stein, and G. Stein, Analysis of histone gene expression during the cell cycle in HeLa cells by using cloned human histone genes, <u>Proc. Natl. Acad. Sci. USA</u> 79:749-753 (1982).

83.  L. Green, G. Stein, and J. Stein, Histone gene expression in human diploid fibroblasts: analysis of histone mRNA levels using cloned human histone genes, <u>Mol. Cell. Biochem.</u> 60:123 (1984).

84.  G. S. Stein, J. L. Stein. W. D. Park, S. Detke, A. L. Lichtler, E. A. Shephard, R. L. Jansing, I. R. Phillips, Regulation of histone gene expression in HeLa S3 cells, <u>Cold Spring Harbor Symp. Quant. Biol.</u> 42:1107-1120 (1977).

85.  S. Detke, A. Lichtler, I. Phillips, J. L. Stein, and G. S. Stein, Reassessment of histone gene expression during the cell cycle in human cells by using homologous H4 histone cDNA, <u>Proc. Natl. Acad. Sci. USA</u> 76:4995-4999 (1979).

86.  G. S. Stein, W. D. Park, C. L. Thrall, R. J. Mans, and J. L. Stein, Regulation of histone gene transcription during the cell cycle by nonhistone chromosomal proteins, <u>Nature</u> 257:764-767 (1975).

87.  J. L. Stein, C. L. Thrall, W. D. Park, R. J. Mans, and G. S. Stein, Hybridization analysis of histone messenger RNA association with polyribosomes during the cell cycle, <u>Science</u> 189:557-558 (1975).

88.  I. Parker and W. Fitschen, Histone mRNA metabolism during the mouse fibroblast cell cycle, <u>Cell Diff.</u> 9:23-30 (1980).

89.  I. M. Chiu, D. Cooper, and W. F. Marzluff, Unscheduled synthesis of histone H1 in isoleucine starved cells, <u>Abstracts of the second</u>

annual meeting of the American Cancer Society (Florida Division), No. 38 (1979).

90.  N. Heintz, H. L. Sive, and R. G. Roeder, Regulation of human histone gene expression:  Kinetics of accumulation and changes in the rate of synthesis and in the half-lives of individual histone mRNAs during the HeLa cell cycle, Mol. Cell Biol. 3:539-550 (1983).

91.  L. M. Hereford, M. A. Osley, J. R. Ludwig, and C. S. McLaughlin, Cell cycle regulation of yeast histone mRNA, Cell 24:367-375 (1981).

92.  M. Plumb, F. Marashi, L. Green, A. Zimmerman, S. Zimmerman, J. Stein, and G. Stein, The cell cycle regulation of human histone H1 mRNA, Proc. Natl. Acad. Sci, USA 81:434-438 (1984).

93.  D. M. Prescott, R. M. Liskay, and G. M. Stancel, The cell life cycle and the G1 period, in:  "Cell Growth, NATO Advanced Study Institutes Series A:  Life Sciences," Volume 38 , C. Nicolini, ed., Plenum Press, New York, pp. 305-314 (1982).

94.  T. W. Borun, F. Gabrielli, K. Ajiro, A. Zweidler, and C. Baglioni, Further evidence of transcriptional and translational control of histone messenger RNA during the HeLa S3 cycle, Cell 4:59-67 (1975).

95.  M. Breindl and D. Gallwitz, Effects of cordycepin, hydroxyurea and cycloheximide on histone mRNA synthesis in synchronized HeLa cells, Mol. Biol. Reports 1:263-268 (1974).

96.  M. Jacobs-Lorena, F. Gabrielli, T. W. Borun, and C. Baglioni, Studies on the transcriptional control of histone synthesis, Biochem. Biophys. Acta. 324:275-281 (1973).

97.  L. Hereford, S. Bromley, and M. A. Osley, Periodic transcription of yeast histone genes, Cell 30:305-310 (1982).

98.  R. P. Perry and D. E. Kelley, Messenger RNA turnover in mouse L cells, J. Mol. Biol. 79:681-696 (1973).

99.  N. S. Kunkel, K. Hemminki, and E. S. Weinberg, Size of histone gene transcripts in different embryonic stages of the sea urchin, Strongylocentrotus purpuratus, Biochemistry 17:2591-2598 (1975).

100.  P. A. Hieter, M. B. Hendricks, K. Hemminki, and E. S. Weinberg, Histone gene switch in the sea urchin embryo:  indentification of late embryonic histone mRNAs and the control of their synthesis, Biochemistry 18:2707-2716 (1979).

101.  R. Maxson, T. Mohun, G. Gormezano, G. Childs, and L. Kedes, Distinct organizations and patterns of expression of early and late gene sets in the sea urchin, Nature 301:120-125 (1983).

102.  R. W. Lennox and L. H. Cohen, The H1 subtypes of mammals:  metabolic characteristics and tissue distribution, in: "Histone Genes," G. S. Stein, J. L. Stein, and W. F. Marzluff, eds., John Wiley and Sons, New York (1984).

103.  A. Zweidler, Core histone variants of the mouse:  primary structure and differential expression, in: "Histone Genes," G. S. Stein, J. L. Stein, W. F. Marzluff, eds., John Wiley and Sons, New York (1984).

104.  H. R. Woodland and E. D. Adamson, The synthesis and storage of

histones during the oogenesis of Xenopus laevis, Develop. Biol. 57:118-135 (1977).

105. A. Skoultchi and P. R. Gross, Maternal histone messenger RNA: Detection by molecular hybridization, Proc. Natl. Acad. Sci. USA 70:2840-2844 (1973).

106. D. E. Woods and W. Fitschen, The mobilization of maternal histone messenger RNA after fertilization of sea urchin eggs, Cell Diff. 7:103-114 (1978).

107. R. Maxson and F. Wilt, Accumulation of the early histone mRNAs during development of S. purpuratus, Dev. Biol. 94:435-440 (1982).

108. H. Stahl and D. Gallwitz, Fate of histone messenger RNAs in synchronized HeLa cells in the absence of initiation of protein synthesis, Eur. J. Biochem. 72:385-392 (1977).

109. M. Breindl and D. Gallwitz, On the translational control of histone synthesis. Eur. J. Biochem. 45:91-97 (1974).

110. D. Gallwitz and G. C. Mueller, Histone synthesis in vitro on HeLa cell microsomes, J. Biol. Chem. 244:5947-5952 (1969).

111. E. A. Shephard, I. R. Phillips, J. Davis, J. L. Stein, and G. S. Stein, Evidence for the resumption of DNA replication prior to histone synthesis in HeLa cells after release from treatment with hydroxyurea, FEBS Lett. 140:189-192 (1982).

112. W. B. Butler and G. C. Mueller, Control of histone synthesis in HeLa cells, Biochim. Biophys. Acta. 294:481-491 (1973).

113. G. Stein, J. Stein, E. Shephard, W. Park, and I. Phillips, Evidence that the coupling of histone gene expression and DNA synthesis in HeLa S3 cells is not mediated at the transcriptional level, Biochem. Biophys. Res. Comm. 77:245-252 (1977).

114. T. W. Borun, M. Scharff, and F. Robbins, Rapidly labeled, polyribosome-associated RNA having the properties of histone messenger, Proc. Natl. Acad. Sci. USA 58:1977-1983 (1967).

115. L. H. Kedes and P. R. Gross, Identification in cleaving embryos of three RNA species serving as templates for the synthesis of nuclear proteins, Nature 223:1335-1339 (1969).

116. N. Craig, D. E. Kelley, and R. P. Perry, Lifetime of the messenger RNAs which code for ribosomal proteins in L-cells, Biochem. Biophys. Acta 246:493-498 (1971).

117. M. Plumb, J. Stein, and G. Stein, Influence of DNA synthesis inhibition on the coordinate expression of core human histone genes during S phase, Nucl. Acids Res. 11:7927-7945 (1983).

118. L. Baumbach, F. Marashi, M. Plumb, G. Stein, and J. Stein, Inhibition of DNA replication coordinately reduces cellular levels of core and H1 histone mRNAs: requirement for protein synthesis, Biochemistry 23:1618 (1984).

119. J. Huberman, New Views of the biochemistry of eucaryotic DNA replication revealed by aphidicolin, an unusual inhibitor of DNA polymerase, Cell 23:647-648 (1981).

120. M. A. Osley and L. Hereford, Identification of a sequence responsible for periodic synthesis of yeast histone 2A mRNA, Proc. Natl. Acad. Sci. USA 79:7689-7693 (1982).

121. C. C. Hentschel, J.-C. Irminger, P. Bucher, and M. L. Birnstiel, Sea urchin histone mRNA termini are located in gene regions downstream from putative regulatory sequences, Nature 285:147-151 (1980).

122. G. S. Stein, J. L. Stein, L. Baumbach, A. Leza, A. Lichtler, F. Marashi, M. Plumb, R. Rickles, F. Sierra, and T. Van Dyke, Organization and cell cycle regulation of human histone genes, in: "Proceedings of the New York Academy of Sciences Conference on Cell Proliferation, Cancer and Cancer Therapy," Volume 397, R. Baserga, ed., pp. 148-167 (1982).

123. G. Childs, C. Nocente-McGrath, T. Lieber, C. Holt, and J. A. Knowles, Sea urchin (L. pictus) late stage histone H3 and H4 genes: Characterization and mapping of a clustered but nontandemly linked multigene family, Cell 31:383-393 (1982).

124. P. C. Turner and H. R. Woodland, Nucl. Acids Res. 10:3769-3780 (1982).

125. A. F. M. Moorman, P. A. J. de Boer, R. T. M. de Laaf, W. M. A. M. Dongen, and O. H. J. Destree, Primary structure of the histone H3 and H4 gene cluster of Xenopus laevis, FEBS Letters 136:45-52 (1981).

126. E. C. Stephenson, H. P. Erba, and J. G. Gall, characterization of a cloned histone gene cluster of the newt Notophthalmus veridescens, Nucl. Acids Res. 9:2281-2293 (1981).

127. M. Grunstein, K. E. Diamond, E. Knoppel, and J. E. Grunstein, Comparison of the early histone H4 gene sequence of Stronglyocentrotus purpuratus with maternal, early, and late histone H4 mRNA sequences, Biochemistry 20:1216-1223 (1981).

# THE tRNA$^{Asp}$-ASPARTYL-tRNA SYNTHETASE SYSTEM FROM YEAST: STRUCTURAL AND FUNCTIONAL STUDIES

J. P. Ebel, P. Dunman, R. Giege, B. Lorber, D. Moras,
P. Romby, J. C. Thierry and E. Westhof

Institut de Biologie Moléculaire et Cellulaire
15, rue René Descartes
67084 Strasbourg, France

## INTRODUCTION

Transfer ribonucleic acids (tRNAs) play a central role in the complex mechanism of protein synthesis. In that process their chief function is to carry amino acids to the ribosomes, to decode the messenger RNA and to incorporate the correct amino acid into the growing polypeptide chain.

The tRNAs fulfill this function through a series of interactions with their biological partners[1]:
- with the aminoacyl-tRNA synthetases, enzymes which catalyze the specific activation of an amino acid and its transfer to the cognate tRNA;
- with elongation factor Tu, which through the ternary complex aminoacyl-tRNA/GTP/EF-Tu, carries the aminoacyl-tRNA to the ribosome;
- with the mRNA involving the codon-anticodon interaction;
- with the ribosome at the A site in the pretranslocation step or at the P site in the posttranslocation step.

Due to these multiple interactions, tRNAs represent a particularly exciting model for the understanding at the molecular level of the mechanisms of recognition between nucleic acids and proteins and of structure-function relationships. In this chapter, we will focus on the tRNA-aminoacyl-tRNA synthetase interaction, which is essential because the correct attachment of amino acids to the 3'-end of tRNA, which is necessary for the fidelity of translation, relies on accurate recognition between these two macromolecules.

We will concentrate on a specific tRNA-aminoacyl-tRNA synthetase system, which has been extensively studied in our Institute: the tRNA$^{Asp}$-aspartyl-tRNA synthetase system from yeast. This system is particularly interesting because both partners, tRNA$^{Asp}$ and aspartyl-tRNA synthetase, have been crystallized in their free and, more important, in their complexed state. In addition, tRNA$^{Asp}$ could be a tempting model for studying tRNA-mRNA interaction, particularly since it has a self-complementary GUC anticodon. The resulting anticodon-anticodon interaction which mimicks the anticodon-codon interaction exists in solution and in the tRNA$^{Asp}$ crystal structure. For all these reasons, the aspartic acid system from yeast is ideal for studying various types of fundamental tRNA recognition processes.

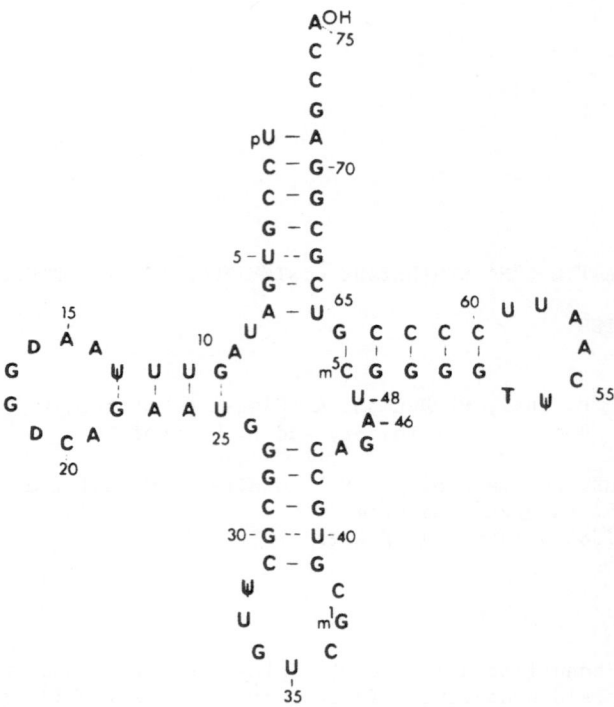

Fig 1:   The nucleotide sequence of yeast tRNA^Asp. For convenience the numbering system of the nucleotides is that of yeast tRNA^Phe; in the 75-nucleotide long tRNA^Asp, position 47 in the variable loop has been omitted.  Non-classical Watson-Crick base pairs are indicated by broken lines.


STRUCTURE OF tRNA

     The three-dimensional structures of two tRNA, yeast tRNA^Phe and tRNA^Asp, have been solved at high resolution.  Both are elongator tRNAs with a short extra-loop.  In this section, we will focus on the structure of tRNA^Asp with reference to that of tRNA^Phe.

Primary structure

     The nucleotide sequence[2] of yeast tRNA^Asp, shown in Figure 1, presents some characteristic features.  It contains a high number of G-C base pairs, except in the D-stem where two G-U base pairs are present.  The variable loop is made of four nucleotides versus five in tTNA^Phe (for convenience of comparison we kept the same numbering, assuming a deletion at position 47). The D-loop has the same length as that of tRNA^Phe but the two conserved Gs, which are crucial for D- and T-loops tertiary interactions, are at positions 17 and 18 instead of 18 and 19, thus making α and β regions of the D-loop quite symmetrical.  Last but not least, the anticodon GUC presents the peculiarity to be self-complementary, with a slight mismatch at the uridine position.  This feature was first noted by Grosjean et al.[3] who showed the existence of a significant interaction in solution and suggested it to be a tempting model to study tRNA-mRNA recognition.

Crystal structure

     For yeast tRNA^Asp two structures have been solved from a multiple

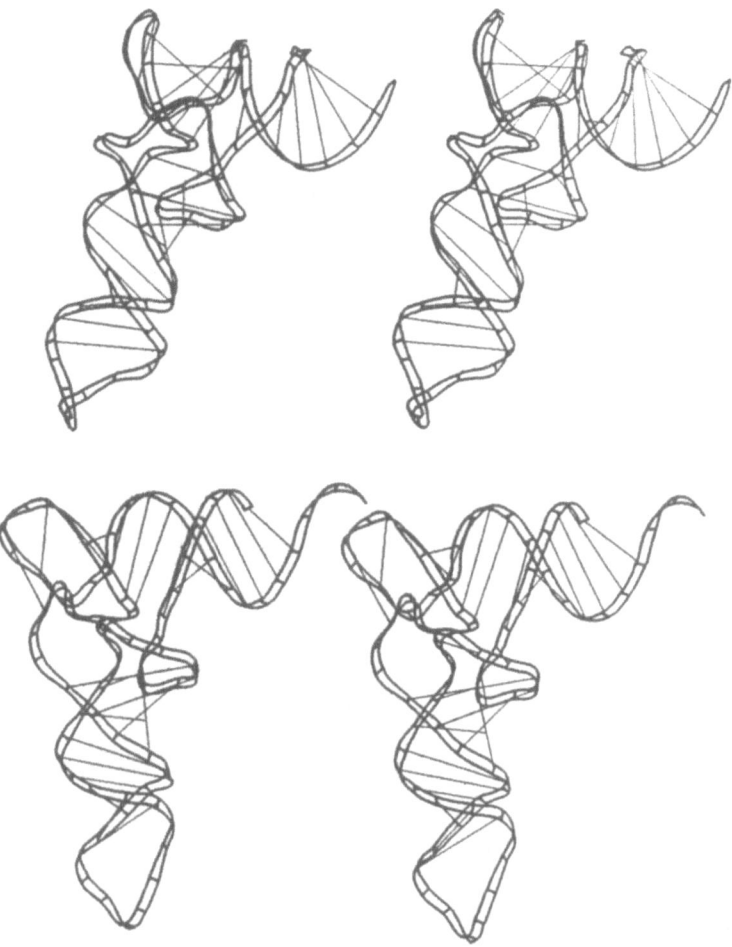

Fig. 2: Two stereo views of the three-dimensional backbones of yeast tRNA
tRNA$^{Asp}$ (top) and tRNA$^{Phe}$ (bottom). The coordinates of tRNA$^{Asp}$
correspond to the refined low temperature form; the R-factor for
these data is presently 23.5% at 3Å resolution. The CCA-end part
however is not fully defined and was set removed. The coordinates
of yeast tRNA$^{Phe}$ are those of the orthorhombic crystal form[8].
Base-pairs are indicated by continuous lines connecting the corresponding backbones.

isomorphous replacement (MIR) X-ray analysis of two crystal forms[4]. The
transition between forms A and B is temperature dependent but it can also
be induced around 20° by pH changes or the addition of some heavy atom
derivatives[5]. The structure of one form, the lower temperature form, has
been refined in reciprocal space using the restrained least-square method
of Konnert and Hendrickson[6] and in real space with the graphic modeling
program FRODO[7]. Both programs were adapted for nucleic acid handling.

Boomerang versus L-shape. A view of the tRNA$^{Asp}$ molecule together
with a similar view of tRNA$^{Phe}$ is shown on Figure 2. The topological
organization of the cloverleaf sequence is similar to that first found for
yeast tRNA$^{Phe}$. This gives the L-shaped structure formed by two units:
vertically the anticodon and the D-stems, horizontally the T- and the amino
acid accepting stems. However, in the case of tRNA$^{Asp}$, the two branches

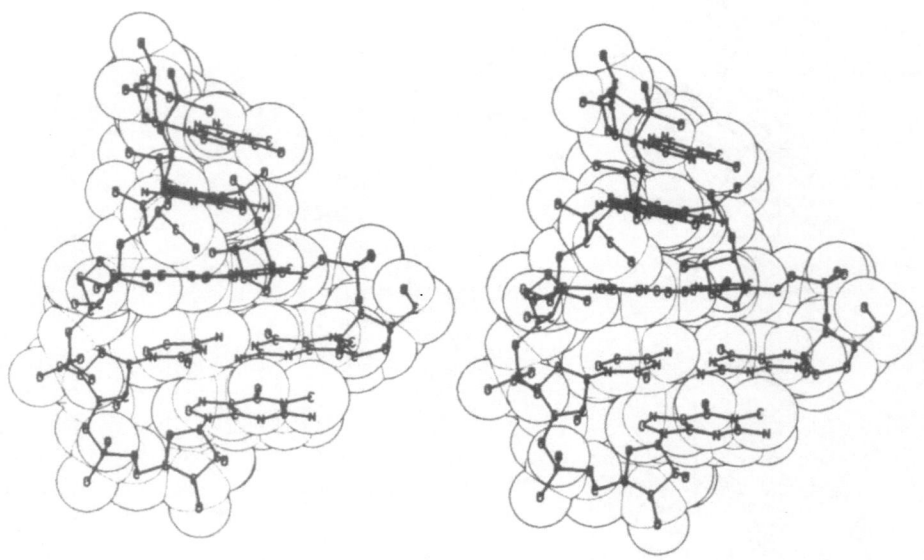

Fig. 3: Stereo views of the anticodon triplet (GUC) base pairing in yeast tRNA$^{Asp}$.

forming the L are more open (by more than 10°) than in tRNA$^{Phe}$, conferring to this tRNA a boomerang-like shape. This results in a different position-ing of the anticodon and of the T-stems and loops with respect to fixed acceptor and D-stems which superpose well to the corresponding part of tRNA$^{Phe}$[4].

Anticodon-anticodon interaction. In the orthorhombic cyrstal lattice (space group C222$_1$) tRNA$^{Asp}$ molecules are associated through a two-fold symmetry axis parallel to the crystallographic b direction by anticodon-anticodon interactions. Figure 3 represents the local conformation[9]. The GUC anticodon triplets of symmetrically related molecules form complementary hydrogen bonded base pairs, arranged in a normal helical conformation. This small helix is stabilized by stacking of the modified base m$^1$G37 on both sides. This packing confers a great stability to the dimeric structure and explains the good quality of the electron density map in the anticodon region. A contact between the anticodon loops of two tRNAs also exists in the orthorhombic form of yeast tRNA$^{Phe}$. In that case, however, the G$_m$AA anticodons cannot be base paired and they are arranged in a stacked con-formation.

Dynamic aspects. Crystallographic refinement leads to the determina-tion of the so-called Debye-Waller temperature factor. Although temperature factors contain various components, it has been shown[10,11] that their variation along a macromolecular backbone has some physical meaning. In Figure 4 are represented the temperature factors of each phosphate along the polynucleotide chain in tRNA$^{Asp}$ and in tRNA$^{Phe}$.

For tRNA$^{Asp}$, it is apparent that the stems are more rigid than the loops, except for the end of the amino acid acceptor stem. This variation is not so apparent for tRNA$^{Phe}$, although the effect is present. Also, in tRNA$^{Asp}$, the T-loop presents higher temperature factors than the anticodon loop. This is in marked contrast to the situation in tRNA$^{Phe}$, where the anticodon loop presents the highest temperature factors and the T-loop the lowest ones. There is a similar but less pronounced reversal in the region

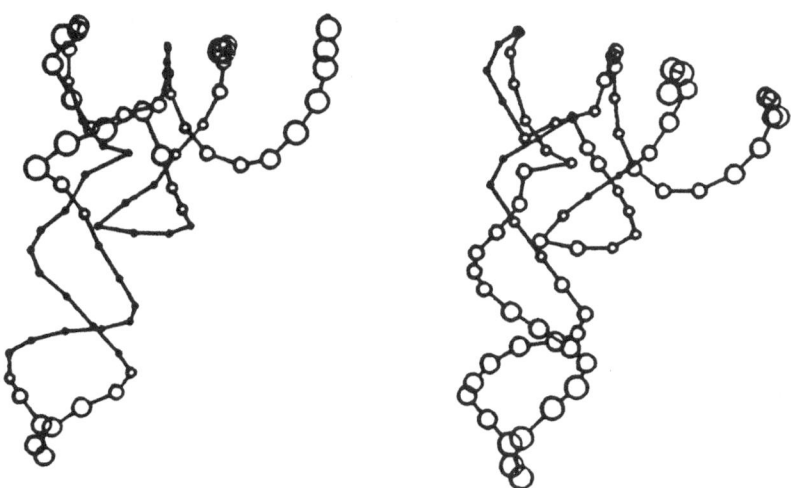

Fig. 4: Thermal vibration of the backbones. Two views of yeast tRNA$^{Asp}$ (left) and tRNA$^{Phe}$ (right) are shown. Each phosphate group is presented by a ball proportional to the value of the temperature factors.

of the P10-loop, where P10 is at a minimum in tRNA$^{Asp}$ and at a maximum in tRNA$^{Phe}$. The origins of these differences are difficult to pinpoint. We think that the different behavior of the "flexibility" of the tRNA molecule in the two crystals arises from the different packing of the molecules in crystals of tRNA$^{Asp}$ and of tRNA$^{Phe}$, since there is anticodon-anticodon base-pairing in the former crystals and not in the latter ones.

To summarize we can say that the structure of tRNA$^{Asp}$ shows the conformational state of a tRNA on the ribosome. In the crystals one GUC triplet from one tRNA molecule mimicks a codon of mRNA interacting with the GUC anticodon of a second molecule. This interaction might act as a signal and trigger conformational changes elsewhere. Influence on the D and T-loop association is strongly suggested by thermal factors. The structure of tRNA$^{Phe}$ would be that of a free tRNA, with flexible anticodon stem and loop.


INTERACTION BETWEEN tRNA AND AMINOACYL-tRNA SYNTHETASE

## Crystallization of the tRNA$^{Asp}$-aspartyl tRNA synthetase complex

Both tRNA$^{Asp}$ and aspartyl-tRNA synthetase could be crystallized in various media including low salt conditions[12],[13]. The best diffracting crystals, however, could only be grown in the presence of ammonium sulfate at 62% saturation for tRNA$^{Asp}$ and at 54% for synthetase. For the complex, crystallization was observed to occur only under high salt conditions, between 48 and 53% saturation of ammonium sulfate depending upon the concentration of macromolecular components and the temperature. The optimal crystallization conditions for the different components of the aspartic acid system are summarized in Table 1. A full account of the crystallization procedure was reported by Giegé et al.[14] and Lorber et al.[15]

For the complex, one of the most important factors in crystal formation is the stoichiometry of the components. No crystals can be grown for a molecular ratio tRNA/enzyme inferior to 1.8 and the quality of the crystals

171

Table 1:  Crystallization conditions of tRNA$^{Asp}$ aspartyl-tRNA synthetase
and the complex formed between these two macromolecules.

| MOLECULES | tRNA | AspRS | COMPLEX |
|---|---|---|---|
| Molecular weight | 24,160 | 125,000 | 175,000 |
| Precipitant Nature | | $(NH_4)_2\,SO_4$ | |
| Concentration | 62% | 54% | 50% |
| Macromolecular concentrations | | $mg.ml^{-1}$ | |
| tRNA | 3–5 | – | 1–5 |
| Enzyme | – | 4 | 3–12 |
| pH | 6.8 | 6.7 | 7.0–8.0 |
| Crystal form | Orthorhombic | Quadratic | Cubic |
| Space group | $C222_1$ | $P4_12_12$ | $I432$ |

degrades when that ratio increases to more than 2.2.  These values only
reflect the experimental uncertainty of the concentration measurements; the
best crystals are obtained when the mother liquor contains two tRNA molecules for one dimeric enzyme.

The first problem to solve in the presence of putative complex
crystals is to ascertain the coexistence, within the crystal, of both the
nucleic acid and the protein.  The presence of tRNA$^{Asp}$ and aspartyl-tRNA
synthetase was tested by gel electrophoresis and by biochemical activity
assays.  All experiments were done with crystals carefully washed so that
the possibility of contamination by non-crystallized material could be
eliminated.  The presence of aspartyl-tRNA synthetase was demonstrated by
the aminoacylation of exogenous tRNA added to the medium.  For the tRNA,
two different experiments demonstrated its presence.  With and without
addition of exogenous enzyme it was possible to recover equivalent amounts
of trichloroacetic acid precipitable radioactivity, clearly establishing
the aspartylation of a significant amount of tRNA.

Crystals belong to the cubic system with a unit cell parameter of
354Å.  The systematic absence of hkl for h + k + l = 2n + 1 leads to the
space group I432, with 48 asymmetric units/cell.  Assuming one molecule of
enzyme and two molecules of tRNA per asymmetric unit, the value of Vm
(crystal volume per unit of macromolecular weight) is a 5.3Å/dalton, outside
the standard range for proteins (1.68 and 3.53).  For a partial specific
volume of 0.7 cm$^3$g$^{-1}$ the solvent content of the crystal would then be 78%,
a large value consistent with the particular softness of the crystals.  For
the best crystals, diffracted intensities extend up to 7.5Å resolution but
routinely the limit of resolution is 8.5Å.

## Solution Studies

One way to determine the part of two macromolecules interacting with
each other is to compare the accessibility of these molecules to a chemical
probe in the free and complexed states.  This can easily be done on tRNA,
a molecule for which many specific chemical reagents are available which

can attack functional groups on the individual nucleotides. The regions interacting with the probe in the free tRNA but not in the complexed molecule can be considered in close contact with the interacting macromolecule, an aminoacyl-tRNA synthetase for example, and thus protected by it.

Here we present results obtained with ethylnitrosourea, an alkylating reagent which essentially ethylates the phosphate residues of nucleic acids[16],[17]. The principle of the method derives from the chemical sequencing methodologies of nucleic acids and relies on statistical and low yield modification at each phosphate in such a way that each tRNA undergoes less than one modification. The tRNA molecules labeled at their 3'- or 5'- end with radioactive ATP are then specifically split at the modified position and the resulting end-labeled oligonucleotides are analyzed by high voltage electrophoresis on sequencing gels followed by autoradiography. Assignment of bands is done by comparing their migrations to ladders obtained after limited T1 RNase digestion or alkaline hydrolysis. In such a way it is possible to probe the entire tRNA molecule in one experiment. In the presence of aminoacyl-tRNA synthetases, experimental conditions must allow both chemical reactivity and good complex formation. Therefore, samples are incubated for 3 hours at pH 8.0 and at 20°C in the presence of magnesium at a rather low ionic strength and with concentrations of tRNA (1.5 μm and enzyme (5 μM) in the range where the complex formation is guaranteed. Detailed experimental procedures were published for experiments with tRNA$^{Asp}$ and tRNA$^{Phe}$[18].

A typical alkylation experiment of 5'-labeled tRNA$^{Asp}$ is shown in Figure 5. This experiment allows us to probe the phosphate groups located between positions 6 to 55. Similar assays with 3'-labeled tRNA probing the phosphates from the 3'- to the 5'-side of the molecule were also carried out. In the presence of aspartyl-tRNA synthetase the splitting at some phosphate positions is nearly suppressed or is strongly reduced (for instance P27 to P33), suggesting that these groups are protected from alkylation by the enzyme and thus most likely are in close contact with the protein. The results are summarized on Figure 5 in which the protected phosphate groups are indicated by arrows on the cloverleaf structure of yeast tRNA$^{Asp}$. Among the parts of the molecule not tested, it is clear that the CCA-end or at least the terminal adenosine, is also in contact with the enzyme for catalytic necessity.

If one compares the protected phosphates in tRNA$^{Asp}$ with results obtained by the same approach in the phenylalanine and valine systems[18], the striking feature which emerges is the large difference between contact areas. In the three systems, the only common contact areas, besides the terminal adenosine, are the variable loop and the neighborhood of P9. Not surprisingly these regions are very close in space. Biochemical experiments have also emphasized the involvement of U8 in a contact interaction of tRNAs with their cognate synthetase[19].

For tRNA$^{Asp}$ one side of the L-shaped molecule is clearly involved in protein-nucleic acid association. This face includes the variable loop, the 5'-end of the anticodon stem and part of the 3'-end of the amino acid arm. The surface involved is quite important, and this observation is consistent with neutron diffraction results which lead to the existence of large contact areas between the protein and the nucleic acid[20]. This interaction differs significantly from the one proposed for tRNA$^{Phe}$ derived from cross-linking experiments[21]. If one assumes a similar folding for tRNA$^{Asp}$, another type of interaction between the enzyme and the tRNA must be postulated.

These observations underline the differences which are likely to exist

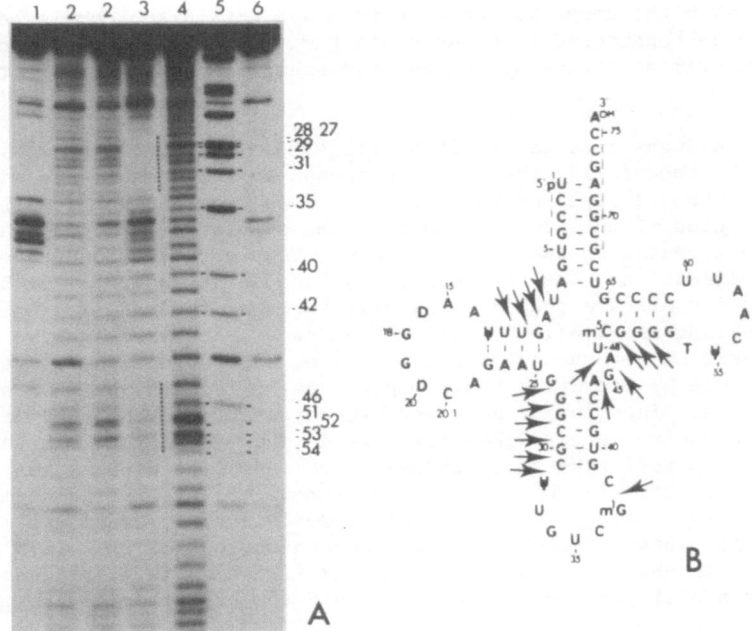

Fig. 5:   A. Autoradiogram of 15% acrylamide gel of a phosphate alkylation
experiment with ENU of 3'-end labeled tRNA[Asp] from yeast in the
presence of yeast aspartyl-tRNA synthetase. Lanes 1, 6:  control
incubations in the absence of reagent (lane 6) and in the presence
of enzyme (lane 1); lanes 2, 4:  alkylation at 20°C (lane 2) and
80°C (lane 4) in the absence of enzyme; lane 3:  alkylation at
20°C in the presence of aspartyl-tRNA synthetase; lane 5:  partial
ribonuclease Tl digest. The phosphates protected against alkylation in the tRNA complexed with its synthetase are indicated by
diamonds.   B. Cloverleaf structure of yeast tRNA[Asp2] with positions
of the phosphates strongly protected by yeast aspartyl-tRNA
synthetase against ENU. Full arrows show the phosphates protected
by the aspartyl-tRNA synthetase, regions not tested for technical
reasons[18] are indicated by dashed line.

in the recognition between tRNAs and their cognate synthetases. It is
worthwhile noticing that the oligomeric structure of the aminoacyl-tRNA
synthetases in the aspartic acid, phenylalanine and valine systems are
quite different:  aspartyl-tRNA synthetase is a dimer ($\alpha_2$) of MW ≅ 125,000
daltons which can bind two tRNA molecules, whereas phenylalanyl-tRNA
synthetase is an $\alpha_2\beta_2$ tetramer (MW ≅ 270,000) which also binds two tRNA[Phe]
molecules and valyl-tRNA synthetase is a large monomer (MW ≅ 130,000) which
binds one tRNA[Val] molecule.


CONCLUSION

The best understood biological role of transfer RNAs is their parti-
cipation in ribosome-mediated protein synthesis. This function leads tRNAs
to many interactions with different proteins and nucleic acids. With
aminoacyl-tRNA synthetases, the molecular recognition must be highly
specific. The same is true for the decoding of the genetic code at the
messenger RNA level. In this report, using both biochemical and crystallographic approaches, we have presented experimental results on yeast tRNA[Asp]

which illustrate these two types of specific interactions.

REFERENCES

1.  P. R. Schimmel, D. Soll, J. N. Abelson, eds., "Transfer RNA Structure, Properties and Recognition," Cold Spring Harbor Laboratory, Cold Spring Harbor, New York (1979).

2.  J. Gangloff, G. Keith, J. P. Ebel, and G. Dirheimer, Structure of aspartate-tRNA from brewer's yeast. Nature New Biol. 230:125-127 (1971).

3.  H. Grosjean, S. De Henau, and D. M. Crothers, On the physical basis in the genetic coding interactions, Proc. Natl. Acad. Sci. USA 75:160-614 (1978).

4.  D. Moras, M. B. Comarmond, J. Fischer, R. Weiss, J. C. Thierry, J. P. Ebel, and R. Giegé, Crystal structure of yeast tRNA$^{Asp}$, Nature 286: 669-674 (1980).

5.  P. V. Huong, E. Audry, R. Giegé, D. Moras, J. C. Thierry, and M. B. Comarmond, Conformational changes in tRNA$^{Asp}$: laser Raman and X-ray crystallographic studies, Biopolymers 23:71-81 (1984).

6.  J. H. Konnert, and O. Hendrickson, A restrained-parameter thermal factor refinement procedure, Acta Cryst. A36:344-350 (1980).

7.  T. A. Jones, FRODO, a graphic modeling program, Appl. Cryst. 11:268-272 (1978).

8.  G. J. Quigley, N. C. Seeman, A. H. T. Wang, F. L. Suddath, and A. Rich, Yeast phenylalanyl transfer RNA: atomic coordinates and torsion angles, Nucl. Acids. Res. 2:2329-2339 (1975).

9.  E. Westhof, P. Dumas, and D. Moras, Loop stereochemistry and dynamics in transfer RNA, J. Biomol. Str. Dyn. 1:337-355 (1983).

10. H. Frauenfelder, G. A. Petsko, and D. Tsernoglou, Temperature-dependent X-ray diffraction as a probe of protein structural dynamics, Nature 280:558-560 (1979).

11. P. J. Artymiuk, C. C. F. Blake, D. E. P. Grace, S. I. Oatley, D. C. Phillips, and N. J. E. Sternberg, Crystallographic studies of the dynamic properties of lysozyme, Nature 280:563-566 (1979).

12. R. Giegé, D. Moras, and J. C. Thierry, Yeast transfer RNA$^{Asp}$: a new high resolution X-ray diffracting crystal form of a transfer RNA, J. Mol. Biol. 115:91-96 (1977).

13. A. Dietrich, R. Giegé, M. B. Comarmond, J. C. Thierry, and D. Moras, Crystallographic studies on the aspartyl-tRNA synthetase-tRNA$^{Asp}$ system from yeast, J. Mol. Biol. 138:129-135 (1980).

14. R. Giegé, B. Lorber, J. P. Ebel, J. C. Thierry, and D. Moras, Crystallization du complexe formé entre l'aspartate de levure et son aminoacyl-tRNA synthétase, C. R. Séances Acad. Sci. Paris Série D 291:393-396 (1980).

15. B. Lorber, R. Giege, J. P. Ebel, C. Berthet, J. C. Thierry, and D. Moras, Crystallization of a tRNA-aminoacyl-tRNA synthetase complex, J. Biol. Chem. 258:8429-8435 (1983).

16. J. T. Kusmierek and B. Singer, Sites of alkylation of polyU by agents of varying carcinogenicity and stability of products, Biochim. Biophys. Acta 142:536-538 (1976).

17. V. V. Vlassov, R. Geigé, and J. P. Ebel, Tertiary structure of tRNAs in solution monitored by phosphodiester modification with ethyl-nitrosourea, Eur. J. Biochem. 119:51-59 (1981).

18. V. V. Vlassov, D. Kern, P. Romby, R. Giegé, and J. P. Ebel, Inter-action of tRNA[Phe] and tRNA[Val] with aminoacyl-tRNA synthetases: a chemical modification study, Eur. J. Biochem. 132:537-544 (1983).

19. R. Starzyk, S. Koontz, and P. Schimmel, A covalent adduct between the uracil ring and the active site of an aminoacyl-tRNA synthetase, Nature 298:136-140 (1982).

20. D. Moras, B. Lorber, P. Romby, J. P. Ebel, R. Giegé, A. Lewitt-Bentley, and M. Roth, Yeast tRNA[Asp]-aspartyl-tRNA synthetase: the crystalline complex, J. Biomol. Str. Dyn. 1:209-223 (1983).

21. A. Rich and P. R. Schimmel, Structural organization of complexes of transfer RNAs with aminoacyl-tRNA synthetases, Nucleic Acids Res. 4:1649-1665 (1977).

# DIFFRACTION STUDIES ON CRYSTALS OF RIBOSOMAL PARTICLES

H. G. Wittmann[1] and A. Yonath[2]

[1]Max-Planck-Institut für Molekulare Genetik
D-1000 Berlin 33, Germany
[2]Department of Structural Chemistry
Weizmann Institute, Rehovot, Israel

## INTRODUCTION

One of the most fascinating biochemical processes is the biosynthesis of protein molecules. This intricate and accurate process takes place in all organisms on their ribosomes in a similar manner. It involves specific interactions of the ribosomes with mRNAs, aminoacyl-tRNAs and a number of proteins such as initiation, elongation and termination factors. During this process the ribosomes dissociate into their two subunits which reassociate after the initiation process. Each of these subunits is a structurally independent distinct assembly of many proteins and several RNA chains.

The structure of ribosomal particles, in particular those from bacterial sources, has been intensively studied during the last two decades by a number of chemical, physical, immunological and genetic methods (for recent reviews see references 1-4). All the ribosomal proteins and RNAs of the Escherichia coli ribosome have been isolated and their primary structures determined. The architecture of the ribosome is currently being investigated by immune electron microscopy, neutron diffraction, chemical cross-linking, and affinity labeling, as well as by fluorescence and other techniques. In spite of the immense progress which has been achieved by these methods, a detailed molecular model for the ribosome has still not been determined.

A few years ago, bacterial ribosomal particles were crystallized in vitro, and diffraction techniques such as X-ray crystallography and three-dimensional image reconstruction from periodically organized specimens have been applied to these crystals. The purpose of this article is to summarize the results of these studies, together with those of diffraction studies on crystalline arrays of ribosomes which occur in vivo in some eukaryotes.

## ONE- AND TWO-DIMENSIONALLY ORDERED FORMS OF RIBOSOMES

Under special conditions (such as suboptimal temperatures, oxygen lack, hibernation, etc.) the ribosomes of several eukaryotic species (lizard, chicken, amoeba and human) associate with each other in vivo to form helices and two-dimensionally ordered layers. Some of these ordered forms have proved useful for low-resolution structural studies.

a) Helices of chromatoid bodies of the protozoan Entamoeba invadens are probably composed of ribosomes or their precursors[5]. Positively stained sections were used to derive a reconstructed body consisting of three regions of unequal size, named: L and S subunits, and X particle, respectively.

b) Membrane bound double layers of ribosomes from the oocytes of the lizard, Lacerta sicula, are formed during hibernation or after prolonged cold treatment. The ribosomes are organized as tetramers in a P4 lattice of a = 59.5 nm. Comparison of three-dimensionally reconstructed models obtained at 6-7 nm resolution from sheets which were contrasted with gold thioglucose or with glucose, showed that the rRNA chains are concentrated in a central core with few accessible sites on the surface; that the ribosomal proteins are located mainly at the periphery; and that the subunit interface is rich in rRNA. However, the shape of the two subunits of the ribosome could be only partially resolved[6].

c) Tetramers of ribosomes have also been observed as the basic building units of the ordered ribosomal sheets in slowly chilled early chick embryos. These sheets are packed with P422 symmetry. A similar organization could be obtained in vitro. In the latter case two-dimensional arrays of ribosomes with the space group $P42_12$ (a = 59.3 nm) and an internal order of 6 nm were produced. The asymmetric unit in these arrays consists of tetramers of whole ribosomes together with four non-ribosomal proteins. Low angle X-ray diffraction patterns of partially oriented gels of these sheets and three-dimensional reconstructions of negatively stained specimens were used to obtain information about the internal packing within these arrays[7].

d) Hirano bodies, which are stacked sheets of membrane bound ribosomal particles, appear in the brains of senile humans[8]. Spatial Fourier filtering of stained sections revealed that the particles are packed in layers of a rhombic lattice with a = b = 13 nm and $\alpha$ = 56° in which the average interparticle distance is 21.5 nm.

These studies on two-dimensional sheets composed of eukaryotic ribosomes have yielded some useful low resolution information about the modes of packing, the interactions between the particles, the outer contour of the ribosomes and the inner distribution of their components. However, the quality of the results is limited by the very nature of the systems. The organization of the sheets is induced by cellular effects and is expressed in only one or two dimensions. Furthermore, the particles are usually packed in rather large unit cells which only permit relatively low resolution studies. Thus, the only suitable diffraction technique to be applied to these systems is three-dimensional image reconstruction from electron micrographs, a technique which has many merits but also severe limitations.

Ribosomes from bacteria are smaller and have been studied biochemically in much greater detail than those from eukaryotes. They can also be produced in high purity and large quantity. Moreover, they provide a system for crystallization which is independent of in vivo events and environmental influences such as hibernation.

Attempts to produce two-dimensional crystalline sheets from bacterial ribosomes in vitro have been successful in a few cases. Helical arrays of E. coli small ribosomal subunits[9] and crystalline sheets of large ribosomal subunits from the same organism[10] have been reported. The building units of these sheets are tetramers which have lattice parameters of a = b = 33 nm and $\alpha$ = 123°, and the space group is most likely $P2_1$.

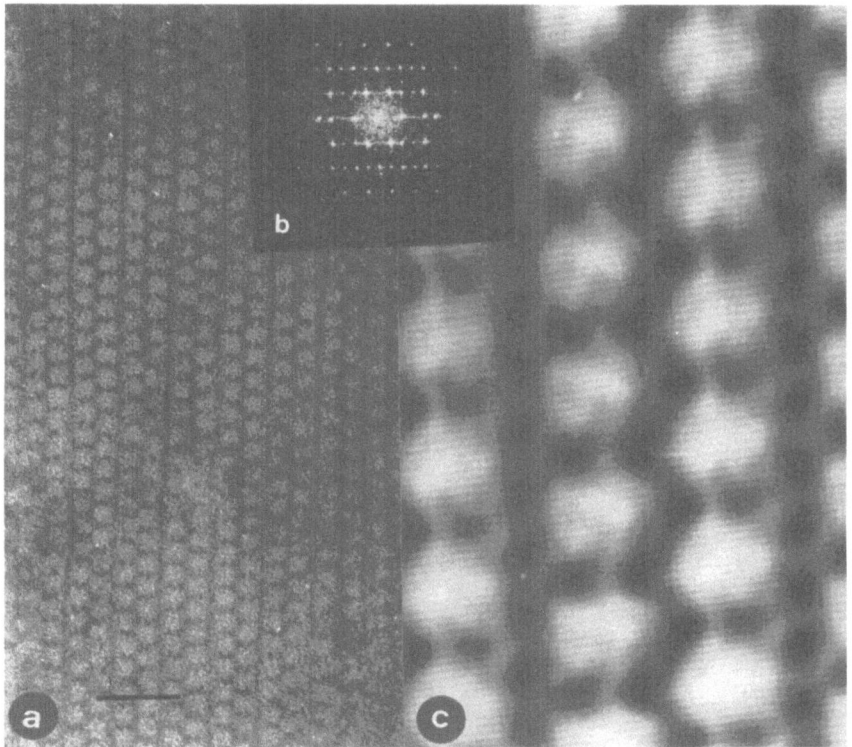

Fig. 1: (a) Electron micrograph of a negatively stained crystalline sheet, (b) its optical diffraction pattern, and (c) its noise filtered image. Bar lengt is 50nm.

Further, two-dimensional crystalline sheets which diffract to the 10th order (3 nm resolution) have been obtained from the large ribosomal subunit of Bacillus stearothermophilus[11] (Fig. 1). In this case two particles related by $P12_1$ symmetry are packed in unit cells with relatively small dimensions (14.5 x 31.1 nm), which agree well with some forms of the three-dimensional crystals of these 50S particles (Table 1). Filtered images of the negatively stained sheets (Fig. 1) show particles with similar dimensions to those revealed by other methods and with the characteristic features that have been detected by electron microscopy of single particles[11].

Table 1: Characterization of crystals of 50S ribosomal particles from B. stearothermophilus using electron microscopy.

| Crystal Form | Cell Parameters (nm) | | |
|---|---|---|---|
| 1* | 13.0; | 25.4 | $\gamma = 95°$ |
| 2* | 15.6; | 28.8 | $\gamma = 97°$ |
| 3 | 26.0; | 28.8 | $\gamma = 104°$ |
| 4 | 40.5; | 40.5; 25.6 | $\gamma = 120°$ |
| 5 | 21.3; | 23.5; 31.5 | $\gamma = 127°$ |

*May be related to each other.

THREE-DIMENSIONAL CRYSTALS OF RIBOSOMAL PARTICLES

The three-dimensional crystallization of bacterial ribosomes was achieved as a result of a systematic exploration of the parameters that control this process and the development of an experimental procedure for fine control of the content of the crystallization medium[12]. Several three-dimensional crystal forms have reproducibly been obtained from the large ribosomal subunits of B. stearothermophilus[13-15] and from E. coli 70S ribosomes[16].

There is a correlation between crystallizability and biological activity since inactive ribosomal particles could not be crystallized. Moreover, in all cases, the in vitro crystalline material retains its biological activity even for as long as several months, in contrast to the relatively short lifetime of isolated ribosomes in solution. This property is in agreement with the hypothesis that periodic organization of ribosomal particles can occur in vivo when external conditions, e.g. hibernation, demand temporary storage of many ribosomes in a cell.

Electron micrographs of positively stained thin sections of embedded three-dimensional crystals show a regular packing of ribosomal particles with dimensions similar to those previously determined for these particles by various physical techniques such as electron microscopy and small angle X-ray scattering. Several crystal forms were suitable for further structural analysis by three-dimensional image reconstruction.

Image Reconstruction from Positively Stained Thin Sections

Since three-dimensional crystals are too thick to be studied directly by electron microscopy they were embedded and sectioned. The thin sections were positively stained with uranyl acetate which reacts mainly with the nucleic acid moiety of the particles. Cell parameters were determined from the optical diffraction patterns of electron micrographs of these sections[13-16].

Microcrystals of 70S E. coli ribosomes are very well organized, and the particles are packed with hexagonal (P63) symmetry in unit cells of a = b = 34 nm, $\gamma$ = 102° and c = 59 nm (Fig. 2). Assuming 50-60% hydration, each asymmetric unit consists of one ribosome for which the approximate dimensions (in two directions) could be estimated. Positively stained sections cut parallel to the 6-fold axis in various positions relative to the AB face (Fig. 3) show several views of the distribution of the stain within the particle (Fig. 4).

For the 50S particles from B. stearothermophilus the cell dimensions are in most cases relatively small. For two crystal forms (#1 and #2 in Table 1) they are in good agreement with the periodic spacings determined from their X-ray patterns (see below).

After staining with uranyl acetate the crystal sections were tilted in the electron microscope, and three-dimensional image reconstruction studies were performed for four forms (#1-#4 in Table 1) of 50S crystals of B. stearothermophilus[17]. All four forms show essentially the same stain distribution within the particle. The model obtained from these studies has dimensions similar to those determined by other physical techniques. It consits of two domains of unevenly distributed density. Comparison of this model obtained by staining with uranyl acetate alone with that obtained from sections stained with uranyl acetate together with phosphotungstic acid, shows that the portion of the subunit that interacts with uranyl acetate (presumably the rRNA) is distributed mainly in the core of the particle, whereas the ribosomal components that interact with phosphotungstic acid

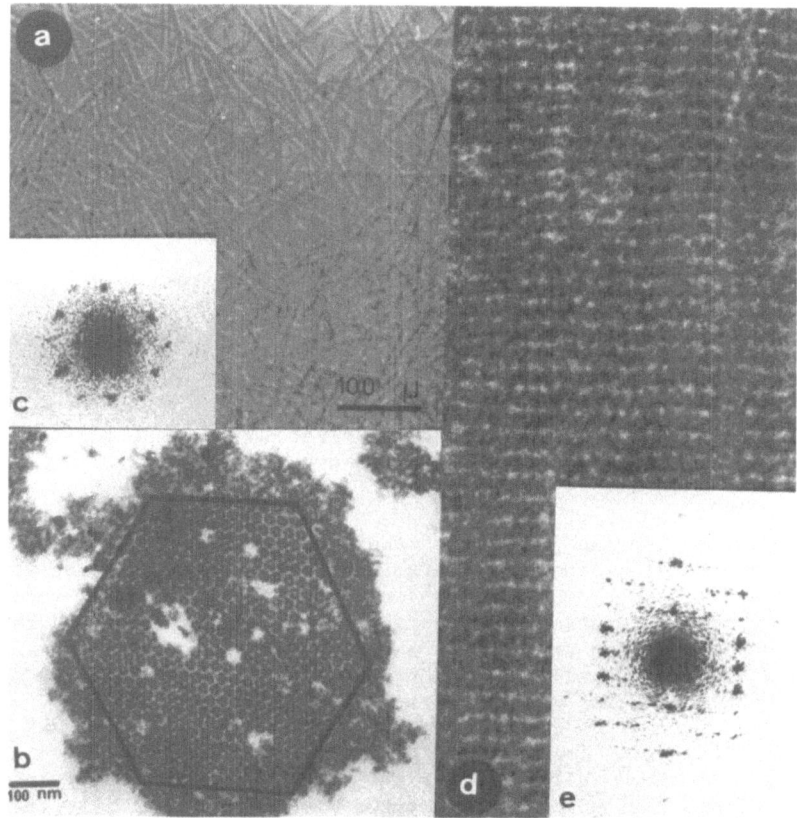

Fig. 2:  (a) Crystals of 70S ribosomes from E. coli as seen by light microscopy.  Growth conditions:  12% methyl pentane diol at pH 8.7.
(b) Electron micrograph of a positively stained thin section
across an embedded crystal, the edges of which are depicted.
(c) Optical diffraction pattern of (b).  (d) Electron micrograph
of a section through another crystal of E. coli 70S ribosomes.
(e) Optical diffraction pattern of (d).

(presumably the proteins) are located closer to the surface and are involved
in interactions between the crystalline particles (unpublished data).

X-Ray Diffraction Studies on Ribosomal Crystals

Preliminary X-ray diffraction patterns have been obtained for crystals
of the large ribosomal subunits of B. stearothermophilus from three types
of specimens:  native single crystals, glutaraldehyde cross-linked single
crystals, and large amounts of microcrystals[18].  These studies include:

a)  Still and 2° oscillation photographs of chunky medium sized crystals
(Fig. 5) and of fragments derived from large (0.9 x 0.25 x 0.15 mm)
crystals (Fig. 6) which are relatively stable in the X-ray beam (more
than three hours in a synchrotron beam of $5 \times 10^8$ photons/sec at 28-35
mA).  The X-ray patterns include reflections to 1.5-1.8 nm resolution
and have periodic spacings of 13.8 ± 0.4 nm and 25.9 ± 0.4 nm (Fig. 7).

b)  Screenless 1° precession photographs of a cross-linked fragile needle-
like thin crystal (0.15 x 0.05 x 0.05 mm) which diffracts to a resolution of 0.95-1.0 nm with periodic spacings of 15.4 nm and 26.1 nm[18].

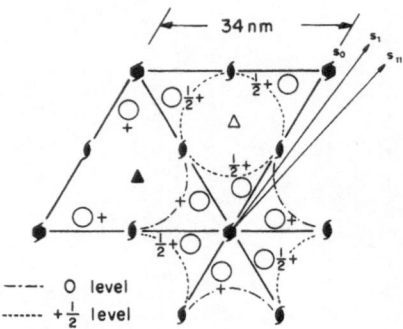

Fig. 3:  A schematic diagram of the AB face of crystals of E. coli ribo-
         somes.  Suggested outer dimensions of the asymmetric units are
         drawn.  $S_0$, $S_1$ and $S_{11}$ define the directions of the sections,
         the filtered images of which are shown in Fig. 4.


The spacings determined in both of these two approaches mentioned are
similar to those obtained by electron microscopy from thin sections of
these crystals and from two-dimensional sheets[11].  The small variations
between the cell constants measured by electron microscopy and the
periodic spacings detected on the X-ray patterns may arise from differences in the crystallization conditions and/or from somewhat different handling during the preparation for electron microscopy.

c)  "Powder" diffraction from samples containing large amounts of micro-
    crystals which gave fairly sharp rings both in high and low resolution.
    Among them are some high angle features with spacings similar to those
    previously reported for gels or ribosomes and extracted rRNA[19,20].  The
    patterns are fairly well oriented, and for aligned crystals the average
    arc length is ± 30°.  Such patterns may arise from partial orientation
    of the nucleic acid component within the particle.  The low angle
    features of these patterns clearly shows two components.  One of these
    arises from the shape of the particles and gives parameters that agree
    well with those measured previously for E. coli 50S non-crystallized
    subunits[21].  The other component consists of some crystalline sharp,
    oriented rings with spacings that probably correspond to a unit-cell
    packing of 14 nm x 26 nm (Fig. 7; Wachtal, Yonath and Wittmann, unpub-
    lished).

Under appropriate crystallization conditions nucleation centers are
formed within aggregates of ribosomal subunits during the initial period
of crystallization[22].  An attempt to increase the size simultaneously with
the order of the crystals by slowing down the crystallization process has
failed, probably due to deterioration of the ribosomes before they began
to aggregate.  However, significantly larger and relatively well-ordered
crystals have been obtained by changing the growth medium from a single
solvent to mixtures of organic materials (Fig. 6).


THE NATURE OF THE INTERPARTICLE CONTACTS WITHIN THE CRYSTALS

Two-dimensional crystalline sheets have been obtained from the large
subunits of B. stearothermophilus ribosomes[11] by essentially the same
crystallization method used for production of three-dimensional crystals.
For this purpose an active, pure preparation of the 50S subunit was used
which had failed to produce three-dimensional crystals detectable by light
microscopy, and further, the relative concentrations of the materials in

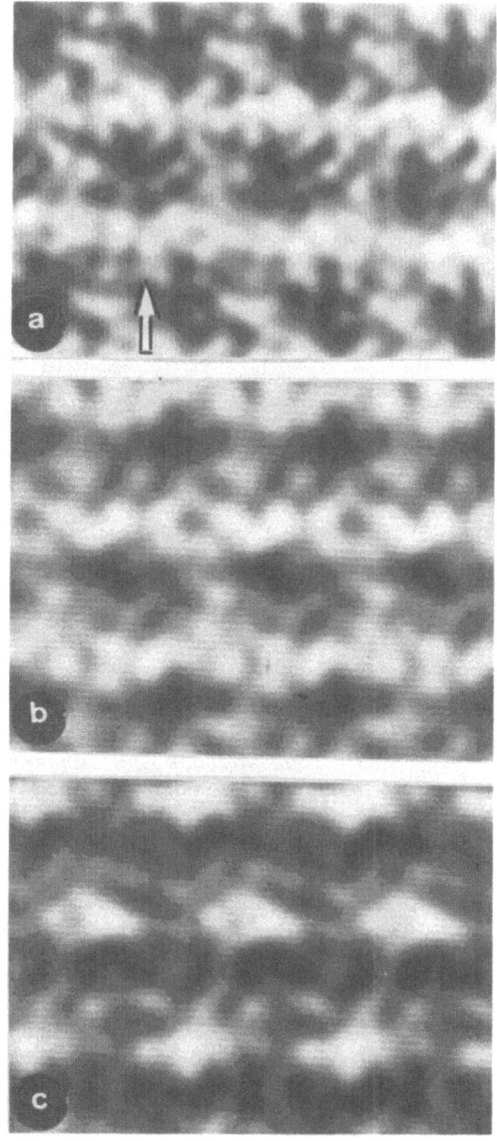

Fig. 4: Filtered images of positively stained thin sections obtained
parallel to the $6_3$-fold axis of crystals of 70S $\underline{E}$. $\underline{coli}$ ribosomes.
(a) (b) and (c) relate to those sections which are marked by $S_0$,
$S_1$ and $S_{11}$ in Fig. 3. The approximate direction of the $6_3$-fold
axis is marked.

the crystallizing medium were altered, e.g. the subunit concentration was
lowered and the $Mg^{++}$ concentration increased.

To characterize the factors that are responsible for the production of
two-dimensional crystals we have investigated the formation of three-dimensional crystals in more detail as a function of the $Mg^{++}$ concentration. 50S
preparations which produce normal three-dimensional crystals at low $Mg^{++}$ concentration were tested for crystal growth over a range of $Mg^{++}$ concentrations. It was found that when the $Mg^{++}$ concentration in the crystallization
medium exceeds 50 mM, in most cases no three-dimensional crystals could be

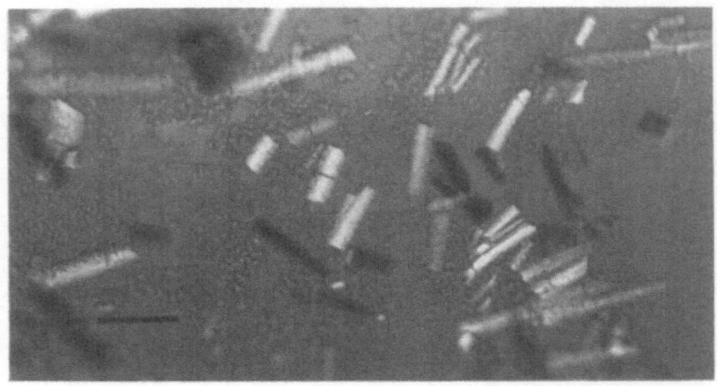

Fig. 5: Crystals of 50S ribosomal subunits of B. stearothermophilus,
grown from 30% methanol at pH 8.6, as seen by polarized light
microscopy. Scale bar = 0.2 mm.


detected by light microscopy. In some experiments small three-dimensional
crystals were produced, but these dissolved within 1-2 days.

A hypothesis to explain these results is that the interparticle
contacts which are created in the two-dimensional plane differ from those
between planes in the three-dimensional crystal. The latter are subjected
to a strong competition with $Mg^{++}$ ions whereas the intra-plane contacts are
either indifferent to, or even enhanced by, the presence of $Mg^{++}$. The
chemical properties of the two types of contact are still unknown.

The two-dimensional sheets were obtained in the presence of ethanol
over the pH-range 5.8-7.2, with optimal size at pH 6.0-6.4. At lower pH-
values (5.4-5.6) a slight tendency for the production of pyramid-like
microcrystals has been observed (Fig. 8), and at higher pH-values (>7.5)
no sheets could be detected. The three-dimensional crystals were grown in
the presence of several alcohols[12] over a wide pH-range (pH 5.6-9), and
those of optimal size were obtained by using 25-30% methanol at pH 7.8-8.7.

The three-dimensional crystals regularly reach their final length and
width in the initial stages of crystal growth. Thus their large face is
almost completely developed within 2-3 weeks. During this period the
crystals are long, very thin and morphologically intact (Fig. 6). Only at
later stages do they become thicker and heavier, thereby sinking to the
bottom of the crystallization drop and developing cracks perpendicular to
their long axes (Fig. 6). Similar fracturing occurs in cross-linked
crystals, regardless of their thickness. It seems probable that the crack-
ing and fracturing of the crystals result from mechanical stress which
originates from accumulating weight or as a result of chemical forces
induced by the cross-linking. For recording X-ray patterns we intended to
expose single separated fragments of these fractured crystals. However,
judging from the nature of the diffraction patterns (Fig. 7), it appears
that we could not detect every crack by visual inspection.

It is of interest to note that all the three-dimensional crystals and
two-dimensional sheets that have so far been obtained both in vivo and in
vitro, are either of the large ribosomal subunits or of whole ribosomes.
There have been many attempts to crystallize the small subunits, and with
the exception of one case in which short helices have been reported[9], no
two-dimensional sheets or three-dimensional crystals have so far been

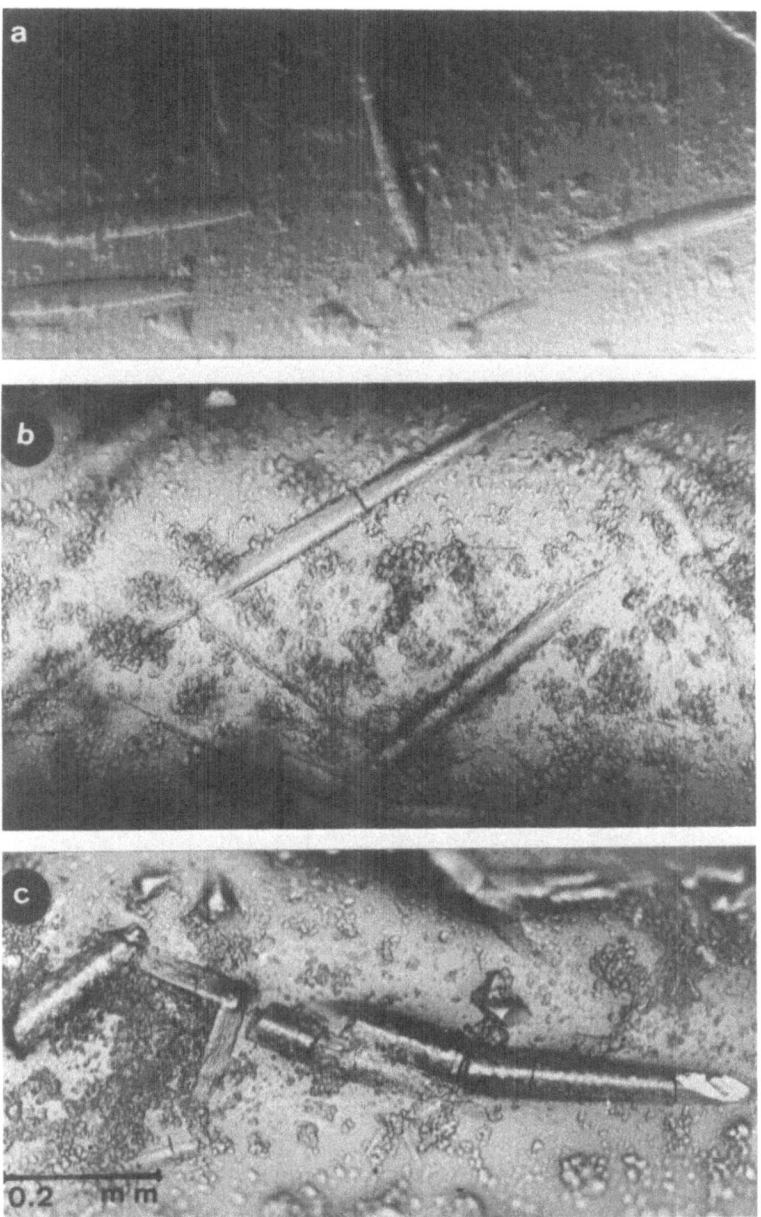

Fig. 6: Crystals of 50S ribosomal subunits of B. stearothermophilus, obtained from 30% methanol at pH 8.4 after (a) 15 days and (b) 30 days. (c) Crystals of the same particles as (a) and (b) but grown from a mixture of 17% ethylene glycol and 17% methanol at pH 8.4.

obtained. Furthermore, the interparticle contacts within the two-dimensional sheets of the whole ribosomes from the oocytes of the lizard Lacerta sicula are formed between the large subunits, and the sheets are stable even when the small subunits are removed[6]. It is not known whether this reflects an inherent flexibility of the small subunits (or a relative rigidity of the large subunits), or whether it is merely coincidence.

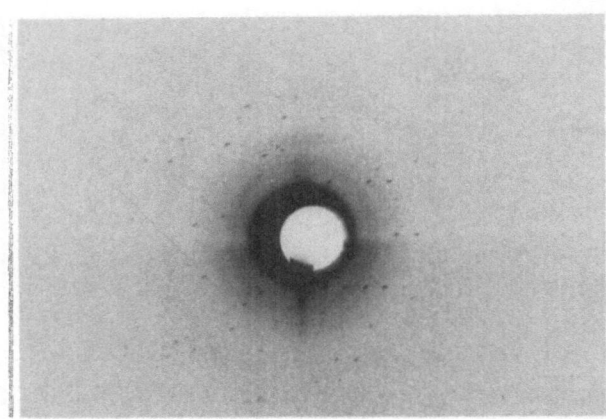

Fig. 7: The central part of a still diffraction pattern obtained with synchrotron radiation. The experimental conditions were: 5 GEV and 22-28 mA with X11/DORIS at DESY in Hamburg, 0.12 mm apperture, 12-15° C for 1 hour. The pattern is from a fragment of the crystal shown in Fig. 6(c). Some low resolution rings probably originated from microcrystals, and a precipitate that was present in the capillary can also be detected.

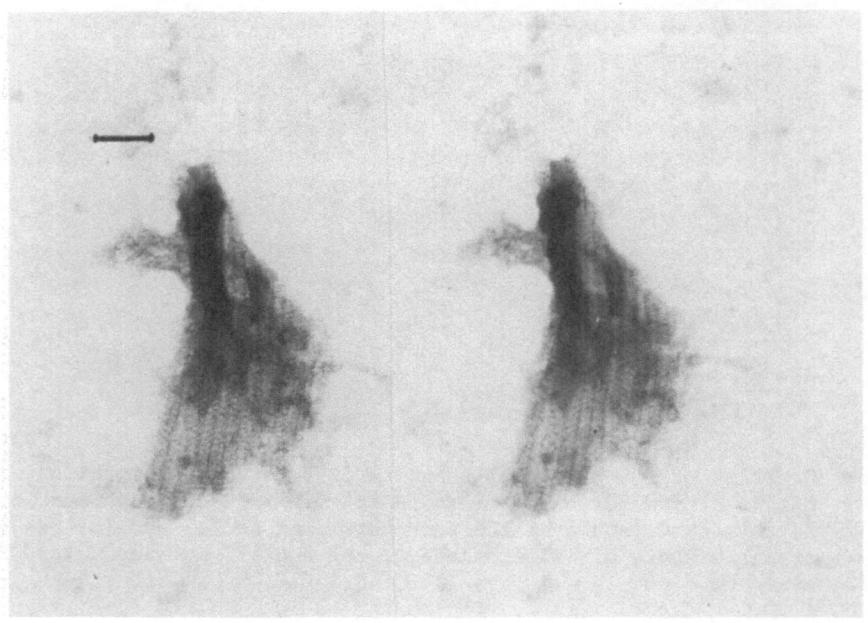

Fig. 8: The development of the growth of a three-dimensional microcrystal from a two-dimensional sheet of 50S particles from B. stearo-thermophilus. The negatively stained (with uranyl acetate) electron micrograph was tilted by ±10° around its axis, and the two views are shown together to enable stereo view representation. Growth conditions: 10% ethanol at pH 5.6. Bar length 100 nm.

## FUTURE PROSPECTS

The ultimate goal of this line of research is to obtain a reliable three-dimensional model for the ribosome which is free from the subjective element inherent in the interpretation of electron micrographs. This model is essential for an understanding of the ribosomal role in protein biosynthesis. The attraction of the scientific problem originates from the immense biological significance of the subject. It is also conditioned by the reasonable expectation that these studies will prove to be feasible, expecially in view of the availability of suitable material, the reproducibility of crystal growth and the quality and the internal order of the crystals. Although the size of the crystals has still to be slightly improved to allow efficient diffraction studies, X-ray data collection from native crystals, using synchrotron radiation and probably newly developed detectors, is not likely to be too difficult. Fortunately, the ribosomal particles are packed in crystals with relatively small unit cells, a reasonable degree of internal order and adequate stability in the X-ray beam.

Phases whose knowledge is important for further progress may be obtained by applying one or more of the following strategies: (1) soaking the crystals in heavy atom cluster derivatives, as used for structure determination of nucleosomes[23]; (2) cocrystallizing of the 50S particles with relatively small molecules which specifically bind to the 50S subunits and to which heavy atoms can be covalently attached; (3) chemical modification of the ribosomes themselves. This might be achieved either by direct interaction of multi-metal containing compounds with the intact ribosome prior to its crystallization or by reconstitution and crystallization of particles in which protein or RNA molecules are loaded with heavy atoms; (4) using information from neutron diffraction studies[24], or from image reconstruction of two-dimensional sheets and of sections through three-dimensional crystals.

Since the ribosomes from "regular" bacteria may disintegrate at high salt concentrations, they have been crystallized from organic solvents. In order to overcome the inconvenience in handling such systems, alternative sources have been considered. One of these is to use halophilic bacteria which contain ribosomes with the unusual property of withstanding and being active at high salt concentrations. This might allow crystallization from salts such as ammonium sulfate instead of alcohols. Three-dimensional crystals of the large subunits of ribosomes from halophilic bacteria have recently been obtained[25].

Much effort and sophistication are still required before the goal of these studies, namely the elucidation of the structure of the ribosome at the molecular level, can be reached. However, the rapid progress and the very promising results achieved so far suggest that this goal is by no means unattainable.

## REFERENCES

1.  G. Chambliss, G. R. Craven, J. Davies, K. Davis, L. Kahan, and M. Nomura (eds), "Ribosomes: Structure, Function and Genetics," University Park Press, Baltimore (1980).

2.  H. G. Wittmann, Components of bacterial ribosomes, Annual Rev. Biochem. 51:155-183 (1982).

3.  A. Liljas, Structural studies of ribosomes, Progr. Biophys. Mol. Biol. 40:161-228 (1982).

4.  H. G. Wittmann, Architecture of prokaryotic ribosomes, Ann. Rev. Biochem. 52:35-65 (1983).

5.  J. Lake and H. S. Slayter, Three-dimensional structure of chromatoid body helix of Entamoeba invadens, J. Mol. Biol. 66:271-282 (1972).

6.  W. Kühlbrandt and P. N. T. Unwin, Distribution of RNA and protein in crystalline eukaryotic ribosomes, J. Mol. Biol. 156:431-448 (1982).

7.  R. A. Milligan and P. N. T. Unwin, In vitro crystallization of ribosomes from chick embryos, J. Cell. Biol. 95:648-653 (1982).

8.  L. O'Brien, K. Shelley, J. Towfighi, and A. McPherson, Crystalline ribosomes are present in brains from senile humans, Proc. Natl. Acad, Sci. USA 77:2260-2264 (1980).

9.  M. W. Clark, M. Hammons, J. A. Langer, and J. A. Lake, Helical arrays of Escherichia coli small ribosomal subunits produced in vitro, J. Mol. Biol. 135:507-512 (1979).

10. M. W. Clark, K. Leonard, and J. A. Lake, Ribosomal crystalline arrays of large subunits from Escherichia coli, Science 216:999-1001 (1982).

11. T. Arad, K. Leonard, H. G. Wittmann, and A. Yonath, Two-dimensional crystalline sheets of Bacillus stearothermophilus 50S ribosomal particles, The EMBO J. 3:127-131 (1984).

12. A. Yonath, J. Müssig, and H. G. Wittmann, Parameters for crystal growth of ribosomal subunits, J. Cell. Biochem. 19:145-155 (1982).

13. A. Yonath, J. Müssig, B. Tesche, S. Lorenz, V. A. Erdmann, and H. G. Wittmann, Crystallization of the large ribosomal subunits from Bacillus stearothermophilus, Biochem. Internat. 1:428-453 (1980).

14. A. Yonath, B. Tesche, S. Lorenz, J. Müssig, V. A. Erdmann, and H. G. Wittmann, Several crystal forms of the Bacillus stearothermophilus 50S ribosomal particles, FEBS Lett. 154:15-20 (1983).

15. A. Yonath, J. Piefke, J. Müssig, H. S. Gewitz, and H. G. Wittmann, A compact three-dimensional crystal form of the large ribosomal subunits from Bacillus stearothermophilus, FEBS Lett. 163:69-72 (1983).

16. H. G. Wittmann, J. Müssig, J. Piefke, H. S. Gewitz, H. J. Rheinberger and A. Yonath, Crystallization of Escherichia coli ribosomes, FEBS Lett. 146:217-220 (1982).

17. K. R. Leonard, T. Arad, B. Tesche, V. A. Erdmann, H. G. Wittmann, and A. Yonath, Crystallization, electron microscopy and three-dimensional reconstruction studies of ribosomal subunits, 10th Internatl. Congr. Electron Microscopy, Hamburg, Vol. 3:9-15 (1984).

18. A. Yonath, H. D. Bartunik, K. S. Bartels, and H. G. Wittmann, Some X-ray diffraction patterns from single crystals of the large ribosomal subunit from Bacillus stearothermophilus, J. Mol. Biol. 177:201-206 (1984).

19. G. Zubay and M. H. F. Wilkins, X-ray diffraction studies on the structure of ribosomes from Escherichia coli, J. Mol. Biol. 2:105-112 (1960).

20. A. Klug, K. C. Holmes, and J. T. Finch, X-ray diffraction studies on ribosomes from various sources, J. Mol. Biol. 3:87-100 (1961).

21. R. Langridge and K. C. Holmes, X-ray diffraction studies of concentrated gels of ribosomes from Escherichia coli, J. Mol. Biol. 5: 611-617 (1962).

22. A. Yonath, G. Khavitch, B. Tesche, J. Müssig, S. Lorenz, V. A. Erdmann, and H. G. Wittmann, The nucleation of crystals of the large ribosomal subunits from Bacillus stearothermophilus, Biochem. Internat. 5:629-636 (1982).

23. T. J. Richmond, J. T. Finch, and A. Klug, Studies on nucleosome structure, Cold Spring Harbor Symp. 47:493-501 (1982).

24. G. A. Bentley, J. T. Finch, and A. Lewit-Bentley, Neutron diffraction studies on crystals of nucleosome cores using contrast variation, J. Mol. Biol. 145:771-784 (1981).

25. A. Shevack, H. S. Gewitz, B. Hennemann, A. Yonath and H. G. Wittmann, Characterization and crystallization of ribosomal particles from Halobacterium marismortui, FEBS Lett. 184:68-71 (1985).

UNDERSTANDING CANCER - THE NEED FOR A BROAD AND INTEGRATED SCIENTIFIC

APPROACH

Anne Brown, Sarah A. Bruce and Paul O.P. Ts'o

Division of Biophysics
School of Hygiene and Public Health
The Johns Hopkins University
Baltimore, Maryland

INTRODUCTION

Understanding and controlling cancer is a challenge to science equal to the challenge of controlling hereditary disorders and understanding the aging process. Several aspects of the disease are considered in making such a comprehensive statement.

First, where adequate medical facilities exist for the prevention and treatment of disease such that the lifespan of the population extends into "old age", cancer is a leading cause of death. In fact, a recent report from the American Cancer Society states that mainly because of increase in life expectancy, the incidence of cancer in people born in 1985 will approach 33%[1]. This is a trend that we can expect to become even more widespread as improved medical facilities contribute to worldwide increases in life expectancy.

Second, the cost of cancer is astronomical with respect to the physical, emotional, and financial demands. Because cancer is incompletely understood, treatment so often traumatic, and the course of the disease so physically extreme, the misery associated with cancer is significantly different from that associated with other diseases or phenomena including old age.

Third, an understanding of carcinogenesis will contribute to our knowledge of normal differentiation and growth control since a normal cell is the precursor of the cancer cell that is no longer subject to regulatory controls governing cell division, tissue specificity, and differentiation. In order to prevent or correct a malignant change, an understanding of the regulatory mechanisms operating during normal cell growth and tissue development may be essential.

APPROACHES TO UNDERSTANDING CARCINOGENESIS

The challenge can be divided into three major areas: 1) evaluation of concepts upon which experiments are designed, 2) application of available technology and development of new technology with which to the implement the design, and 3) design of experimental approaches.

The direction of molecular biology in the last two decades is an example of the influence of concept on the experimental and technological direction of science. Through the period from the late 1950s to the late 1970s, it was widely accepted that knowledge of the primary structure of macromolecules would elucidate the mechanisms of their regulation. Great progress was made in understanding enzyme catalysis, the genetic code and protein synthesis, tRNA structure and function, Hn RNA processing and many aspects of gene expression such as the molecular lesions involved in thalessemia. But we now realize that control of gene expression resides not only in primary sequences but also in secondary, tertiary and higher order structure. We know now that DNA exhibits conformational polymorphism (A, B, Z conformers) and that the conformational state may influence the interaction of DNA with regulatory proteins[2]. DNase I sensitivity studies[3] have shown that gene expression depends upon partial unwinding of the helix undoubtedly assisted by a subset of proteins or other macromolecular complexes.

Another influential idea was the concept that a genome is composed of an unchanging linear array of nucleotides. The first observation that challenged this concept was that DNA rearrangement occurs during the ontogeny of an active immunoglobulin-secreting cell[4]. Since Hozumi and Tonegawa made this landmark discovery, we have witnessed not only the molecular verification of the work of McClintock who proposed, in the 1950s, the existence of mobile controlling genetic elements in maize[5], but also the discovery of mobile genetic elements in virtually every organism[6]. Moreover, there is accumulating evidence that DNA sequences rearrange not only within a single genome but also between the nuclear genome and the genomes of subcellular organelles such as mitochondria and chloroplasts[7]. Reports have also been presented of DNA transfer between different sea urchin species and between feline and primate species[8,9]. No specific function has been assigned to most DNA rearrangement events and in many cases rearrangement is associated with a pathological state, including cancer. However, with the discovery of DNA rearrangements in genesis of the T-cell receptor[10], one can speculate that as yet unknown rearrangements are involved in biological processes that require a complex response to environmental challenge.

While our concepts about the fluidity of the genome are changing, our concepts about the dimensionality of gene control are also changing. Until recently, minimal experimental effort was made to explore the three-dimensional arrangement of nuclear components and the possible function that spatial arrangements might have in the regulation of gene expression (see chapter by K.J. Pienta and D.S. Coffey). However, in the last several years the concept and definition of a nuclear matrix have evolved, and experimental data from several laboratories suggest that DNA replication and RNA transcription are intimately associated with the matrix[11,12]. These data suggest that nuclear compartmentalization within the matrix may be involved in the specificity of genetic control in growth and differentiation. Thus, the concept of the genetic apparatus has evolved from that of a linear, one-dimensional regulatory apparatus to that of a multidimensional, dynamic array. The possibility that genes may be an integral part of complex, three-dimensional structures should be kept in mind when formulating hypotheses of molecular mechanisms of cancer and differentiation and when interpreting data in those areas.

With respect to the technology (ie., instrumentation and biological material) with which we carry out the experimental design, much of our knowledge of the biological processes of cancer and differentiation is derived from a biochemical approach that reflects statistical averages of cellular populations. Now, however, we may be on the threshold of a revolution in defining populations by observing individual cells, both fixed and living, within the population. The coupling of fluorescence-labeled antibodies and fluorescence-labeled nucleic acid probes with computer assisted microphotometry introduces the possibility of studying the spatial location of macromolecules (proteins, mRNA, DNA), the interaction of two or more macromolecules, and the movement of cellular components in a living cell. While antibodies would allow us to specifically tag a protein component of interest, nucleic acid probes[13] would allow us to localize individual genes and mRNA. This in situ approach is particularly valuable in the study of cancer where biochemical heterogeneity is characteristic of tumor cell populations. The ability to monitor (at the single cell level) changes in a population should allow us to answer questions about carcinogenesis (initiation and promotion) and about the later stages of tumor progression. We could document the earliest biochemical changes which occur in cells in response to external chemicals (growth factors, hormones, tumor promoters, carcinogens, etc.) and identify the affected subset(s) of cells which progressively acquires preneoplastic properties and malignancy. And because only small numbers of cells are required for analysis, cells of limited availability from different tissues and ages not otherwise amenable to biochemical studies could be analyzed.

Through the use of in vivo nucleic acid hybridization we might be able not only to observe but also to control the expression of specific genes[13] and subsequently examine the effect of experimentally-imposed changes in gene expression on cellular populations. The development of these tools is in its infancy, but when this technology is perfected, it will allow us to explore the little known parameters of cellular population biology and the pattern of macromolecular changes in biological processes such as carcinogenesis.

The conceptual training and specialization of the investigator influences experimental design and choice of experimental model. For example, since the discovery of the homology between viral oncogenes and cellular proto-oncogenes, there has been a movement to conceptualize cancer as changes in the expression or function of a small subset of genes (proto-oncogenes). Such reduction can be productive since questions can be better defined and variables limited. For example, aberrant proto-oncogene expression, although perhaps not an early event in cancer, may still serve as an assay to identify more fundamental cellular changes associated with the temporal acquisition of neoplasia-related phenotypes.

Through the reductionist approach we have gained insight into the mechanisms by which growth control may be disrupted in cancer cells. Two recent observations have provided an explanation of the observation that proliferation of cancer cells is not always dependent upon the presence of exogenous growth factors. The discovery that the v-sis oncogene sequence is homologous to cellular sequences for platelet-derived growth factor[14] immediately suggested a mechanism by which tumor cells could autonomously regulate their own proliferation. Following this discovery it was found that the ros oncogene of the UR2 retrovirus and the src oncogene of Rous sarcoma virus could phosphorylate plasma membrane inositides and that this phosphorylation caused a sequence of biochemical events that resulted in stimulation of a cellular enzyme involved in cell proliferation[15,16]. Thus the reduction of cancer biology to the study of gene function contributed to the elucidation of the biochemical basis of an empirical conclusion, the mechanistic understanding of which may be essential in designing effective therapeutic agents.

Despite advantages of the reductionist approach, studies of isolated cellular components will not be adequate unless the studies are designed with an appreciation of the biological milieu of which the component is a part. One could call such an approach 'constructionist'. Obtaining meaningful data about the mechanisms of carcinogenesis from cellular and molecular experiments requires knowledge of the biology of the source of the experimental material. The components (macromolecules and subcellular structures) must be considered in the context of cells and tissues; cells and tissues must be considered in the context of the physiological state of the tissue or organism. For example, because oncogene expression may be related to differentiation, meaningful interpretation of the relationship between Philadelphia chromosome-positive (Ph+) chronic myelocytic leukemia and c-abl proto-oncogene expression can be made only if the clinical manifestations of the leukemia (eg. the differentiation stage of the Ph+ peripheral leukocytes in each particular patient) are known.

Consideration of the cell type, source and system used to explore carcinogenesis is crucial and will be addressed again in the following sections where we review work accomplished in our laboratory and by others, consider the relevance of this work to carcinogenesis, and explore molecular models of carcinogenesis and tumor progression.

MECHANISM OF CARCINOGENESIS - RELATIONSHIP BETWEEN SOMATIC MUTATION AND

CANCER

Since Boveri[17] first postulated the somatic mutation theory of carcinogenesis, considerable evidence has accumulated to indicate a genetic or mutational basis for the heritable alterations exhibited by neoplastic cells. This evidence includes the aneuploid character of most tumors[18], the dominantly inherited familial cancers such as retinoblastoma[19], genetic defects affecting DNA damage repair such as xeroderma pigmentosum[19], and the observation that most carcinogens are mutagenic[20]. However, arguments against a simple mutational mechanism for carcinogenesis have also been presented, including the clear distinction between the one step nature of somatic mutation and the progressive multistep nature of carcinogenesis[21-25], and the ability of the microenvironment to modulate tumorigenic potential as exemplified by embryonal carcinoma cells which can develop alternatively into normal tissue or into teratocarcinomas depending on their environment[26]. Thus, both mutational (genetic) and non-mutational (epigenetic or developmental) mechanisms have been implicated in carcinogenesis.

To examine more critically the relationship between somatic mutation and carcinogenesis, our laboratory has developed a cell culture system in which somatic mutation and neoplastic transformation can be analyzed simultaneously[27]. In these analyses, in which the intent is also to extrapolate the in vitro data to in vivo carcinogenesis, the choice of the experimental system is crucial. In this regard, normal diploid cell strains have a distinct advantage over aneuploid, established cell lines because the former are a better approximation of normal diploid cells in vivo. In our laboratory, we have chosen to use the Syrian hamster embryo (SHE) fibroblastic cell system originally developed by Berwald and Sachs[28,29], and DiPaolo and colleagues[30,31]. These cells are generated from normal 13 day gestation fetal tissue, generally maintain their diploid character in culture and exhibit in vitro cellular senescence with a very low frequency of spontaneous neoplastic transformation[32,33].

Using this in vitro cell system, we have shown that DNA is a critical cellular target of carcinogenic attack. Three types of experiments designed to perturb DNA alone without altering any other cellular macromolecules have shown that neoplastic transformation can be induced by DNA-specific perturbations. These include incorporation of 5-bromodeoxyuridine into DNA followed by near-UV irradiation[34,35], incorporation of tritiated thymidine with incorporation of tritiated-uridine as a control[36], and treatment with pancreatic DNase I encapsulated in phosphatidylserine liposomes[37]. These experiments clearly indicate the direct involvement of DNA damage in carcinogenesis but do not define the relationship between somatic mutation and cancer.

A second set of experiments showed that _in vitro_ neoplastic transformation of SHE cells is a multistep, progressive phenomenon characterized by the temporal acquisition of neoplasia-related phenotypes, e.g. morphological transformation, enhanced fibrinolytic activity, contact-insensitivity, anchorage independence, and ultimately tumorigenicity[37,38]. _In vitro_ neoplastic transformation is similar to the progressive development of tumors _in vivo_ as described by Foulds[20,21].

Other experiments directly compared the induction of somatic point mutation to the acquisition of neoplasia-associated phenotypes[23]. Point mutations induced by benzo(a)pyrene (B(a)P) and N-methyl-N'-nitro-N-nitroso-guanidine (MNNG) at the HPRT (6-thioguanine resistance) and $Na^+/K^+$ ATPase (ouabain resistance) loci were quantitated and compared to the acquisition of morphological transformation and anchorage-independence which is highly correlated to tumorigenicity in the Syrian hamster system (Kendall coefficient of rank correlation = 0.986)[40]. Both cellular transformation phenotypes have characteristics distinct from the somatic mutation phenotypes observed at the two loci. Morphological transformation was observed after an expression time comparable to somatic mutation but at a 25 to 540-fold higher frequency. Anchorage independent transformants were detected at a frequency of $10^{-5}$-$10^{-6}$ but not until 32-75 population doublings after carcinogen treatment. Although this frequency of transformation to anchorage independence is comparable to that of somatic mutations, the expression time for this transformation is much longer than the optimal expression time of conventionally studied somatic mutations. One reason for this difference is that somatic point mutation involves a one-step change but neoplastic transformation is a multistage phenomenon.

However, the analysis of the role of somatic mutation in neoplastic initiation or progression is complicated by the phenomenon of progression itself. Therefore, the involvement of mutation must be analyzed separately at each of the various steps between the stages of neoplastic progression. Fluctuation analysis of the progressive acquisition of anchorage independence by clonally derived, preneoplastic, subtetraploid SHE cells indicated that variants with this phenotype are generated randomly at a rate of $10^{-8}$-$10^{-7}$ variant/cell/generation, a rate similar to the rate of codominant somatic mutation at the $Na^+/K^+$ ATPase locus in these cells[41]. However this rate could not be increased by treatment of the cells with known point, frameshift or deletion mutagens[42]. The inability of these mutagens to increase the rate of appearance of anchorage-independent variants along with the inability of mutagens to induce recessive mutations at the HPRT locus can be explained by the subtetraploid nature of these cells, and suggests the ploidy dependent, recessive nature of the anchorage-independent phenotype. The observed spontaneous rate of emergence of anchorage independent variants can, however, be explained by chromosomal nondisjunction resulting in the conversion of heterozygous preneoplastic cells to anchorage-independent homozygotes[42,43].

Two other types of experiments provide additional evidence for the recessive nature of anchorage independence and tumorigenicity. First, near diploid clones of SHE cells treated with chemical carcinogens (MNNG or ethyl methane sulfate) acquire anchorage independence and tumorigenicity while similarly treated near tetraploid clones of SHE cells do not[44]. Thus neoplastic transformation is ploidy or gene-dosage dependent. Second, intraspecies somatic cell hybrids between normal diploid, anchorage-dependent SHE cells and anchorage independent, highly tumorigenic BP6T cells[45] initially exhibit a suppression of the anchorage independent phenotype. However, both anchorage independence and tumorigenicity are reexpressed after further passage in culture and the rate of reemergence of the anchorage independent phenotype approximates the rate of chromosomal segregation thus implicating chromosome loss in the reexpression of these traits[42].

Lastly, several studies have shown that SHE cells can be neoplastically transformed by non-mutagenic treatments such as diethylstilbesterol (DES)[46], sodium bisulfite[47], L-ethionine[48], and colcemid[49]. Although no single gene mutations were detected at the HPRT or $Na^+/K^+$ ATPase loci in these experiments, some of these treatments, such as DES and colcemid, did induce aneuploidy[49,50].

Taken together, these studies show that a single-gene somatic point mutation model is inadequate to explain the complex process of neoplastic transformation, which requires a long expression time and appears to involve a cascading series of changes in cellular processes eventually leading to tumorigenicity and metastasis. Although single-gene mutation may not adequately explain the frequency and onset of neoplastic transformation of normal cells in vitro, it may be an integral part of the process. Simple mutation could lead to progressive genetic or epigenetic changes. For example, a mutation in a DNA repair enzyme could lead to the accumulation of subsequent oncogenic mutations, or a mutation in a structural gene for DNA methylation enzymes could lead to hypomethylation and subsequent expression of oncogenic DNA sequences. The challenge remains to determine the role, if any, of mutation in neoplastic transformation and the nature of the mutation(s) involved.

MORE COMPREHENSIVE MOLECULAR HYPOTHESIS OF CARCINOGENESIS

The exploration of the progressive nature of neoplastic transformation could benefit from a hypothesis that extends beyond single-gene point mutation to explain how oncogenic cellular sequences could become inappropriately expressed. Two general observations form the foundation of an alternative hypothesis of neoplastic transformation: (i) progressive karyotypic abnormalities parallel the progression to malignant phenotypes and (ii) mobile genetic elements can act as agents of genetic instability and chromosome changes and can activate proto-oncogene expression in eucaryotic cells.

Aberrations such as aneuploidy, deletions, translocations, inversions, amplifications, and chromosome fragmentation characterize most advanced malignancies, particularly sarcomas and carcinomas[18,51-52]. Some acute leukemias have been notable exceptions, but recently, high resolution chromosome banding techniques have revealed small chromosomal aberrations even within this group of leukemias[53,54]. Such observation, based on chromosome banding, may eventually be extended to all advanced tumors, although with some tumors, molecular analysis (Southern blot, DNA sequence) may be required to reveal rearrangements.

The crucial question is whether rearrangements are causally related to carcinogenesis or neoplastic progression. Several observations demonstrate that karyotypic abnormalities precede cancer. First, analysis of the karyotypic changes that occurred during the spontaneous acquisition of tumorigenicity by euploid Chinese hamster embryo cells in culture showed that aneuploidy preceded the early stages of transformation and that progression of the culture to later stages was paralleled by increasing chromosome aberrations[25]. Second, premalignant lesions which occur in progression of cervical carcinoma and carcinoma of the large bowel contain chromosome aberrations which become more prevalent in the fully invasive lesions[55]. In the case of cervical carcinoma where multiclonal preinvasive lesions are eventually superseded by monoclonal malignancy, it appears that the genetic instability that can initially give rise to karyotypically distinguishable clones may also serve as the mechanism that produces the surviving malignant clone. Third, as mentioned above, malignancies previously regarded as diploid actually contain chromosome abnormalities, and it is likely that with improved resolution this observation will be extended. Fourth, non-random chromosomal aberrations are associated with specific forms of cancer, and in the case of double minute chromosomes, homogeneously staining regions, deletions, and translocations, the aberration is specifically associated with proto-oncogene sequences ([54],[56-64]).

If we accept the hypothesis that continuous large and small scale genetic rearrangements are an integral part of malignant progression, we might then explore the possible mechanism(s) that facilitate the instability and generate the rearrangements. We might ask, for example, whether there is a normal basal level of chromosome aberration analogous to a basal level of DNA replication error or replicon misfiring[65]. Alternatively, specific organismal or cellular changes may initiate aberrations. Several mechanisms can be envisioned. Examples include (i) unregulated expression of meiotic recombination enzymes; (ii) mutations in proteins that govern chromatid pairing, condensation, or movement during mitosis; (iii) activation and transposition of endogenous mobile elements and/or retroviruses. The latter example is particularly attractive since there is extensive experimental evidence that mobile genetic elements (including RNA and DNA viruses) can act as agents of genetic instability[66-72] and in some cases have been implicated in cancer.

Mobile genetic elements were first cloned, sequenced, and explored in procaryotes, where they act as agents of host gene rearrangements and as insertional mutagens[67,68]. Structurally there are several forms with respect to size, sequence, and mode of transposition[68,70-75]. Lower and higher eucaryotes also contain endogenous mobile elements, some of which are structurally similar to procaryotic elements and others of which are unique (P elements of _Drosophila_[73] and the _Alu_ elements of primates)[74]. Functionally, however, there is overlap in different species since current evidence suggests that all elements can transpose and act as insertional mutagens. Mobile eucaryotic DNA sequences, both exogenous and endogenous, can facilitate host gene rearrangement, as do the procaryotic elements.

The endogenous mammalian retroviruses are structurally related to bacterial transposable elements and can transpose and act as insertional mutagens[76,77]. Although there is no evidence as yet that they can rearrange cellular DNA sequences (as can mammalian DNA viruses) this is a viable possibility. Because exogenous retroviruses induce many kinds of chromosomal aberrations which are identical to those observed in tumors, it is possible that endogenous retroviruses might induce similar damage if they were activated in normal or initiated cells. It is worth noting here that normally transcriptionally silent endogenous viral sequences are expressed in experimental tumors and transformed cell lines obtained by exposure to diverse carcinogens[78-81].

In addition to the possibility that the transposition of endogenous mobile elements (including endogenous retroviruses) facilitates the rearrangement of other host DNA sequences, the movement per se of the elements could be relevant to cancer and particularly to progression. Activation of normally repressed elements could lead to successive transpositions which have oncogenic consequences; for example, the elements could integrate between a silent proto-oncogene and a repressor DNA sequence thus releasing the structural sequence from regulatory control. Alternatively, the strong promoters or enhancers contained in retroviruses and transposable elements could activate the transcription of a proto-oncogene in whose proximity the element has integrated. This kind of program operates during oncogenesis by weakly oncogenic retroviruses such as the virus that causes avian lymphomas. Bursal lymphomas in chickens do not appear until months (latent period) after infection with the exogenous leukosis virus. When tumor DNA is examined, the integration site of the virus is next to or near the cellular gene homologous to the myc gene of the MC29 avian retrovirus. The hypothesis is that the virus initially integrates at many sites but may not integrate near an oncogenic sequence (myc) until subsequent transposition occurs[82]. It is this rare transposition event which results in malignancy. The important idea is that there is no a priori reason to suppose that the molecular consequences of endogenous viral activation would be vastly different from the consequences of exogenous viral infection. In fact, several investigations have shown that endogenous viruses are rearranged, sometimes next to cellular proto-oncogenes, in tumors and tumor cell lines[82-84]. These viruses can facilitate transcription of flanking genes. The relevance of these observations to human cancer should be considered in light of the discovery of endogenous retroviruses and transposon-like sequences in the human genome[85-87].

In summary, an alternative model to simple somatic mutation for neoplasia involves (i) random progressive genome instability initiated by endogenous mobile elements and resulting in activation of cellular oncogenic sequences or (ii) direct promotion of oncogenic sequences as a result of transposition of an endogenous element to the site of the cellular oncogenic sequence, and in the absence of major genome changes. The rationale for the first alternative is the chromosomal aberrations incurred after infection with eucaryotic exogenous viruses or after movement of endogenous elements in lower eucaryotes. The rationale for the second alternative is the so-called "latent period" and subsequent oncogene activation associated with infection by the chronic retroviruses such as the avian leukosis viruses.


MECHANISM OF CARCINOGENESIS - RELATIONSHIP BETWEEN CANCER AND CELLULAR

DIFFERENTIATION

Carcinogenesis can also be considered as an aberration of normal cellular differentiation. In order to investigate the relationship between the potential for carcinogenesis and the stage of differentiation, we need to identify which cells in vivo are the crucial cells for carcinogenic attack. Are the consequences of carcinogenic attack equal for all cells, or are the consequences greatest for a subset of cells? If a carcinogen-initiated cell does not divide and hence does not progress to neoplasia, the consequences of the carcinogenic attack are minimal. Thus, although a non-proliferative, differentiating or terminally differentiated cell may be attacked by a carcinogen, the crucial target cell may be a

less differentiated cell such as a stem cell or a progenitor cell that is
capable of cell division. Thus, the developmental stage and/or differentiation state of the target cell may be crucial in determining the
cell's response to perturbation.

A working hypothesis on the relationship between neoplasia and
cellular differentiation is shown in Figure 1. Stem cells and progenitor
cells have at least two possible pathways which they can follow. One
pathway is the progressive development of an undifferentiated, slowly
proliferating stem cell to a committed progenitor cell with high proliferative capacity, to a less proliferative differentiating cell and,
finally, to a generally non-proliferative, fully differentiated cell. In
this case, cell division is tightly controlled and coupled to the differentiation sequence[88]. An alternative pathway is one characterized by
continued cell division and the progressive acquisition of altered growth
properties including tumorigenicity. This pathway produces neoplastic
cells which appear to have infinite proliferative capacity and, as a population, lack the ability to terminally differentiate although individual
tumor cells within the population may cease dividing and differentiate or
die. Thus, neoplastic transformation can be viewed as an uncoupling of
cell division from differentiation.

Several studies from our laboratory suggest that a subset of cells is
more susceptible to carcinogen-induced neoplastic transformation and that
susceptibility to transformation is greatest at earlier stages of development and differentiation. A subpopulation of cells has been identified
in primary and low passage cultures of SHE cells[89]. This subpopulation,
identified by its lack of post-confluence inhibition of cell division
(i.e. contact-insensitivity, $CS^-$), could be quantitated by measuring the
ability of cells to form colonies on irradiated confluent monolayers of
contact-sensitive ($CS^+$) cells (cell mats). It was also shown that the
frequency of $CS^-$ cells decreased from ~10-20% at passage 1 to less than
0.001% by passage 6 (population doubling level, PDL 16-20) and that these
$CS^-$ cells were lost by conversion to $CS^+$ cells[90].

The initial frequency of these transient $CS^-$ cells and the rate of
their loss appear to be directly related to the proliferative capacity of
untreated mass cultures. The PDL at which a given primary culture
senesces shows a positive correlation to the frequency of $CS^-$ cells
present at passage 1. In addition, treatments, such as continuous exposure to tumor promoters from passage 1, which retard the rate of loss of
$CS^-$ cells, extend the in vitro proliferative life span of the mass
culture. This is true both for different preparations of 13 day gestation
fetal cell cultures which show some variation in their initial frequency

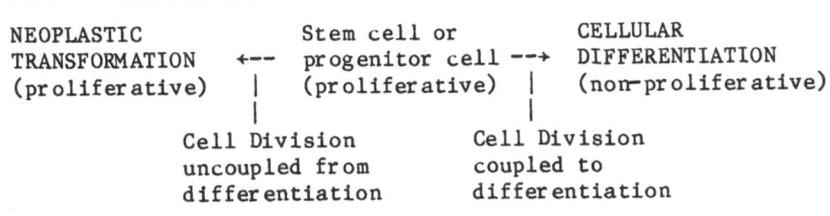

NEOPLASTIC          Stem cell or       CELLULAR
TRANSFORMATION  ←-- progenitor cell --→ DIFFERENTIATION
(proliferative) |   (proliferative)  |  (non-proliferative)
                |                     |
         Cell Division        Cell Division
         uncoupled from       coupled to
         differentiation      differentiation

FIG. 1.  Working hypothesis on the relationship between
         differentiation, proliferation and neoplasia.

of CS⁻ cells[90], and for fetal cell cultures (high initial CS⁻ frequency)[91]. Our hypothesis is that the transient CS⁻ cells in low passage cultures are less differentiated progenitor-like cells and that the CS⁻ → CS⁺ conversion may represent an early stage of differentiation characterized by an altered control of proliferation acquired prior to the appearance of a terminally differentiated phenotype. Purified populations of CS⁻ cells are being isolated in order to define more critically the role of these cells in differentiation and cellular senescence.

To determine whether these CS⁻ cells are more sensitive to carcinogenic and/or mutagenic perturbation, the susceptibility to neoplastic transformation and somatic mutation induced by MNNG was examined in clonally isolated cell cultures containing various proportions of CS⁻ cells (4% - 0.02%)[92]. The frequencies of MNNG-induced morphological transformation, focus formation and neoplastic transformation were 20-40 fold higher in CS⁻ enriched cultures (4%) compared to CS⁻ depleted cultures (0.02%). In contrast, the frequency of MNNG-induced somatic mutation at the Na⁺/K⁺ ATPase locus was similar among cultures varying in their proportion of CS⁻ cells. These data suggest that the transient CS⁻ cells in primary Syrian hamster cell cultures are more susceptible to neoplastic transformation although equally susceptible to induced point mutation when compared to CS⁺ cells. If CS⁻ cells are indeed progenitor cells, these data show that less differentiated cells are more susceptible to carcinogenic transformation than their more differentiated progeny.

Preliminary experiments comparing the susceptibility of fetal, young adult, and aged adult dermal fibroblasts to carcinogen-induced neoplastic transformation also show an inverse correlation between transformation frequency and donor age. In response to B(a)P or MNNG, fetal cell cultures escape senescence and acquire anchorage independence and tumorigenicity. Similarly treated young adult cell cultures exhibit an altered in vitro senescence pattern but have a reduced frequency of progression to anchorage independence and tumorigenicity. Treated aged adult cell cultures also show a perturbed in vitro senescence pattern but rarely progress to anchorage independence. Young and aged adult cells that do not acquire these neoplastic phenotypes with continued passaging eventually senesce but do so at a higher PDL than their untreated control (Bruce, et al., unpublished data). These data suggest that fetal cells are more susceptible than adult cells to carcinogen-induced neoplastic transformation.

More recently, we have begun to study the in vitro behavior of cells derived from 9 day gestation embryos (E9 cells). Nine day gestation was chosen because it is the earliest stage in gestation at which the formed embryo can be isolated readily from the maternal tissue. In addition, 9 to 10 days represents the end of embryonic development in the Syrian hamster with the remaining 5-1/2 to 6-1/2 days representing fetal development[93-94]. Most E9 cell cultures exhibit cellular senescence and the pattern of alterations in morphology and proliferation is similar to fetal and adult cells. However, E9 cell cultures exhibit a greater frequency (~20%) of spontaneous escape from senescence relative to fetal and adult cells (<5%); and whereas continuous exposure to tumor promoters can extend the proliferative lifespan of fetal cells, similar treatment of E9 cells with tumor promoters or epidermal growth factor results in a significant increase in the frequency of escape from senescence (50-80% of treated cultures)[95]. Thus, cells from earlier stages of gestation are more easily perturbed even by non-carcinogenic treatment. Further, these established E9 cell lines appear to follow one of two alternative paths, either becoming a relatively stable preadipocyte or premyoblast progenitor cell line or progressing to anchorage independence and tumorigenicity[96].

| DIFFERENTIATION AND/OR PHYSIOLOGICAL STATE | SUSCEPTIBILITY TO SPONTANEOUS AND/OR CARCINOGEN-INDUCED NEOPLASTIC TRANSFORMATION | DEVELOPMENTAL STAGE OR AGE |
|---|---|---|
| Stem cell | high frequency short progression | Embryonic |
| Progenitor cell | intermediate frequency intermediate progression | Fetal/ Neonatal |
| Differentiating cell | low frequency long progression | Young adult |
| Fully differentiated (non-proliferative) cell | non-responsive | Aged adult |

FIG. 2.   Possible interrelationships among neoplastic transformation, differentiation and aging.

Taken together, all of these experiments indicate that the developmental stage, age and/or physiological state of the target population has a significant influence on that population's susceptibility to neoplastic transformation (Figure 2).

SPECIFIC GENETIC CHANGES IN CANCER:  HISTORY AND RESEARCH POTENTIAL

The recent discovery of cellular transforming genes and proto-oncogenes has led to the development of a promising avenue of cancer research. This discovery of DNA sequences specifically involved in neoplastic transformation and tumor formation allows us to interrelate several independent observations in cancer biology, genetics, and virology.

DNA sequences in acute transforming viruses, such as the sarc sequence of Rous sarcoma virus and the myc sequence of the avian myelocytomatosis virus MC29, were known for many years to be oncogenic before their significance in non-viral cancer was appreciated.  The existence of proto-oncogenes, the genomic homologs of viral oncogenes, was postulated in the 1960s[97] and oncogene homologs not connected to viral structural genes[98] were subsequently found in the genomes of diverse eucaryotic organisms.

A unification in cancer virology came about when Neel et al.[99] discovered that tumors caused by the chronic (non-oncogene-containing) avian leukosis virus contained transcripts of the cellular myc gene which had been activated by the viral promoter in the long terminal repeat (LTR). Similar molecular events have been observed with several other avian and mammalian retrovirus LTRs and other proto-oncogenes[100-103].

These observations demonstrated that oncogenesis by chronic and acute transforming retroviruses involves the expression of homologous DNA sequences either located in the viral genome or located in the host genome and activated by the virus.

The evidence that proto-oncogenes are significant in tumorigenesis was strengthened by the discovery that genomic DNA sequences from human tumors that transform NIH 3T3 cell lines (cellular transforming genes) are the cellular homologs of the ras oncogene of the Harvey and Kirsten murine sarcoma viruses[104]. Subsequent studies designed to identify other transforming genes revealed that several cellular genes with no viral oncogene counterparts could transform NIH 3T3 cells[105]. These transforming genes were altered by specific point mutations in tumor DNA but not in other somatic DNA of the same patient[106-108]. Although the normal gene could induce cellular transformation of NIH 3T3 cells when linked to a strong transcriptional promoter (such as a viral LTR), the mutated gene exerted its effect without overexpression.

Proto-oncogenes were implicated again in neoplasia by the discovery that they are involved specifically in diverse chromosomal rearrangements. Chromosomal translocation breakpoints in Burkitt's lymphoma and chronic granulocytic leukemia contain the cellular myc and abl genes respectively[54]. Diverse proto-oncogenes are associated with specific translocation breakpoints and proto-oncogenes are also amplified on the double minute chromosomes and the homogeneously staining regions often observed in human tumors and tumor cell lines[54,61,62].

Proto-oncogenes are also implicated in the genesis of familial tumors of childhood. The deletion at both Rb alleles on chromosome 13 in primary retinoblastoma cells, for example, is associated with elevated expression of the N-myc gene. In this case, the deleted DNA sequence is not itself a proto-oncogene but may be involved in proto-oncogene regulation[63]. Data from related studies support the hypothesis that a similar mechanism operates in the genesis of childhood Wilms' tumor[109,110].

Perhaps the most pivotal observations that related proto-oncogenes to neoplasia were those that established a direct relationship between oncogenes and growth control. Comparison of DNA sequence information in computer data banks with the amino acid sequence of platelet derived growth factor (PDGF) demonstrated that portions of the v-sis oncogene are homologous to the PDGF gene[14]. Subsequently, homology of the erb-B oncogene with the gene for epidermal growth factor (EGF) was demonstrated[111]. Prior to these demonstrations it had been known that the src gene product, pp60, could phosphorylate tyrosine residues in proteins[112]. It had also been postulated that tumor cells escape external growth control (for example, low serum requirement) by producing endogenous growth factors, thereby bypassing the growth factor-receptor pathways that control normal cell proliferation[113]. Furthermore, phosphorylation of tyrosine residues was associated with membrane receptor signal transduction by the EGF and PDGF[114-117].

Thus, these previously existing observations could be unified following the identification of specific genes whose products in tumor cells are altered components of the normal growth control apparatus. And because several other oncogene products have tyrosine kinase activity, perhaps these genes are also homologous to cellular growth factors, possibly tissue specific growth factors. Furthermore, tyrosine phosphorylation is implicated in differentiation[118], so it is possible that proto-oncogenes may also affect normal cellular development. If this is the case, then proto-oncogenes are implicated in yet another cellular process known to be disrupted in tumors and tumor cell lines.

In addition to tyrosine kinase activity, oncogenes can function in growth control by other biochemical pathways: it was recently demonstrated that the ros oncogene product of the avian virus UR2 phosphorylates the inositides whose subsequent breakdown initiates a cascade of biological responses that culminate in the activation of protein kinase C which stimulates cell division[15,16]. And recently, it was shown that the GTPase activity of the ras gene product is linked to cAMP-dependent control of cell proliferation[119,120]. Thus it appears that at least some of the proto-oncogenes may allow a cell to escape growth control by providing their own normal or altered growth factors or growth factor receptors.

It is revealing that the experimental findings just cited were made, in a sense, by 'reducing cancer to the level of genes'. One looks where the light is and sometimes the lost article is indeed under the streetlamp. The oncogene hypothesis existed for many years but became significant when a molecular genetic approach, first used in procaryotic systems (DNA transfection), was applied to eucaryotic cells[121,122]. The tumor DNA sequences that caused transformation in transfection experiments were the very sequences that were known as oncogenic viral genes[123].

On the other hand, the significance of oncogenes in gene rearrangements was confirmed by molecular analysis only after presentation of a hypothesis based on observations of clinical manifestations of tumor progression such as recurrent non-random chromosomal aberrations in hematopoietic tumors[124]. The power to predict is strongest in those disciplines which deal with direct study of clinical aspects of oncogenesis, experimental tumorigenesis, or neoplastic transformation. It is with guidance and direction from veterans in these fields that the tools of molecular biology can be maximally used. Presently, we have strong evidence for the involvement of specific genes in cancer, but our challenge is to determine the most productive experimental direction for the future. Input should be derived from cell biologists, oncologists, and epidemiologists. For example, cellular transforming genes were initially identified by transfection of tumor cell line DNA into NIH 3T3 established cell lines. The initial interpretation was that the activation by point mutation or overexpression of specific cellular sequences was sufficient to cause cancer. Enthusiasm for this interpretation was tempered by the reminder from cancer cell biologists that NIH 3T3 cells are not normal cells because they are aneuploid, do not exhibit cellular senescence, and have a high rate of spontaneous transformation. In addition, tumor cell line DNA is not necessarily equivalent to tumor DNA. These caveats were well-heeded by molecular biologists who then proceeded to study proto-oncogene function by transfecting tumor DNA into normal diploid cell strains or other established cell lines[125-127]. By this method they found that at least two oncogenic sequences were required for transformation and tumorigenicity. Thus, the concept of the multi-hit requirement for transformation became incorporated into the molecular genetic experiments where several independent experiments now support the concept that single alterations of single proto-oncogenes are not sufficient for neoplastic transformation.

Recently, oncogenic DNA sequences joined to manipulatable regulatory sequences were transfected into fertilized mouse eggs so that these sequences were present in all cells of the adult organism[128]. It must be acknowledged that this current technique does not yet place the genes in their normal genomic context, so care is required in the interpretation of these kinds of experiments. Nonetheless, with this technique we can begin to ask questions about proto-oncogene 'complementation' groups, the effect on proto-oncogene expression of tissue specificity, developmental stage, sex and age, as well as the effects of endocrine and immunological changes, and exposure to various external carcinogens.

The discovery of oncogenic sequences is very promising because if expression of these defined gene sequences indeed proves necessary for tumor formation, we can then explore the parameters involved in activating the expression of these genes. We can also define their activation with respect to the temporal events in neoplasia, for example normal tissue versus benign lesions or preneoplastic lesions, and preneoplastic lesions versus tumors with various metastatic potential. It is the cancer biologists who can help direct proto-oncogene research by emphasizing the maximally relevant experimental systems in which to study these genes. Molecular biology can define the specific genetic changes and then the challenge is to uncover the natural agents which effect those changes and to work with biological material having minimal experimental artifact and maximal relevance to natural tumorigenesis. For example, in a study in which human gliomas were established in culture, only 7-25% of the original karyotypes were present in the cultured population. Therefore, data derived from such cell cultures is based on a limited, selected subpopulation of cells which may not include the biologically relevant cells[129]. In vitro selection must be taken into account; meaningful karyotypic data may need to be derived from studies of the original tumor.

The immediate considerations facing cancer researchers are to choose the most relevant sources of in vivo biological material, to be aware of cell culture selection and other such potential artifacts, and to extrapolate neoplastic transformation data to in vivo biological phenomena. Therefore, it would be most helpful if there were an informational fusion of the disciplines of cancer epidemiology, pathology, and oncology, with cell and molecular biology. In this way, the precise tools and defined questions of molecular biology can be utilized maximally in deriving relevant biological information for the understanding and treatment of cancer. The major challenge, therefore, is to increase the opportunities for cross-disciplinary interaction and to encourage a more comprehensive exchange of ideas and information among those committed to understanding and controlling cancer.

REFERENCES

1.  E. Silverberg, Cancer statistics, Ca. A Cancer Journal for Clinicians, 35:19 (1985).

2.  A. Nordheim and A. Rich, Negatively supercoiled SV40 DNA contains Z DNA segments within transcriptoinal enhancer sequences, Nature 303:674 (1983).

3.  S. Weisbrod, Active chromatin, Nature 297:289 (1982).

4.  N. Hozumi, and S. Tonegawa, Evidence for somatic rearrangement of immunoglobulin genes coding for variable and constant regions, Proc. Natl. Acad. Sci. USA, 73:3628 (1976).

5.  B. McClintock, The significance of responses of the genome to challenge, Science 226:792 (1984).

6. "Symposia on Quantitative Biology", Vol. 45, Part 2, The Cold Spring Harbor Laboratory, New York (1981).

7. R. Lewin, No genome barriers to promiscuous DNA, Science 224:970 (1984).

8. R. Lewin, Can genes jump between eukaryotic species? Science 217:42 (1982).

9. R. Jaenisch, Endogenous retroviruses, Cell 32:5 (1983).

10. Y. Chien, N. R. J. Gascoigne, J. Kavaler, N. E. Lee, and M. M. Davis, Somatic recombination in a murine T-cell receptor gene, Nature 309:322 (1984).

11. M. Bouteille, D. Bouvier, and A. P. Seve, Heterogeneity and territorial organization of the nuclear matrix and related structure, Int. Rev. Cyt. 83:135 (1983).

12. B. Vogelstein, D. M. Pardoll, D. S. Coffey, Supercoiled loops and eucaryotic DNA replication, Cell 22:79 (1980).

13. P. S. Miller, C. H. Agris, L. Aurelian, K. R. Blake, A. Murakami, M. P. Reddy, S. A. Spitz, and P. O. P. Ts'o, Control of ribonucleic acid function by oligonucleoside methylphosphonates, Biochimie, in press (1985).

14. M. D. Waterfield, G. T. Scrace, N. Whittle, P. Stroobant, A. Johnsson, A. Wasteson, B. Westermark, C. H. Heldin, J. S. Huang, and T. F. Deuel, Platelet-derived growth factor is structurally related to the putative transforming protein p28-sis of simian sarcoma virus, Nature 304:35 (1983).

15. Y. Sugimoto, M. Whitman, L. C. Cantley, and R. L. Erikson, Evidence that the Rous sarcoma virus transforming gene product phosphorylates phosphatidylinositol and diacylglycerol, Proc. Natl. Acad. Sci. USA 81: 2117 (1984).

16. I. G. Macara, G. V. Marinetti, and P. C. Balduzzi, Transforming protein of avian sarcoma virus UR2 is associated with phosphatidylinositol kinase activity: Possible role in tumorigenesis, Proc. Natl. Acad. Sci. USA 81:2728 (1984).

17. T. Boveri, "Zur Frage der Entstehung Maligner Tumoren,", Fisher, Jena (1914).

18. J. German, ed., "Chromosomes and Cancer," John Wiley and Sons, New York (1974).

19. A. G. Knudson, Mutation and human cancer, Adv. Cancer Res. 17:317 (1973).

20. B. N. Ames, W. E. Durston, E. Yamasaki and F. D. Lee, Carcinogens are mutagens: A simple test system combing liver homogenates for activation and bacteria for detection, Proc. Natl. Acad. Sci. USA 70:2281 (1973).

21. L. Foulds, "Neoplastic Development," Volume 1, Academic Press, London (1969).

22.  L. Foulds, "Neoplastic Development," Volume 2, Academic Press, London (1975).

23.  J. C. Barrett and P. O. P. Ts'o, Relationship between somatic mutation and neoplastic transformation, Proc. Natl. Acad. Sci. USA 75:3761 (1978).

24.  P. M. Kraemer, G. L. Travis, F. A. Ray, and L. S. Cram, Spontaneous neoplastic evolution of Chinese hamster cells in culture: Multistep progression of phenotype, Cancer Res. 43:4822 (1983).

25.  L. S. Cram, M. F. Bartholdi, F. A. Ray, G. L. Travis, and P. M. Kraemer, Spontaneous neoplastic evolution of Chinese hamster cells in culture:  Multistep progression of karyotype, Cancer Res. 43:4828 (1983).

26.  B. Mintz, Genetic mosaicism and in vivo analysis of neoplasia and differentiation, in:  "Cell Differentiation and Neoplasia," G.F. Saunders, ed., Raven Press, New York (1978).

27.  J. C. Barrett, N. E. Bias and P. O. P. Ts'o, A mammalian cellular system for the concomitant study of neoplastic transformation and somatic mutation, Mutation Res. 50:121 (1978).

28.  Y. Berwald and L. Sachs, In vitro cell transformation with chemical carcinogens, Nature 200:1182 (1963).

29.  Y. Berwald and L. Sachs, In vitro transformation of normal cells to tumor cells by carcinogenic hydrocarbons. J. Natl. Cancer Inst. 35:641 (1965).

30.  J. A. DiPaolo and P. J. Donovan, Properties of Syrian hamster cells transformed in the presence of carcinogenic hydrocarbons, Exptl. Cell Res. 48:361 (1967).

31.  J. A. DiPaolo, P. Donovan and R. Nelson, Quantitative studies of in vitro transformation by chemical carcinogens, J. Natl. Cancer Inst. 42:867 (1969).

32.  S. A. Bruce, S. F. Deamond, and P. O. P. Ts'o, In vitro senescence of Syrian hamster mesenchymal cells of fetal to aged adult origin. Inverse relationship between in vivo donor age and in vitro proliferative capacity, Mech. of Ageing and Devel., in press (1985).

33.  J. C. Barrett, A preneoplastic stage in the spontaneous neoplastic transformation of Syrian hamster embryo cells in culture, Cancer Res. 40:91 (1980).

34.  J. C. Barrett, T. Tsutsui and P. O. P. Ts'o, Neoplastic transformation induced by a direct perturbation of DNA, Nature 274:229 (1978).

35.  T. Tsutsui, J. C. Barrett and P. O. P. Ts'o, Morphological transformation, DNA damage, and chromosomal aberrations induced by a direct DNA perturbation of synchronized Syrian hamster embryo cells, Cancer Res. 39:2356 (1979).

36. S. L. Lin, M. Takii and P. O. P. Ts'o, Somatic mutation and neoplastic transformation induced by [methyl-$^3$H] thymidine, <u>Radiation Res.</u> 90:142 (1982).

37. M. Zajac-Kaye and P. O. P. Ts'o, DNAse I encapsulated in liposomes can induce neoplastic transformation of Syrian hamster embryo cells in culture, <u>Cell</u> 39:427 (1984).

38. J. C. Barrett and P. O. P. Ts'o, Evidence for the progressive nature of neoplastic transformation <u>in vitro</u>, <u>Proc. Natl. Acad. Sci. USA</u> 75:3761 (1978).

39. S. Nakano, S. A. Bruce, H. Ueo, and P. O. P., A qualitative and quantitative assay for cells lacking postconfluence inhibition of cell division: Characterization of this phenotype in carcinogen-treated Syrian hamster embryo cells in culture, <u>Cancer Res.</u> 42:3132 (1982).

40. J. C. Barrett, B. D. Crawford, L. O. Mixter, L. M. Schechtman, P. O. P. Ts'o and R. Pollack, Correlation of <u>in vitro</u> growth properties and tumorigenicity of Syrian hamster cell lines, <u>Cancer Res.</u> 39:1504 (1979).

41. B. D. Crawford, J. C. Barrett and P. O. P. Ts'o, Neoplastic conversion of pre-neoplastic Syrian hamster cells: Rate estimation by fluctuation analysis, <u>Molec. and Cell. Biol.</u> 3:931 (1983).

42. B. D. Crawford, Cellular and somatic genetic aspects of neoplastic transformation <u>in vitro</u>, Ph.D. Thesis, The Johns Hopkins University, Baltimore (1981).

43. A. R. Kinsella and M. Radman, Tumor promoter induces sister chromatid exchanges: Relevance to mechanisms of carcinogenesis, <u>Proc. Natl. Natl. Acad. Sci.</u> USA 75:6149 (1978).

44. D. Morry, Gene dosage dependence of mutation, cellular senescence and transformation related phenotypes, Ph.D. Thesis, The Johns Hopkins University, Baltimore (1980).

45. R. Moyzis, D. Grady, D. Li, S. Mirvis and P. Ts'o, Extensive homology of nuclear ribonucleic acid and polysomal poly(adenylic acid) messenger ribonucleic acid between normal and neoplastically transformed cells, <u>Biochemistry</u> 19:821 (1980).

46. J. C. Barrett, W. Wong and J. A. McLachlan, Diethylstilbesterol induces neoplastic transformation without measurable gene mutation at two loci. <u>Science</u> 212:1402 (1981).

47. J. A. Dipaolo, A. J. DeMarinis and J. Doniger, Neoplastic transformation of Syrian hamster embryo cells by bisulfite is accompanied with a decrease in the number of functioning replicons, <u>Cancer Lett.</u> 12:203 (1981).

48. K. K. Gyi, Non-mutational induction of transformation-associated phenotypes in Syrian hamster fibroblasts by L-ethionine, <u>Proc. Amer. Assoc. for Cancer Res.</u> 23:77 (1982).

49.  T. Tsutsui, H. Maizumi and J. C. Barrett, Colcemid-induced neoplastic transformation without and aneuploidy in Syrian hamster embryo cells, Carcinogenesis 5:89 (1984).

50.  T. Tsutsui, H. Maizumi, J. A. McLachlan and J. C. Barrett, Aneuploidy induction and cell transformation by diethylstilbesterol:  A possible chromosome mechanism in carcinogenesis, Cancer Res. 43:3814 (1983).

51.  "Genes, Chromosomes, and Neoplasia," F. E. Arrighi, P. N. Rao, and E. Stubblefield, eds., Raven Press, New York, (1980).

52.  "Precancerous States," R. L. Carter, ed., Oxford University Press, London (1984).

53.  J. J. Yunis The chromosomal basis of human neoplasia, Science 221:227 (1983).

54.  J. D. Rowley, Biological implications of consistent chromosome rearrangements in leukemia and lymphoma, Cancer Res. 44:3159 (1984).

55.  N. B. Atkin, Cytogenetic studies on human tumors and premalignant lesions:  The emergence of aneuploid cell lines and their relationship to the process of malignant transformation in man, in:  "Genetic Concepts and Neoplasia, Williams and Wilkins Co., Baltimore (1970).

56.  P. E. Barker, Double minutes in human tumor cells, Canc. Genet. Cytogenet. 5:81 (1982).

57.  G. R. Stark and G. M. Wahl, Gene amplification, Ann. Rev. Biochem. 53:447 (1984).

58.  G. Balaban and F. Gilbert, Homogeneously staining regions in direct preparations from human neuroblastomas, Cancer Res. 42:1838 (1982).

59.  A. Levan, G. Levan and F. Mitelman, Chromosomes and cancer, Hereditas 86:15 (1977).

60.  F. Mitelman, Restricted number of chromosomal regions implicated in aetiology of human cancer and leukemia, Nature 310:325 (1984).

61.  M. Schwab, K. Alitalo, K. H. Klempnauer, H. E. Varmus, J. M. Bishop, F. Gilbert, G. Brodeur, M. Goldstein, and J. Trent, Amplified DNA with limited homology to myc cellular oncogene is shared by human neuroblastoma cell lines and a neuroblastoma tumor, Nature 305:245 (1983).

62.  N. E. Kohl, N. Kanda, R. R. Schreck, G. Bruns, S. A. Latt, F. Gilbert and F. W. Alt, Transposition and amplification of oncogene-related sequences in human neuroblastomas, Cell 35:359 (1983).

63.  W. H. Lee, A. L. Murphree, and W. F. Benedict, Expression and amplification of the N-myc gene in primary retinoblastoma, Nature 309:458 (1984).

64.  J. D. Rowley, Human oncogene locations and chromosome aberrations, Nature 301:  290 (1983).

65. A. Varshavsky, On the possibility of metabolic control of replicon "misfiring": Relationship to emergence of malignant phenotypes in mammalian cell lineages, Proc. Natl. Acad. Sci. USA 78:3673 (1981).

66. W. W. Nichols, Viral interactions with the mammalian genome relevant to neoplasia in: "Chromosome Mutation and Neoplasia, J. German, ed., Alan R. Liss, Inc., New York (1983).

67. M. P. Calos and J. H. Miller, Transposable elements, Cell 20:579 (1980).

68. P. Nevers and H. Saedler, Transposable genetic elements as agents of gene instability and chromosomal rearrangements, Nature 268:109 (1977).

69. M. M. Green, Genetic instability in Drosophila melangaster: Deletion induction by insertion sequences, Proc. Natl. Acad. Sci. USA 79:5367 (1982).

70. W. McGinnis and S. K. Beckendorf, Association of Drosophila transposable element of the Roo family with chromosomal deletion breakpoints, Nucleic Acids Res. 11:737 (1983).

71. G. S. Roeder, P. J. Farabaugh, O. T. Chaleff, and G. R. Fink, The origins of gene instability in yeast, Science 209:1375 (1980).

72. B. Calabretta, D. L. Robberson, H. A. Barrera-Saldana, T. P. Lambron, and G. F. Saunders, Genome instability in a region of human DNA enriched in Alu repeat sequences, Nature 296:219 (1982).

73. W. R. Engels and C. R. Preston, Identifying P factors in Drosophila by means of chromosome breakage hotspots, Cell 26:421 (1981).

74. G. W. Schmid and W. R. Jelinek, The Alu family of dispersed repetitive sequences, Science 216:1065 (1982).

75. M. F. Singer, SINES and LINES: Highly repeated short and long interspersed sequences in mammalian genomes, Cell 28:433 (1982).

76. R. A. Weinberg, Origins and roles and endogenous retroviruses, Cell 22:643 (1980).

77. H. M. Temin, Origin of retroviruses from cellular moveable genetic elements, Cell 21:599 (1980).

78. K. J. McCormick and J. J. Trenton, Tumor-associated viruses of the Syrian hamster, Prog. Exp. Tumor Res. 23:13 (1979).

79. F. Kelly and H. Condamine, Tumor viruses and early mouse embryos, Biochim. Biophys. Acta 651:105 (1982).

80. W. Bernhard, Electron microscopy of tumor cells and tumor viruses, Cancer Res. 18:491 (1958).

81. Y. Ohtsuki, G. Seman, L. Dmochowski, J. M. Bowen and D. E. Johnson, Virus-like particles in a case of human prostate carcinoma, J. Natl. Cancer Inst. 58: 1493 (1977).

82. W. S. Hayward, B. G. Neel and S. M. Astrin, Activation of cellular onc gene by promoter insertion in ALV-induced lymphoid leukosis, Nature 290: 475 (1981).

83. E. Canaani, O. Dreazen, A. Klar, G. Rechavi, G. Ram, J. B. Cohen, and D. Givol, Activation of the c-mos oncogene in a mouse plasmacytoma by insertion of an endogenous intracisternal A-particle gene, Proc. Natl. Acad. Sci. USA 80:7118 (1983).

84. I. B. Weinstein, S. Gattoni-Celli, P. Kirschmeier, M. Lambert, W. Hsiao, J. Backer, and A. Jeffrey, Multistage carcinogenesis involves multiple genes and multiple mechanisms, in: "Cancer Cells/1 The Transformed Phenotype," A.J. Levine, G.F. Vande Woude, W.C. Topp, and J.D. Watson, eds., Cold Spring Harbor Laboratories, New York (1984).

85. A. B. Rabson, P. E. Stelle, C. F. Garon, M. A. Martin, mRNA transcripts related to full-length endogenous retroviral DNA in human cells, Nature 306:604 (1983).

86. S. S. Potter. Rearrangement sequences of a human Kpn I element, Proc. Natl. Acad. Sci. USA 81:1012 (1984).

87. C. D. O'Connell and M. Cohen, The long terminal repeat sequences of a novel human endogenous retrovirus, Science 226: 1204 (1984).

88. L. Sachs, Normal development programmes in myeloid leukaemia: Regulatory proteins in the control of growth and differentiation, Cancer Survey, Vol. 1, (1982).

89. S. Nakano and P. O. P. Ts'o, Cellular differentiation and neoplasia: Characterization of subpopulations of cells that have neoplasia-related growth properties in Syrian hamster embryo cell cultures, Proc. Natl. Acad. Sci. USA 78:4995 (1981).

90. H. Ueo, S. A. Bruce, S. Nakano and P. O. P. Ts'o, Tumor promoters retard the loss of a transient subpopulation of cells in low passage Syrian hamster fetal cell cultures and extend the in vitro proliferative life span of the cultures, J. Cell Physiol., in press (1985).

91. S. Bruce, S. Deamond, H. Ueo and P. O. P. Ts'o, Age-related differences in promoter-induced extension of in vitro lifespan of Syrian hamster cells, J. Cell Biol. 97:346a (1983).

92. S. Nakano, H. Ueo, S. A. Bruce and P. O. P. Ts'o, A contact-insensitve subpopulation in Syrian hamster cell cultures with a greater susceptibility to chemically induced neoplastic transformation, Proc. Natl. Acad. Sci. USA, in press (1985).

93. C. C. Boyer, Embryology, in: "The Golden Hamster", R.A. Hoffman, P.F. Robinson and H. Magalhaes, eds., Iowa State Press, Ames (1968).

94. S. A. Bruce, K. K. Gyi, S. Nakano, H. Ueo, M. Zajac-Kaye and P. O. P. Ts'o, Genetic and developmental determinants in neoplastic transformation, in: "Biochemical Basis of Chemical Carcinogenesis," H. Greim, R. Jung, M. Kramer, H. Marquardt and F. Oesch, eds., Raven Press, New York, (1984).

95.  T. Okeda, S. A. Bruce, M. A. Bury and P. O. P. Ts'o, Tumor promoters and epidermal growth factors increase the frequency of conversion of Syrian hamster embryonic cell cultures to permanent progenitor cell lines, Manuscript in preparation.

96.  T. Okeda, H. Ueo, Y. Yokogawa, S. A. Bruce, M. A. Bury, and P. O. P. Ts'o, Characterization of an establshed pre-adipocyte Syrian hamster embryonic cell line, Manuscript in preparation.

97.  H. Temin, On the origin of the genes for neoplasia, Cancer Res. 34: 2835 (1974).

98.  P. H. Duesberg, Retroviral transforming genes in normal cells, Nature 304:219 (1983).

99.  B. G. Neel, W. S. Hayward, H. L. Robinson, J. Fang and S. M. Astrin, Avian leukosis virus-induced tumors have common proviral integration sites and synthesize discrete new RNAs: Oncogenesis by promoter insertion, Cell 23:323 (1981).

100. Y. T. K. Fung, W. G. Lewis L. B. Crittenden, H. J. Kung, Activation of the cellular oncogene c-erb B by LTR insertion: Molecular basis for induction of erythroblastosis by avian leukosis virus, Cell 33:357 (1983).

101. R. Nusse, A. Ooyen, D. Cox, Y. K. T. Fung, and H. Varmus, Mode of proviral activation of a putative mammany oncogene (int-1) on mouse chromosome 15, Nature 307:131 (1984).

102. C. D. Dickson, R. Smith, S. Brookes, and G. Peters, Tumorigenesis by mouse mammary tumor virus: Proviral activation of a cellular gene in the common integration region int-2, Cell 37:529 (1984).

103. G. L. C. Shen-Ong, M. Potter, J. F. Mushinski, S. Lavu and E. P. Reddy, Activation of the c-myb locus by viral insertional mutagenesis in plasmacytoid lymphosarcomas, Science 226:1077 (1984).

104. C. J. Der, T. G. Krontiris, and G. M. Cooper, Transforming genes of human bladder and lung carcinoma cells lines are homologous to the ras genes of Harvey and Kirsten sarcoma viruses, Proc. Natl. Acad. Sci. USA 79:3637 (1982).

105. G. M. Cooper, Cellular transforming genes, Science 218:801 (1982).

106. L. A. Feig, R. C. Bast, P. C. Knapp and G. M. Cooper, Somatic activation of ras$^k$ gene in a human ovarian carcinoma, Science 223:698 (1984).

107. J. Fujita, O. Yoshida, Y. Yuasa, J. S. Rhim, M. Hatanaka, and S. A. Aaronson, Ha-ras oncogenes are activated by somatic alterations in human urinary tract tumors, Nature 309:464 (1984).

108. I. Guerrero, A. Vilasante, V. Corces, and A. Pellicer, Activation of a c-K-ras oncogene by somatic mutation in mouse lymphomas induced by gamma radiation, Science 225:1159 (1984).

109. S. H. Orkin, O. S. Goldman, and S. E. Sallan, Development of homozygosity for chromosome 11p markers in Wilms' tumor, Nature 309:172 (1984).

110. E. R. Fearon, B. Vogelstein, and A. P. Feinberg, Somatic deletion and duplication of genes on chromosome 11 in Wilms' tumours, Nature 309:176 (1984).

111. J. Downward, Y. Yarden, E. Mayes, G. Scrace, N. Totty, P. Stockwell, A. Ullrich, J. Schlessinger, and M.D. Waterfield, Close similarity of epidermal growth factor receptor and v-erb-B oncogene protein sequences, Nature 307:521 (1984).

112. T. Hunter and P. M. Sefton, Transforming gene product of Rous sarcoma virus phosphorylates tyrosine, Proc. Natl. Acad. Sci. USA 77:1311 (1980).

113. M. B. Sporn and G. J. Todaro, Autocrine secretion and malignant transformation of cells, New Engl. J. Med. 303:878 (1980).

114. H. Ushiro and S. Cohen, Identification of phosphotyrosine as a product of epidermal growth factor - activated protein kinase in A-431 cell membranes. J. Biol. Chem. 255:8363 (1980).

115. J. A. Cooper, D. F. Bowen-Pope, E. Raines, R. Ross, and T. Hunter, Similar effects of platelet-derived growth factor and epidermal growth factor on the phosphorylation of tyrosine in cellular proteins, Cell 31:263 (1982).

116. B. Ek and C. H. Heldin, Characterization of a tyrosine-specific kinase activity in human fibroblast membranes stimulated by platelet-derived growth factor, J. Biol. Chem. 257:10486 (1982).

117. J. Nishimura, J. S. Huang, and T. F. Deuel, Platelet-derived growth factor stimulates tyrosine-specific protein kinase activity in Swiss mouse 3T3 cell membranes, Proc. Natl. Acad. Sci. USA 79:4303 (1982).

118. J. M. Hutson, M. E. Fallat, S. Kamagata, P. K. Donahoe, and G. P. Budzik, Phosphorylation events during Mullerian duct regression, Science 223:586 (1984).

119. J. L. Marx, Oncogene linked to cell regulatory system, Science 226:527 (1984).

120. J. B. Hurley, M. I. Simon, D. B. Teplow, J. D. Robishaw and A. G. Gilman, Homologies between signal transducing G proteins and ras gene products, Science 226:860 (1984).

121. F. L. Graham and A. Van der Eb, A new technique for the assay of human adenovirus 5 DNA, Virology 52:456 (1973).

122. M. Wigler, A. Pellicer, S. Silverstein, and R. Axel, Biochemical transfer of single-copy eucaryotic genes using total cellular DNA as donor, Cell 14:725 (1978).

123. C. Shih, B. Shilo, M. P. Goldfarb, A. Dannenberg and R. A. Weinberg, Passage of phenotypes of chemically transformed cells via transfection of DNA and chromatin, Proc. Natl. Acad. Sci. USA 76:5714 (1979).

124. G. Klein, The role of gene dosage and genetic transpositions in carcinogenesis, Nature 294:313 (1981).

125. R. F. Newbold and R. W. Overell, Fibroblast immortality is a prerequisite for transformation by EJ c-Ha-ras Oncogene, <u>Nature</u> 304:648 (1983).

126. H. Land, L. F. Parada and R. A. Weinberg, Tumorigenic conversion of primary embryo fibroblasts requires at least two cooperating oncogenes, <u>Nature</u> 304:596 (1983).

127. H. E. Ruley, Adenovirus early region 1A enables viral and cellular transforming genes to transform primary cells in culture, <u>Nature</u> 304:602 (1983).

128. T. A. Stewart, P. K. Pattingale, and P. Leder, Spontaneous mammary adenocarcinomas in transgenic mice that carry and express MTV/<u>myc</u> fusion genes, <u>Cell</u> 38:627 (1984).

129. J. R. Shapiro, W. K. A. Yung, and W. R. Shapiro, Isolation, karyotype and clonal growth of heterogeneous subpopulations of human malignant gliomas, <u>Cancer Res.</u> 41:2349 (1981).

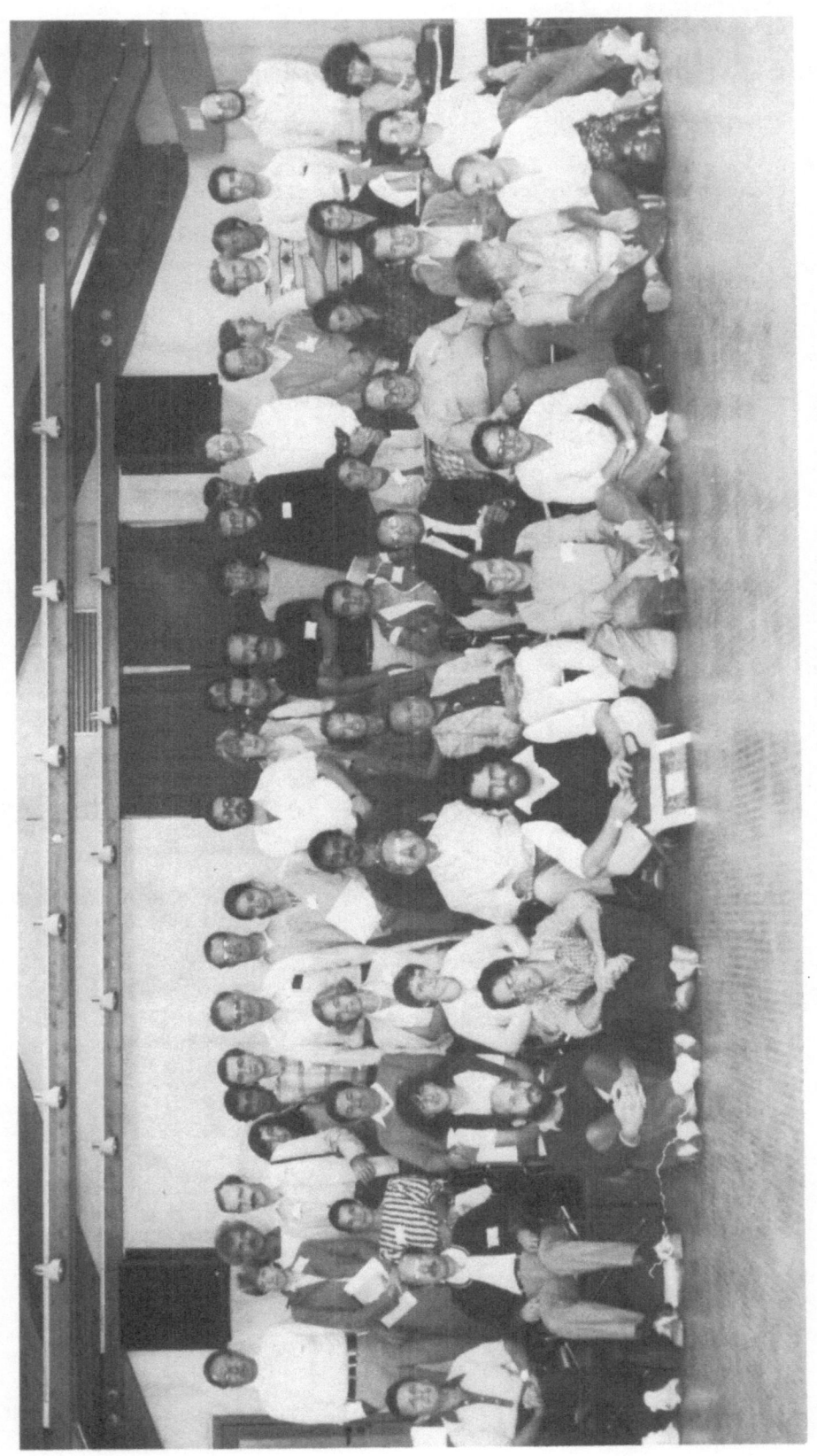

NATO ADVANCED STUDY INSTITUTE, September 18-30, 1983
Erice, Italy

## PARTICIPANTS

Ida ALBANESE

Istituto di Anatomia Comparata
Universita Palermo
Via Archirafi 22
Palermo, Italy

Letizia ANELLO

Instituto Biologia dello Divluppo
Via Archirafi 20
Palermo, Italy

Gulseren BAGCI

Akdeniz Universitesi
Tip Fakultesi Tibbi Biyoloji
Bolumu Arastirma Gorevlisi
Antalya, Turkey

Huseyin BAGCI

Addeniz Universitesi
Tip Fakultesi Tibbi Biyoloji
Bolumu Arastirma Gorevlisi
Antalya, Turkey

Agnieszka BARTOSZEK

Dept. of Pharmaceutical Technology
    and Biochemistry
Technical University of Gdansk
80-952 Gdansk, Poland

Andrew BELMONT

Division of Biophysics
School of Hygiene and Public Health
The John Hopkins University
615 North Wolfe Street
Baltimore, Maryland 21205   USA

Jordi BERNUES

Universitat Autonoma de Barcelona
Institut de Biologia Fonamental
Vincent Villar Palasi
Molecular Biology Group
Barcelona, Spain

Franco Armando BIGNONE

Division of Biophysics
School of Hygiene and Public Health
The Johns Hopkins University
615 North Wolfe Street
Baltimore, Maryland 21205   USA

Max BIRNSTIEL

Zurich University
Zurich, Switzerland

Andrea BOICELLI

Istituto di Anatomia Umana Normale
      dell'Universita di Bologna
Bologna, Italy

William BONNER

National Cancer Institute
Building 37, Room 5D19
National Institutes of Health
Bethesda, Maryland 20892   USA

E. Morton BRADBURY

Department of Biological Chemistry
School of Medicine
University of California
Davis, California 95616   USA

Anne BROWN

Division of Biophysics
School of Hygiene and Public Health
The Johns Hopkins University
615 North Wolfe Street
Baltimore, Maryland 21205   USA

Elisa CAFFARELLI

Molecular Biology Laboratory
University of Rome
Rome, Italy

S. CAPITANI

Istituto di Anatomia Umana Normale
      dell'Universita di Bologna
Bologna, Italy

Caterina CASANO

Istituto di Anatomia Comparata
Universita Palermo
Via Archirafi 22
Palermo, Italy

Allessandro CESTELLI

Istituto de Anatomia Comparata
Universita Palermo
Via Archirafi 22
Palermo, Italy

Donald S. Coffey

Department of Urology
School of Medicine
The Johns Hopkins University
720 Rutland Avenue
Baltimore, Maryland 21205   USA

Massimo P. CRIPPA

Department of Plant Genetics
The Weizmann Institute of Science
76100 Rehovot, Israel

Donald CROTHERS

Department of Chemistry
Yale University
225 Prospect Street
New Haven, Connecticut 06520   USA

Marta CZUPRYN

Institute of Biochemistry
Al. Zwirki i Wigury 93
02-089 Warsaw, Poland

Axel DEHN

Veterinary School
Institute of Parasitology
D-3000 Hanover
Federal Republic of Germany

Maria Teresa Rangel DE FIGUIREDO

Instituto Universitario de Tras-Os-
    Montes E Alto Douro
Vila Real, Portugal

Luciano DE PETROCELLIS

Istituto di Cibernetica
Consiglio Nazionale delle Richerche
80072 Arco Felice
Napoli, Italy

Pilar DIAZ

Departmento de Bioquimica
Facultad de Ciencias
Universidad Autonoma
Bellaterra, Barcelona, Spain

Italia DI LIEGRO

Istituto di Anatomia Comparata
Universita di Palermo
Via Archirafi 22
Palermo, Italy

Philippe DUMAS

Centre Nationale de la Recherche
    Scientifique
Institut de Biologie Moleculaire et
    Cellulaire
15, rue Rene Descartes
67084 Strasbourg Cedex
France

Jean Pierre EBEL

Centre Nationale de la Recherche
    Scientifique
Institut de Biologie Moleculaire et
    Cellulaire
15, rue Rene Descartes
67084 Strasbourg Cedex
France

Endre EGYHAZI

Karolinska Institute
Department of Histology
P.O. Box 60400
S-104 01 Stockholm, Sweden

Henryk EISENBERG

Polymer Research Department
Weizmann Institute of Science
Rehovot 76100, Israel

Mine ENGINUN

University of Istanbul
Faculty of Engineering
Department of Chemistry
Istanbul, Turkey

Gary FELSENFELD

Laboratory of Molecular Biology
National Institutes of Health
Building 2, Room 301
Bethesda, Maryland 20892   USA

Karl Otto GREULICH

Weizmann Institute of Science
P.O. Box 26
Rehovot 76100, Israel

Rodney E. HARRINGTON

Department of Biochemistry
University of Nevada at Reno
Reno, Nevada 89557-0046    USA

Richard HERZOG

Dipl.-Biochemistry
Gmelinstrasse 68
7400 Tubingen 1
Federal Republic of Germany

Ru-Chih HUANG

Department of Biology
School of Arts and Sciences
The Johns Hopkins University
34th and Charles Streets
Baltimore, Maryland 21218   USA

J. Gordon KAPLAN

Department of Biochemistry
The University of Alberta
Medical Sciences Building
Edmonton T6G 2H7
Canada

Tibor IGO-KEMENES

Institut fur Physiologische Chemie,
    Physikalische Biochemie und
    Zellbiologie der Universitat Munchen
Goethestrasse 33
D-8000 Munchen 2
Federal Republic of Germany

Ilana KEPTEN

Department of Biology
Israel Institute of Technology
Haifa, Israel

Sung-Hou KIM

Department of Chemistry
University of California
Berkeley, California 94720   USA

Patrizia LAVIA

Universita degli Studi di Roma
Istituto de Genetica
Faculta di Scienze
00185 Roma, Italy

Ulrich LAEMMLI

University of Geneva
30 Quai Ernest-Ansemeet
Geneva CH-1211, Switzerland

Michele LO CASTO

Universita Palermo
Via Archirafi 22
90127 Palermo, Italy

Dennie E. LOHR

Chemistry Department
Arizona State University
Tempe, Arizona 85287 USA

A. MACIEIRA-COELHO

Institut de Cancerologie
et d'Immunogenetique
14 & 16 Avenue Paul-Vaillant-Couturier
94800 Villejuif, France

Nadir MARALDI

Consiglio Nazionale dell Ricerche
Istituto di Citomorfologia Normale
e Patologica
S. Maria Imbaro
Chieti, Italy

Jose MARIA

University of Manchester
Department of Botany
Manchester M13 9PL
United Kingdom

Daniel B. MATLOK

Biology Department
Southern Utah State College
Cedar City, Utah 84720 USA

Galina MENGERITSKY

Polymer Research Department
Weizmann Institute of Science
76100 Rehovot, Israel

B. MERTENS

Katholieke te Leuven
Rega-Institut
Lab. voor Experimentele Geneeskunde
3000 Leuven, Belgium

Gioacchino MICHELI

Dipartimento de Genetica e Biologia
Molecolare
Universita "La Sapienza"
Piazzale Aldo Moro 5
00185 Roma, Italy

Rodolfo NEGRI

Centro Acidi Nucleari C.N.R.
Istituto di Fisiologia
Universita di Roma
Piazzale Aldo Moro 5
00185 Roma, Italy

Claudio NICOLINI

Temple University
Health Sciences Center
Philidelphia, Pennsylvania 19140 USA

Franco PALLA

Istituto Biologia dello Dviluppo
Universita Palermo
Via Archirafi 20
Palermo, Italy

Silvio PARODI       Istituto Scientifico per la Ricerca
              sul Cancro
             Viale Benedetto XV-10
             16132 Genova, Italy

Sari PENNINGS       Institut voor Molekulaire Biologie
             VRIJE Universiteit
             Paardenstraat 65
             1640 St. Genesius-Rode
             Brussels, Belgium

George SCANGOS       Department of Biology
             School of Arts and Sciences
             The Johns Hopkins University
             34th and Charles Streets
             Baltimore, Maryland 21218   USA

Joy SCHOCHET        Roosevelt University
             430 South Michigan Avenue
             Chicago, Illinois   USA

Mario SOUMPASIS       Institute of Theoretical Physics
             Freie Universitat Berlin
             Arnimallee 1000
             Berlin 33, Federal Republic of Germany

Giovanni SPINELLI      Istituto di Anatomia Comparata
             Universita Palermo
             Via Archirafi 20
             Palermo, Italy

Gary STEIN         Department of Biochemistry & Molecular
              Biology
             College of Medicine
             University of Florida
             Gainesville, Florida 32610   USA

Paul O.P. TS'O        Division of Biophysics
             School of Hygiene and Public Health
             The Johns Hopkins University
             615 North Wolfe Street
             Baltimore, Maryland 21205   USA

Levy ULANOVSKY       Department of Polymer Research
             The Weizmann Institute of Science
             P.O. Box 26
             76100 Rehovot, Israel

Kensal VAN HOLDE      Department of Biochemistry and
              Biophysics
             Oregon State University
             Corvallis, Oregon 97331   USA

J.H. WATERBORG       Cell and Molecular Biology Laboratory
             University of Sussex
             Brighton, BN1 90G
             United Kingdom

Eric WESTHOF

Centre Nationale de la Recherche
    Scientifique
Institut de Biologie Moleculaire et
    Cellulaire
15, rue Rene Descartes
67084 Strasbourg Cedex, France


Ilga WINICOVC

Department of Biochemistry
University of Nevada at Reno
Reno, Nevada 89557   USA


H. G. Wittmann

Max Planck Institut fur Molekulare
    Genetik
Ihnestrasse 63-73
D-1000 Berlin 33 (DAHLEM)
Federal Republic of Germany


Jan M. WOYNAROWSKI

Department of Pharmaceutical Technology
    and Biochemistry
Technical University of Gdansk
80-952 Gdansk, Poland


Thomas D. YAGER

Department of Biochemistry and
    Biophysics
Oregon State University
Corvallis, Oregon 97331   USA


Stacieann YUHASZ

Division of Biophysics
School of Hygiene and Public Health
The Johns Hopkins University
615 North Wolfe Street
Baltimore, Maryland 21205   USA